Between Zeus and the Salmon

THE BIODEMOGRAPHY OF LONGEVITY

Kenneth W. Wachter and Caleb E. Finch, Editors

Committee on Population

Commission on Behavioral and Social Sciences and Education

National Research Council

NATIONAL ACADEMY PRESS
Washington, D.C.   1997

NATIONAL ACADEMY PRESS • 2101 Constitution Avenue, NW • Washington, D.C. 20418

NOTICE: The project that is the subject of this report was approved by the Governing Board of the National Research Council, whose members are drawn from the councils of the National Academy of Sciences, the National Academy of Engineering, and the Institute of Medicine. The members of the committee responsible for the report were chosen for their special competences and with regard for appropriate balance.

This report has been reviewed by a group other than the authors according to procedures approved by a Report Review Committee consisting of members of the National Academy of Sciences, the National Academy of Engineering, and the Institute of Medicine.

The National Academy of Sciences is a private, nonprofit, self-perpetuating society of distinguished scholars engaged in scientific and engineering research, dedicated to the furtherance of science and technology and to their use for the general welfare. Upon the authority of the charter granted to it by the Congress in 1863, the Academy has a mandate that requires it to advise the federal government on scientific and technical matters. Dr. Bruce M. Alberts is president of the National Academy of Sciences.

The National Academy of Engineering was established in 1964, under the charter of the National Academy of Sciences, as a parallel organization of outstanding engineers. It is autonomous in its administration and in the selection of its members, sharing with the National Academy of Sciences the responsibility for advising the federal government. The National Academy of Engineering also sponsors engineering programs aimed at meeting national needs, encourages education and research, and recognizes the superior achievements of engineers. Dr. William A. Wulf is president of the National Academy of Engineering.

The Institute of Medicine was established in 1970 by the National Academy of Sciences to secure the services of eminent members of appropriate professions in the examination of policy matters pertaining to the health of the public. The Institute acts under the responsibility given to the National Academy of Sciences by its congressional charter to be an adviser to the federal government and, upon its own initiative, to identify issues of medical care, research, and education. Dr. Kenneth I. Shine is president of the Institute of Medicine.

The National Research Council was organized by the National Academy of Sciences in 1916 to associate the broad community of science and technology with the Academy's purposes of furthering knowledge and advising the federal government. Functioning in accordance with general policies determined by the Academy, the Council has become the principal operating agency of both the National Academy of Sciences and the National Academy of Engineering in providing services to the government, the public, and the scientific and engineering communities. The Council is administered jointly by both Academies and the Institute of Medicine. Dr. Bruce M. Alberts and Dr. William A. Wulf are chairman and vice chairman, respectively, of the National Research Council.

This study was supported by Contract No. N01-OD-4-2139 between the National Academy of Sciences and the National Institute on Aging. Any opinions, findings, conclusions, or recommendations expressed in this publication are those of the author(s) and do not necessarily reflect the view of the organizations or agencies that provided support for this project.

Library of Congress Catalog Card No. 97-33767
International Standard Book Number 0-309-05787-6

This book is available for sale from the National Academy Press, 2101 Constitution Avenue, N.W., Box 285, Washington, D.C. 20055. Call 800-624-6242 or 202-334-3313 (in the Washington Metropolitan Area). Order electronically via Internet at http://www.nap.edu.

COMMITTEE ON POPULATION

RONALD D. LEE (*Chair*), Department of Demography and Economics, University of California, Berkeley
CAROLINE H. BLEDSOE, Department of Anthropology, Northwestern University
JOSÉ LUIS BOBADILLA,* Inter-American Development Bank, Washington, D.C.
JOHN BONGAARTS, The Population Council, New York
JOHN B. CASTERLINE, The Population Council, New York
LINDA G. MARTIN, RAND, Santa Monica, California
JANE MENKEN, University of Pennsylvania
ROBERT A. MOFFITT, Department of Economics, Johns Hopkins University
MARK R. MONTGOMERY, The Population Council, New York
W. HENRY MOSLEY, Department of Population Dynamics, Johns Hopkins University School of Hygiene and Public Health
ALBERTO PALLONI, Department of Sociology, University of Wisconsin, Madison
JAMES P. SMITH, RAND, Santa Monica, California
BETH J. SOLDO, Department of Demography, Georgetown University
MARTA TIENDA,** Population Research Center, University of Chicago
AMY O. TSUI,** Carolina Population Center, University of North Carolina, Chapel Hill

JOHN G. HAAGA, Director
BARNEY COHEN, Program Officer
TRISH DeFRISCO, Senior Project Assistant
KAREN A. FOOTE, Program Officer (to July 1996)
JOEL A. ROSENQUIST, Senior Project Assistant

---

* deceased October 1996
** through October 1996

iii

CONTRIBUTORS

STEVEN N. AUSTAD, University of Idaho
JAMES R. CAREY, University of California, Davis
CALEB E. FINCH, University of Southern California
CATHERINE GRUENFELDER, University of California, Davis
THOMAS E. JOHNSON, University of Colorado
HILLARD KAPLAN, University of New Mexico
RONALD D. LEE, University of California, Berkeley
LINDA PARTRIDGE, University College London
MICHAEL R. ROSE, University of California, Irvine
DAVID R. SHOOK, University of Colorado
SHRIPAD TULJAPURKAR, Mountain View Research, California, and
   Stanford University
JAMES W. VAUPEL, Max Planck Institute for Demographic Research,
   Rostock, Germany
KENNETH W. WACHTER, University of California, Berkeley
ROBERT B. WALLACE, University of Iowa
JOHN R. WILMOTH, University of California, Berkeley

Preface

The Committee on Population was established in 1983 by the National Research Council, under the charter of the National Academy of Sciences, to bring the knowledge and methods of the population sciences to bear on major issues of science and public policy. Much of the committee's work has concerned the demography and health of aging populations. Together with the Committee on National Statistics and the Institute of Medicine, the Committee on Population sponsored a Workshop on Forecasting Survival, Health, and Disability in 1992. Also in 1992, the committee organized a Workshop on the Demography of Aging covering a range of topics, from household and family demography, to work and retirement, intergenerational transfers, and health (*Demography of Aging*, 1994). A 1994 workshop examined the reasons for continued racial and ethnic differences in health and survival at older ages (*Racial and Ethnic Differences in the Health of Older Americans*, 1997). It was clear from all these efforts that future work on the progress of life expectancy at older ages would require genuine interdisciplinary communication between (and within) the social and life sciences.

This concern led the committee, with funding from the National Institute on Aging (NIA), to organize a series of planning and discussion meetings, culminating in a workshop in Washington in April 1996, at which demographers, evolutionary theorists, genetic epidemiologists, anthropologists, and biologists from many different scientific taxa could meet and share contributions to the understanding of human longevity. These were exciting occasions, as I believe this volume, consisting of revised versions of some papers originally presented at the April workshop, attests.

The call for interdisciplinary communication is often just a polite but inconsequential line in conclusions or book reviews, or a grandiose promise in conference proposals. Making it happen productively requires a good deal of preparation and commitment on the part of scholars, all with competing demands on their time and attention. The committee was especially fortunate to get advice and help from thoughtful and busy individuals. We would like to thank Richard Suzman of NIA, who saw the need, shared his ideas, and infected all of us with his enthusiasm. Kenneth Weiss of Pennsylvania State University was especially helpful; he was uniquely qualified to tell us what would interest scientists working in a whole range of fields, and what they knew that would interest the rest. We thank Richard Hodes of NIA for his interest and support. Harold Morowitz of George Mason University, Richard Sprott, Richard Havlik, and Evan Hadley (all of NIA), and Eric Fischer of the NRC Board on Biology gave us sound advice in the design stages and good ideas in the discussions. Elizabeth Corder of Duke University and the Stockholm Gerontology Research Center, Marcus Feldman of Stanford University, Trudy Mackay of North Carolina State University, Jennifer Madans of the National Center on Health Statistics, Randolph Nesse of the University of Michigan, Alan Rogers of the University of Utah, Burton Singer of Princeton University, and Robert Willis of the University of Michigan were generous with their ideas at the workshops and afterward.

Our greatest debt is to Kenneth Wachter of the University of California, Berkeley, and Caleb Finch of the University of Southern California, who devoted time and energy to planning and chairing the workshop, guiding authors in their revisions, and editing this volume. The success of the project depended on their ability to listen and read carefully and critically, and discern what each speaker and author had to contribute to those working in different areas.

Thanks also are due to Beth Soldo, who reviewed the manuscript on behalf of the committee. Colene Walden gave a helpful copy editing of the report and drafted the Glossary. Christine McShane guided the manuscript through the publication process. Karen Foote was diligent and thorough in handling the organization of the workshop and the review process. Trish DeFrisco handled all the administrative tasks for the workshop and manuscript production with her customary efficiency and good grace. Trang Ta helped with manuscript preparation and citation checking in the final stages. John Haaga, the committee staff director, wrote the proposals, supervised the process between meetings, and ably replaced Karen as project officer when she moved to the University of Illinois.

Most of all, of course, we appreciate the contributions of authors and workshop participants. We trust that this volume will inspire others to join in their valuable work.

Ronald D. Lee
Chair, Committee on Population

Contents

vii

Between Zeus and the Salmon

1

Between Zeus and the Salmon: Introduction

Kenneth W. Wachter

This volume takes stock of what biology and demography have to tell and ask each other about human longevity as we move into the Third Millennium. The timing is auspicious. First, recently published works have made the base of accumulated biological knowledge accessible. Finch (1990) has written an authoritative summary of the comparative biology of senescence. Charlesworth (1994) and Rose (1991) have covered evolutionary theory for aging, and Stearns (1992) has covered organism life-history analysis. A historical perspective has been given by Olshansky and Carnes (1997). Second, the initial harvest of results from program projects combining biology and demography sponsored by the U.S. National Institute on Aging has just reached the scientific literature. The remarkable hazard functions for a million Mediterranean fruit flies (Carey et al., 1992) and for genetically uniform populations of *Drosophila* (Curtsinger et al., 1992) are prominent examples. Now is the moment for planning the next waves of joint research. Third, forecasting survival and health for the oldest-old over the next 50 years has become an urgent political need, as developed societies try to plan for avoiding bankruptcy for their social insurance and medical systems. Our uncertainty as to whether current trends will continue or taper is bound up with our uncertainty about the general nature of biological limits to longevity.

This introductory chapter is a personal overview from the vantage point of a demographer. A balancing perspective from the vantage point of a biologist appears in Caleb Finch's concluding chapter. As I see it, for demographers today, the golden challenge is to make the right judgment call predicting our children's life spans. Will the recent pace of gains in life expectancy and active life expectancy extend to the next generation, or are we approaching the point of diminishing returns? The deep theoretical questions in the demography of mortality and aging—including the proper framework for incorporating genetic variables and cofactors into demographic models—cluster around this very practical question of prediction, whose answer some of us may live to know.

Confronting this question, the in-house tools of traditional demography— accurate accounting of vital trends and descriptive modeling of variability across time and circumstances—are indispensable but inconclusive. Knowledge of detailed mechanisms is too patchy for causal models with aggregate implications. Thus demographers are thrown back on a search for analogues. Biology is our cornucopia of analogues.

I do not want to overstate the relevance of biology to demography. Biology will not settle demographic questions directly. Finding the causes behind the leveling out of fruit-fly hazard functions after 100 days will not disclose the causes behind any leveling out of human hazard functions after 100 years. Genes promoting survival at advanced ages may be found in nematode worms without giving us any right to expect usefully close counterparts in people. Darwinian theory, for all its triumphs, is a poor basis for predicting whether women's advantage in life expectancy over men will be increasing or decreasing in 2047.

Nonetheless, biology is definitive. Experiments with laboratory organisms, genetic mapping, natural history, and evolutionary theory are defining the intellectual landscape within which demographic arguments and forecasts gain or lose their appeal. Uncertainties are so great and mortality prediction is so much a matter of bets and guesses that the powerful analogies provided by biology are the best guides we have. These analogies offer a basis for implicit choices about what to regard as ad hoc and what to regard as general, what forms of models to try, what kinds of data to put in the foreground. Biological analogies raise or lower our comfort level with particular kinds of scientific explanations. It seems to me, as I shall describe, that the newest work in biodemography is lowering our comfort level with accounts involving limits to life expectancy and programmed senescence and enhancing our openness to models and hunches that treat life spans as highly plastic.

I begin by reviewing ideas from the evolutionary theory of longevity that have coexisted amicably with a pessimistic demographic stance in regard to open-ended further progress against old-age mortality. I then turn to new empirical results that are reviving an optimistic stance, to studies of the role of the elderly in nature, and to new theoretical departures. I conclude with a look at the immediate future and the knowledge we can hope to gain from further joint work in biodemography.

STERN THEORIES

The emphasis on limits and tradeoffs in biologists' discourse about longevity goes far back, and still predominates. In the 1960s, when a plateau seemed to be appearing in progress against human mortality at older ages in developed societies, the climate of biological opinion made it natural for demographers to see the plateau as a long-term phenomenon. Diminishing returns at older ages fitted into the broad-brush theoretical picture and made it reasonable to discount the likelihood of that resumption of progress that did, as it turned out, actually occur.

Evolution coddles you when young and forsakes you when old. This central idea can be traced back more than a century to Alfred Russel Wallace (Rose, 1991:4); the evolutionary theory of senescence that has grown from it is described by Shripad Tuljapurkar, Linda Partridge, and Michael Rose in Chapters 4, 5, and 6, respectively. Natural selection clears away genes that compromise reproduction or survival to and through the ages of reproduction. Natural selection leaves to their own devices genes with bad effects at ages that no longer matter as far as the propagation of progeny is concerned. In most mathematical implementations of this kind of theory, "ages that no longer matter" have been equated to postreproductive ages of zero fertility; the efficacy of natural selection on mortality as a function of age has been taken to decline smoothly throughout the reproductive period, reaching zero at its end. These ideas have ramified into two intertwining but distinguishable theories, the "mutation-accumulation theory" and "antagonistic pleiotropy."

The mutation-accumulation theory recognizes that most mutations are unfavorable. Some portion of mutations elude repair. Suppose there are genes that specifically impair survival at some range of older ages without substantially reducing net reproduction. Suppose that the structures affected by the genes and the environmental preconditions for their actions have been in place for a very long time and that what is bad for survival stays bad in the face of surrounding change. Then mutations deleterious to survival at older, postreproductive or postnurturant ages should accumulate over eons, since selection is not clearing them away. Genes predisposing to cancers are often adduced as examples. In its simple forms, this mutation-accumulation theory predicts sharply rising hazard functions beyond some threshold age.

Antagonistic pleiotropy, as it pertains to senescence, occurs if there are genes that have positive effects on net reproduction and negative effects on postreproductive survival. If such genes exist, then organisms would be making a tradeoff between investments in younger-age reproductive fitness, which matters to natural selection, and older-age viability, which does not matter to natural selection. Kirkwood's (1977) "disposable soma theory" sees tradeoffs of this kind as a general phenomenon arising as organisms allocate limited energy between functions of reproduction and functions of somatic—bodily—maintenance. Like mutation accumulation, antagonistic pleiotropy and the tradeoffs posited by the disposable soma theory are reasons for hazard rates to rise with age.

Sustaining these considerations is the timeless observation that life in the wild is, as Hobbes put it, "nasty, brutish, and short"—in the wild few creatures survive to old age, so genes governing late-age processes have had little opportunity to matter. The higher the background frequency of deaths from predators or accidents, the more this should be so. Evolutionary theory successfully predicts an association between greater vulnerability and more rapidly rising age-specific mortality. Small insects are an example. Small, exposed, ground-dwelling mammals are another example, contrasting with safer, tree-dwelling mammals and birds (see Charlesworth, 1994:247-248). Finch (1990:22-25 and throughout) sets out an impressive array of evidence from modest samples from many species displaying rising and often accelerating hazard rates with age. Ever-accelerating hazard rates with age imply de facto limits on later life expectancy, and if the observed accelerations with age do share a common general evolutionary origin, that would be a rationale for expecting genetically preprogrammed limits to longevity.

Alongside these ideas from evolutionary biology, there is the mystique of the "Hayflick limit" from cell biology (see Hayflick, 1994:111-136). Certain types of mammalian cells transplanted to cultures only divide up to a limited number of times. The limits correlate roughly with the typical life spans of the organisms from which the cells come. The cells that have stopped dividing often continue to survive in less-than-prime condition. While this process may be implicated in some localized phenomena of aging, any pervasive role for the Hayflick limit on cells in determining the senescent mortality of organisms remains uncertain, as Caleb Finch discusses in the concluding chapter. Nonetheless, as the most frequently cited result in all of gerontology, the Hayflick limit has contributed powerfully to a general sense that the study of longevity is a study of limits, tradeoffs, and diminishing returns.

The ideas that lead to the theories of mutation accumulation and antagonistic pleiotropy are very general principles of evolution. They serve as a paradigm for thinking more broadly—transcending specific reference to genes—about the investments reflected in the ways we and other creatures are designed. Nature puts a premium on solving problems of the kind that show up early in the life course. Organ systems need not be constructed to implement repairs or withstand cumulating challenges late in life.

Out of this essentially pessimistic view, however, has come a simile with an optimistic turn. In this volume, James Vaupel develops it in Chapter 2. The body is likened to a planetary space probe like the Pioneer mission to Mars. The Pioneer's engineers worked through all the problems and built in all the safeguards needed to be sure that the Pioneer probe would reach Mars and complete its mission. Just so, the body must be engineered to complete its evolutionary mission—produce and nurture its young and pass on its genes. After its mission is accomplished, it is disposable. No special provisions for longer operation or late-stage repair are advantageous. But the Pioneer space probe was still functioning as it left the Solar System. The same mechanisms built in to guarantee fail-safe completion of the mission may endow the body, as they did the Pioneer, with residual post-completion life.

This simile is optimistic, for it emphasizes the degree to which we and other creatures may be preadapted for late-life survival. Preadaption means that a system honed by evolution to solve one problem turns out, serendipitously, to be a full-fledged good start on the solution to another problem. For longevity, the idea is that Murphy's Law functions in our favor. Most of the things that can go wrong do, early in life, during development or on its heels, and the list of specifically late-life major problems that evolution was able to leave unsolved is not endless but finite.

Nature provides us with examples of preprogrammed senescence in its most dramatic form—hazard rates that rise abruptly toward infinity at the end of reproduction. Shripad Tuljapurkar, in Chapter 4, points to the most famous example, the salmon, struggling upstream, in Robert Lowell's words, "... alive enough to spawn and die."

For an image of the opposite alternative, we may turn to the Greek gods on Mount Olympus. The gods are born and go through infancy. Hermes carries the infant Dionysus. The gods grow up. Each develops up to his or her own characteristic age. Artemis grows into a young woman, Apollo into a young man, Zeus into a patriarch in the prime of life, Hephaistos into middle age. When development is complete, aging stops. The Olympian gods stay the same age forever after. Their genes, as it were, specify their developmental stages. Programmed aging occurs up through the intervals of development. But then, when development is complete, aging is over. In the favorable environment of Mount Olympus, with the favorable nutrition of nectar and ambrosia, the organism simply goes on surviving. The gods become no frailer with further age. (They also become no wiser.) The celestial genome, as it were, has no genes with specific effects for late-age changes, and nothing stands obdurately in the way of uncurtailed longevity.

The title of this book comes from the thought that the mission of biodemography is to find for us our proper place between Zeus and the salmon.

EMPIRICAL CHALLENGES

The ideas that emphasize limits have been challenged in the last decades by new empirical results and by new theoretical departures. In this section I review the new empirical results.

First is the discovery that hazard functions measured at extreme ages in large populations from several profoundly different species do not rise indefinitely with age. In some other cases, they rise, but at decreasing rates. These results come from the first wave of studies sponsored by the U.S. National Institute on Aging's initiative on the oldest-old, principally from the program project led by James Vaupel, and he sums them up in Chapter 2. The million Mediterranean fruit flies (medflies) and the genetically homogeneous populations of Drosophila flies mentioned at the outset of this introduction have been joined by nematode worms and

Mexican fruit flies and millions more medflies. Controlled experiments have established that the leveling is not an effect of decreasing density. Some leveling-off of the hazard function at extreme ages has been detected in the best-recorded recent data on human populations, and decreasing hazards at extreme ages are implied by the survival of the world's oldest well-documented individuals.

A second set of empirical results that challenge the ethos of limit theories are careful measurements that show human death rates in developed societies to be falling even among the oldest of the oldest-old. John Wilmoth describes these trends in Chapter 3. He shows how gains against mortality over age 80 and even over age 90 have been accelerating since 1960 in nine countries with high-quality data. Wilmoth's own studies of Swedish deaths show an aging of mortality decline; the ages at which one finds the most rapid improvements have been moving up. The graph of maximum reported age at death for each calendar year has a visible upward trend. Wilmoth brings some order into the grab bag of definitions people have given for what "limits to longevity" might mean and infers, on the basis of a cross-national comparison, that advanced societies are unlikely to be approaching any such limits at the present time.

A third set of empirical results come from laboratory experiments with the selective breeding of flies, mice, and other laboratory animals. These have re-vealed an extraordinary plasticity of life span in the face of selection. An account of these studies, including many performed in his own laboratory, is given by Michael Rose in Chapter 6. Under favorable conditions in the laboratory, as has long been known, some individuals live many times as long as their typical life spans in the wild. There turns out to be enough genetic variability for traits related to longevity that artificial selection for late reproduction in the laboratory over 50 generations can increase average life spans by 80 percent. Genes have also been identified, preeminently in nematodes, with special alleles that increase average life spans up to severalfold. These "longevity assurance genes" are discussed by Thomas Johnson and David Shook in Chapter 7. All this research suggests impressive genetic potential for enhanced longevity. Caleb Finch makes plasticity his theme in the concluding chapter of this volume.

A fourth set of empirical results focus on the relationship between heteroge-neity and hazard rates at extreme ages. They come from the studies of *Droso-phila* and nematodes by James Curtsinger's and Thomas Johnson's groups. These studies indicate that the observed leveling of hazards at advanced ages is not produced solely by the selective effect of genetically frailer individuals dying earlier, leaving genetically more robust individuals to die at lower rates at later ages. The leveling occurs in pure-bred strains, among populations of individuals who are nearly genetically identical.

A critical open question is whether selectivity in the face of developmental and environmental heterogeneity can account for all the leveling not attributable to genetic heterogeneity. James Vaupel debates this question in Chapter 2 and cites one calculation indicating that some part of the leveling is not a selectivity effect but is built into the life course of individuals. This calculation is preliminary and is uncomfortably closely tied to particular mathematical forms for the hazard function. If further research, however, does compel us to invoke a complicated dynamic of individual life-course changes at extreme ages for comparatively simple species of flies and worms, then we shall find ourselves prepared to expect it in ourselves.

THE ELDERLY IN NATURE

These new empirical results promote a sense of a genetic heritage produced by evolution that is permissive or even positive, as far as old-age survival is concerned, in contrast to the sense of limits characteristic of earlier writings in the evolutionary theory of senescence. Paralleling this work is a renewed appreciation of the roles of the elderly in nature.

The middle chapters of this volume shift attention away from the common case of species in which elderly individuals are hardly to be found alive in nature to the interesting exceptional cases in which postreproductive individuals are to be found. In Chapter 8, James Carey and Catherine Gruenfelder challenge the assumption that postreproductive years make little contribution to fitness in the face of natural selection. They draw on recently enriched natural histories and observational studies of elephants, toothed whales, and primates to document contributions of the elderly in social species that might be important in evolutionary terms. Demographers of aging will encounter in this chapter remarkable precedents in nature for human social roles. There are male dolphins of grandparental age babysitting the young in sheltered coves while parents cruise the coast for food. There are elephant matriarchs serving as the seasoned executives of their herds. Effects on fitness are difficult to quantify, but such a variety of contributions can be identified that substantial total effects are plausible.

Kin selection is nothing new to Darwinian theory. But the mathematical theory for age-structured populations, taking off from Norton (1928) and developed by Charlesworth (1994), has been preoccupied with direct contributions to reproduction as reflected in Lotka's net maternity function. Expressions with grandparental and other postreproductive terms in them have been relegated to the background, and, for the most part, "out of sight is out of mind." The new interest in the elderly in nature reflected in this volume calls for a redeployment of mathematical attention.

In thinking about biodemography, we have to remind ourselves continually that day by day we are not seeing humans within the relevant evolutionary environment. Neither, however, are the conditions under which humans evolved entirely a black box. Close observation of the small remaining groups of hunter-gatherers on the planet and of the small remaining groups of primates in unruined habitats can stretch our minds in an imaginative reconstruction of the constraints and opportunities our ancestors may have faced. The coming decade or two may be the last opportunity to gather priceless knowledge.

Hillard Kaplan writes from personal experience and published studies in Chapter 10 about the demography and life-course patterns of hunter-gatherers. He singles out the skill-intensive food niche that these humans occupy in comparison with primates as a decisive evolutionary factor. This situation implies a long provisioning period for the young. High returns to investments in slowly acquired skills go in tandem with high returns to prolonged adult survival. Kaplan estimates that couples begin reproducing at ages when they are first able to support themselves alone. Food for their offspring must come initially as transfers from older members of the group, such as grandparents. Meticulous field work has given us estimates of interage and intergenerational transfers in several hunter-gatherer societies. Ronald Lee shows in Chapter 11 that these estimates fit in well with the patterns of downward age-specific resource flows measured by himself and others in agricultural societies, which have given way to upward flows in economically more developed societies.

The theme of intergenerational transfers is probably the closest meeting ground between biodemography and the rest of contemporary demographic research. Steve Austad surveys precedents among other species in Chapter 9, including mother kangaroo rats who bequeath to their daughters mounds with food stores. There is a tantalizing circularity to intergenerational transfers. Downward age-specific flows imply a higher contribution of older individuals to Darwinian fitness, through the net reproduction of their descendants, letting evolution encourage older survival. Upward resource flows, however, help keep older individuals alive. Ronald Lee imagines what would happen if there were a gene governing behavior impelling offspring to take care of their parents in old age. The parents could then confidently sacrifice their own reproduction on behalf of their offspring's reproduction, having guaranteed that their offspring could not go back on the bargain, having endowed them already with the hypothetical "take-care-of-us" gene.

The evolutionary role of the elderly is intertwined with the question of adaptive menopause. Steve Austad sets out the issues in Chapter 9. In those select species like our own with substantial postreproductive life, menopause might have evolved in response to tradeoffs favoring the cessation of one's own reproduction and the channeling of effort into protecting and endowing the reproductive chances of one's offspring, via the kinds of transfers emphasized in Chapters 8, 10, and 11 respectively by Carey and Gruenfelder, Kaplan, and Lee. On the other hand, menopause could be a somewhat accidental outcome of removing species from their stringent evolutionary environments, in our case taking us out of the wild and into our global zoo. A female's initial endowment of egg cells (oocytes) together with the depletion rate of egg cells over time determine the age when no more egg cells remain, which appears to be the age of menopause. The initial endowment and the rate of depletion could have been fine-tuned to match the life spans existing over evolutionary time in the wild and then stayed constant as life spans increased with the development of sociality or the adventure of civilization.

The population age pyramid of prehistoric men and women is a crucial unknown in this debate. Ethnographers studying the remaining hunter-gatherer populations of today find significant postreproductive survival. Paleo-demographers studying skeletons from prehistory estimate survival curves that drop quickly toward zero at ages like 50. Which is the better guide to human experience over evolutionary time? Ronald Lee provides a demographic analysis in Chapter 11. The ethnographic estimates are of debatable relevance, given the altered environments and impacts of contact that make the hunter-gatherers of today not wholly like our ancestors. The paleo-estimates suffer from selection biases in skeletal remains and difficulties in skeletal-age attributions. Carey and Gruenfelder, Kaplan, and Lee appear more comfortable with the ethnographic estimates. Austad is unconvinced. If postreproductive survival were a feature of our evolutionary past, then, as Lee points out, the question of whether the postreproductive elderly were net economic contributors remains distinct from the question of whether they contributed enough to their descendants' reproduction to make menopause an adaptive trait.

Much that bears on the debate over adaptive menopause remains uncertain. The age of menopause may have changed, possibly under the influence of genes regulating gene expression. Genetic drift may be significant along with selective pressure. The narrow range of ages of menopause observed across human cultures today could bespeak detailed genetic programming, or it could be a shallow consequence of oocyte depletion. We do not know whether to think primarily about time scales of a hundred thousand years or a million years when we think about evolutionary changes relevant to menopause or longevity.

The adaptive status of menopause has medical implications. Austad mentions its bearing on potential side effects of hormone-replacement therapy for postmenopausal women. Randy Nesse and George Williams in their book, *Why We Get Sick: The New Science of Darwinian Medicine* (1994), argue for the relevance of an adaptive evolutionary perspective in understanding a variety of acute and chronic conditions that now affect us. Questions that arise in this book with regard to death and survival are mirrored in their book with regard to morbidity and health. These parallels will need to be pursued in coming years. Biodemography has not yet come to grips very fully with diverse pathologies and causes of death. As Robert Wallace has often pointed out, medflies, *Drosophila*, and nematodes are not just dying, with a certain hazard function. Each is dying of something, although we can hardly say of what. Intelligent speculation about commensurable causes of death will be needed to strengthen the analogy with humans. Among humans, causes of death are more specifiable among the younger-old than among the oldest-old. It might follow that arguments from general principles should be more relevant to the oldest-old. The thinking I have been describing about the elderly in nature, however, is relevant as yet mainly to the younger-old.

THEORETICAL DEPARTURES

The new empirical findings and broader studies of the elderly in nature are providing a powerful stimulus for new theoretical departures.

James Vaupel introduces one of the main new movements in Chapter 2. He shows that automobiles resemble humans, medflies, and nematodes inasmuch as their rising "mortality" rates ultimately also taper with age. Theorists are looking beyond biology to general properties of modes of failure in complex systems. Just as Gauss's normal distribution in statistics arises as a limit under a wide range of basic probability laws, so a tapered modification of the Gompertz (exponential hazard) distribution might be shown to arise as a limiting form of hazard function for organisms with a wide range of detailed mortality dynamics. The trouble so far with complex-system models is that their assumptions can be fairly freely chosen to produce any desired hazard function. We need sharper biological constraints on the assumptions to dispel unpleasant feelings of "ad-hocracy."

In the realm of mathematical models for evolutionary processes, the great challenge is for modeling that gives pride of place to the features—absent from Lotka's equation—bearing directly on the evolutionary role of the elderly. I have already mentioned grandparental and multigenerational terms. Two further features are critical—homeostatic feedback and fluctuating environments.

The word "homeostasis" has different connotations in demography than it has in medicine and physiology, although the root meaning is the same. A homeostatic process in demography is one that tends to drive the population size or growth rate back toward some equilibrium level through some feedback mechanism. Fertility or survival rates that fall at higher family sizes or population densities and rise at lower ones are examples. In demographic homeostasis, it is the population that is subject to regulation; in medicine, it is the physiological state of the organism or the cell. Demographers view homeostatic models as one of the chief common interests uniting biology and demography (see R.D. Lee, 1987). Simple density-dependent models, formulated in terms of disjoint aggregate carrying capacities, have been treated in the evolutionary literature (see Charlesworth, 1994:54-56, 146-154), but more versatile models with intersecting response functions admitting cyclic as well as convergent solutions now deserve energetic study.

For the biodemography of longevity, homeostatic processes that operate at the level of the family or small group are more interesting than population-wide density dependence. Contemporary demography emphasizes tradeoffs between quantity and quality of children, as does Kaplan in Chapter 10. Maximal family sizes are not optimal family sizes, just as with the great tits of Wytham Wood mentioned by Austad and by Partridge in Chapters 9 and 5. Splitting parental investment among too many offspring may compromise their long-term chances to command resources through times of scarcity. Fertility is well below its physiological maximum in hunter-gatherers today, and aggregate growth rates over human prehistory seem to have been fine-tuned remarkably close to zero. There may, therefore, have been little marginal cost to foregoing extra births and high marginal returns to parental survival and investment, especially in the face of recurrent scarcity. Calculations done without assuming homeostasis, cited in Chapter 9, have suggested that the help provided by postmenopausal human females to their kin is not sufficient to offset the losses to their own reproductive potential imposed by menopause. It is imperative to revisit such calculations within the context of homeostatic models.

Fluctuating environments are another critical component of models for the evolution of senescence. Shripad Tuljapurkar has pioneered this subject and addresses it briefly in Chapter 4. When conditions are variable, there are advantages to the ability to prolong or postpone reproduction, wait out times of hardship, and generate families in times of plenty. This is an effect on reproductive spans. But the idea also fits together neatly with Carey's and Gruenfelder's emphasis in Chapter 8. They stress the protective role of surviving parents and parental ability to confer status on their offspring that translates into claims on resources under conditions of scarcity. These factors probably express themselves mainly in cultural and social arrangements, but those then change the parameters for further biological evolution. There is a fuzzy boundary between factors that can plausibly affect our evolving gene pool and factors that operate through culturally transmitted practices, and there is a potent analogy between genetic evolution and cultural evolution.

The evolutionary theory of senescence is itself undergoing rapid evolution. The simple form of mutation-accumulation theory, with its stark force, is giving place to versions with escape clauses, fitter to survive in the face of new empirical evidence. Recent moves in this direction are found in Curtsinger's study of postreproductive mortality rates (unpublished work). As James Vaupel points out in Chapter 2, the mutations at stake in the theory may be rarities. They have to have two quite special properties. They must have specific bad effects on survival at ages unimportant for reproductive fitness. They also have to lack any generalized bad effects on development and viability at earlier ages, so as to accumulate despite natural selection. Genes with both these properties could be exceptional. Mutation accumulation may be just one among several of the stories evolution has to tell. The effect may be most relevant to immediately postreproductive years rather than to extreme ages, and it may imply a relatively short, rather than a nearly endless, list of pathologies and failure modes.

Demographers delving into biological literature are apt to be struck by the frequent assumption that populations will be in genetic equilibrium. The physiological mechanisms that are specifically vulnerable to old-age, postreproductive decay or failure only come into being or salience at some stage in an organism's evolutionary development and only with the inauguration of some set of background environmental and interactive conditions. Mutations with deleterious specific effects on old-age survival have not been accumulating since forever. I miss in biological writing on the evolution of senescence the comparisons of competing time scales that are so common and so helpful in astronomical writing on the evolution of the physical universe.

New theory is giving new emphasis to the historically contingent character of evolutionary change. Mutations produce incremental changes in preexisting physiological structures, gradually suiting them to new functions and purposes. Traits and structure may typically evolve because of one set of advantages and then prove to be preadapted for other advantageous uses. The playing field on which natural selection plays its role is always shifting. James Carey, Catherine Gruenfelder, and Hillard Kaplan discuss this theme in Chapters 8 and 10.

To my mind, nutrition presents us with a mystery of preadaption. In work not well-represented in this volume but central to biodemography, Robert Fogel and his colleagues (see Fogel and Costa, 1997) ascribe a substantial portion of the gains in longevity over the last few centuries to improvements in net nutritional status. Fogel sees a long-term process of "technophysio" evolution that produces nongenetic biological change, such as increasing stature and body mass, translated via relationships called "Waaler surfaces" into gains in health and survival. The mystery is that the nutritional "improvements" should be improvements— taking us, as they do, so far outside the range of nutritional experience to which our bodies could have been adapting over evolutionary time. Of course, our recent diets are not unambiguously beneficial, and the point of diminishing returns may be approaching with nutrition or, indeed, with longevity. But Fogel is looking at the broader sweep of long-term trends. From this perspective, we seem to be preadapted to make use of the quantities of calories and varieties of nutrients that civilization has provided. We reach unprecedented average sizes, as well as unprecedented average life spans, perhaps in concert.

This phenomenon is easier to understand if evolution has been selecting for plasticity of response to times of feast and times of famine, rather than for optimum vigor under fixed conditions. In Chapter 10, Hillard Kaplan writes:

> Recently, the concepts of phenotypic plasticity and evolved norms of reaction have become increasingly important in biologists' understanding of adaptation. Under many conditions genotypes are thought to code for mechanisms that translate environmental inputs into phenotypic outputs rather than for an invariant response... . The ability to alter allocations to survival, maintenance, reproductive effort, fertility, and parental investment in response to changing net energy intake rates must have been under selection.

These ideas accord well with the central role that Caleb Finch assigns to plasticity in the conclusion of this volume.

I have been describing new empirical results and theoretical departures that seem to me to be shifting the scientific ambience of ideas in the biology of longevity away from their longstanding emphasis on limits and tradeoffs. None of the new developments are so tightly connected with demographic processes in humans that they compel the adoption of different models or forecasts. But if further results and theoretical developments in biology in the next few years reinforce the recent developments described in this volume, then I think that demographers will find themselves far less at ease with models that posit strongly diminishing returns in the near future in progress against old-age mortality.

THE PROMISE OF FUTURE RESEARCH

Many chapters in this book point directly toward the future, to kinds of research that should come into their own in the next few years. Chief among these is quantitative trait locus (QTL) analysis of the kind discussed in Chapter 7 by Thomas Johnson and David Shook. We should learn soon how easy it is, in an organism like the elegantly named nematode worm *C. elegans*, to find genes or portions of the genome that do have specific effects on old-age survival. It is tempting for demographers who model hazard rates as functions of age to imagine that genes "know about" ages beyond development and reproduction. In caricature, it is tempting to imagine a set of genes influencing the probability of dying between 50 and 55 and another set influencing the probability of dying between 80 and 85. Results that bolster or undermine this picture will shape the next generation of demographic models.

Tests of predictions from the evolutionary theory of senescence are beginning to capitalize on the quantitative specificity permitted by QTL analysis. We should soon be learning, for some laboratory organisms, whether it is commonplace for portions of the genome that correlate positively with net reproduction to correlate negatively with older-age survival rates, as antagonistic pleiotropy posits. We should be learning systematically about the genetic variance in portions of the genome correlated with older-age hazard rates, and whether the variance increases with age in accordance with mutation-accumulation theory.

QTL analysis, like most of genetics, focuses on polymorphic genes, genes for which two or more forms or alleles remain present in the population despite the ages-long operation of natural selection. However, most genes responsible for structures that promote longevity are doubtless not polymorphic. They have been selected and become fixed in the population. This is less of a worry for geneticists, who are interested in the persistence of genetic variation in its own right, than for demographers. Inducing mutations in genes that have become fixed may sometimes allow QTL analysis to circumvent this limitation, and any such results will be particularly intriguing to demographers. Necessarily, our speculations about fixed genetic components of programmed aging will continue to rely on qualitative comparisons among species, the outcomes of nature's own experiments. But there are enough polymorphic genes to produce nontrivial heritability in human life expectancy at older ages, and QTL analysis of laboratory organisms may guide our understanding of these influences.

Central to my own thinking are a pair of questions that I call the "hundreds-thousands-tens-of-thousands" questions. The first question is this: How many genes should I imagine there being whose specific effects on old-age survival are strong enough to be noticeable in a population? The second question is the converse: How many genes should I imagine typically having to act in concert to produce any one noticeable effect on old-age survival in a population?

I used to think that the answers to these questions were likely to be at the tens-of-thousands end of the scale of orders of magnitude and that the biodemography of longevity would have to become a sort of statistical mechanics before it could make sense. But I have been strongly impressed by the life of Madame Calment and the data on survival at extreme age discussed by Jim Vaupel and John Wilmoth in Chapters 2 and 3. Humans who make it to 110 years of age appear to have truly better further survival rates than those who make it to 95 or 100. No obvious behavioral and environmental determinants of extreme survival have turned up as yet. It therefore seems as if there could be a relatively small number of bad genes—hundreds, not tens-of-thousands—which one has to not have in order to survive ad extrema.

I have already mentioned the hope that research will soon sort out the roles of environmental heterogeneity and individual life-course dynamics in the observed leveling of hazard functions. In the last generation of demographic models, treatment of heterogeneity (the frailty specification) has come first, and life-course dynamics reflected in a changing mix of causes of death by age has come distinctly second. What we learn about the sources of hazard-function leveling in flies and worms is likely to influence the balance of attention in the next generation of demographic models.

In most practical demographic work, genetic heterogeneity is lumped together with a range of omitted variables under the rubric of "unobserved heterogeneity." The new technology of genetic mapping, however, holds out promise of converting some of the unobserved heterogeneity to observed predictor variables. We still have very little insight into the proper ways to incorporate such variables into demographic models. Besides its potential value in predictive models of health status, survival, and other outcomes, individual-level genetic information provides a remarkable source for the reconstruction of the history of population groups.

Parametric models for aggregate hazard functions are at one end of a continuum of modeling in demography. At the other end of that continuum are multiparameter stochastic risk-factor models that derive estimates of transition rates from detailed national surveys with socioeconomic, behavioral, and medical information. In Chapter 12, Robert Wallace discusses the problems and prospects associated with collecting genetic information on specific alleles in conjunction with one or more existing national surveys. Until now, there has been a dearth of thinking on how genetic variables are best introduced into sophisticated mortality models. The availability of even a few genetic markers in large health and demographic data sets would be likely, in my view, to generate rapid improvements in the repertory of models. The central technical problem in recent survey-based research on the impact of health services, interventions, and behavioral changes has been the problem of self-selection bias. Approaches that come under the broad heading of "instrumental variable techniques" are enjoying a vogue in econometrics but remain substantively questionable, because convincing instrumental variables, actually satisfying the statistical assumptions of the models, are hardly to be found. Genetic indicators offer the best hope for obtaining usable instrumental variables and so for beginning to sort out the tangle of selection bias and causation.

The most urgent need for genetic indicators in large national surveys is for confirmatory studies of causal effects of genes on medical conditions. The epidemiological samples on which searches for genes with causal influences are conducted are almost inevitably subject to grave potential selection biases and a large variety of potential confounding factors. Control groups are difficult to arrange. Population-based surveys rich in socioeconomic and demographic background information are going to be essential to confirm the effects on longevity, disability, dementia, and other health-status outcomes as candidate genes are identified. This research will not be easy, because many hard-to-measure factors like dietary patterns are likely to interact with and overshadow the genetic variables. The essential contribution is not to help in the process of screening for candidate genes but rather to detect spurious candidates and sort out the gene-environment-behavior interactions that must underlie many of the observable effects. The inclusion of biomarkers in nationally representative surveys with control variables for potential confounding factors is an essential step in confirming the true role in longevity and health of isolable genetic influences.

The title *Biodemography* is meant to evoke the idea of a marriage of the disciplines of biology and demography. A mixer of metaphors might reasonably ask whether this marriage is to be grounded in mutual affection and commitment or is to be more in the nature of a practically advantageous but cautious arrangement for cohabitation. For neither partner is this a first union. The theories and findings from each discipline discussed in this book are bound to be somewhat in the nature of stepchildren to the other partner. But stepchildren are increasingly central to families in the world around us. The ideas about longevity put forward from the perspectives of biology and demography in the following pages deserve committed nurturance and promise lasting rewards.

REFERENCES

Carey, James R., P. Liedo, D. Orozco, and J. Vaupel
  1992   Slowing of mortality rates at older ages in large medfly cohorts. *Science* 258:457-461.
Charlesworth, Brian
  1994   *Evolution in Age-Structured Populations*, 2nd ed. Cambridge: Cambridge University Press.
Curtsinger, J.W., H. Fukui, D. Townsend, and J.W. Vaupel
  1992   Demography of genotypes: Failure of the limited life-span paradigm in *Drosophila melanogaster. Science* 258:461-463.
Finch, Caleb E.
  1990   *Longevity, Senescence, and the Genome.* Chicago: University of Chicago Press.
Fogel, Robert, and D.L. Costa
  1997   A theory of technophysio-evolution, with some implications for forecasting population, health care costs, and pension costs. *Demography* 34:49-66.
Hayflick, Leonard
  1994   *How and Why We Age.* New York: Ballantine Books.
Kirkwood, B.L.
  1977   Evolution of aging. *Nature* 270:301-304.
Lee, Ronald D.
  1987   Presidential address: Population dynamics of humans and other animals. *Demography* 24:443-466.
Nesse, R., and G. Williams
  1994   *Why We Get Sick: The New Science of Darwinian Medicine*, 1st ed. New York: Times Books.
Norton, H.T.J.
  1928   Natural selection and Mendelian variation. *Proceedings of the London Mathematical Society* 28:1-45.
Olshansky, S.J., and B. Carnes
  1997   Ever since Gompertz. *Demography* 34:1-15.
Rose, M.R.
  1991   *The Evolutionary Biology of Aging.* Oxford: Oxford University Press.
Stearns, S.C.
  1992   *The Evolution of Life Histories.* Oxford: Oxford University Press.

2

Trajectories of Mortality at Advanced Ages

Benjamin Gompertz (1825) proposed that the force of mortality—the hazard of death—increased exponentially with age for humans, at least as a serviceable approximation over the range of adult ages for which he had data. Various subsequent researchers, especially in biology and gerontology, have viewed Gompertz' observation as a law that describes the process of senescence in almost all multicellular animals at all ages after the onset of reproduction. As a rough approximation at younger adult ages, Gompertz' exponential formula does capture the rise in mortality in a great variety of species (Finch, 1990).

Until recently, it was impossible to determine whether this exponential rise continued to advanced ages. For humans, the scattered data available suggested that mortality decelerated at the highest ages, but questions about data reliability precluded strong conclusions. For other species, virtually nothing was known about mortality at advanced ages because the populations studied had been too small to permit dependable estimates of death rates at ages that only a small fraction of the starting cohort reached (Carey et al., 1992).

A research team of demographers and biologists—including James R. Carey, James W. Curtsinger, Thomas E. Johnson, Vaino Kannisto, Pamela Larsen, Hans Lundström, A. Roger Thatcher, Anatoli I. Yashin, myself, and others—has now succeeded in peering into the remote regions of survival for five species—*Homo sapiens, Drosophila melanogaster, Ceratitis capitata* (better known as the medfly), *Anastrepha ludens* (the somewhat larger Mexican fruit fly), and *Caenorhabditis elegans* (a nematode worm). This chapter summarizes the key research findings that pertain to the trajectory of mortality at advanced ages.

The basic finding is that mortality decelerates at older ages. For some species, such as humans, death rates keep on going up with age up to advanced ages but the rate of increase slows down. For other species, such as medflies, death rates reach a plateau and then fall dramatically. Why mortality decelerates at older ages, in all the species for which large, careful studies have been conducted, is a puzzle. The chapter concludes with an explanation of why this is a puzzle and what might be the key to an answer.

The research reported here is based on collaborative efforts by scientists from different backgrounds. Hence, the chapter constitutes a case study of the topic I was asked to address—namely, "demographers, ecologists, and evolutionary biologists: what can we learn from each other?"

THEORIES ABOUT MORTALITY AT ADVANCED AGES

Medvedev (1990) reviews more than 300 theories of aging; most could be used to derive testable predictions about the trajectory of mortality at advanced ages. These theories, however, are, for the most part, simply sets of ad hoc assertions derived from or consistent with a few observations and largely based on strongly held prior beliefs. For example, Buffon, the eighteenth century French naturalist, hypothesized that each species has a characteristic maximum life span and that this maximum life span is six or seven times the duration of the period of growth. A long stream of variants on this theme culminated with Fries (1980), who popularized the conjecture that all individuals are born with a genetically determined maximum life span. Individuals who do not die prematurely die of senescence shortly before their fixed allotment of life.

In the 1950s and 1960s, Medawar (1952), Williams (1957), and Hamilton (1966) developed a more cogent theory, based on evolutionary arguments, of why mortality increases at adult ages. Partridge (in this volume) and Rose (1991) review the development of this theory. Charlesworth (1994) summarized it as follows: at older ages "mutation pressure overpowers selection," leading to "mutational collapse." The basic idea is that there will be little or no pressure of evolutionary selection against mutations that have detrimental effects at older ages but neutral or positive effects at younger ages. The elderly have little impact on evolution because only a fraction of a cohort live to old age and few, if any, of them produce offspring. For humans and other species that care for their children and grandchildren, the elderly may have some evolutionary role, but this role diminishes with advancing age. The prediction of this line of thinking is that the age-trajectory of mortality should shoot up at postreproductive ages, especially for species in which parents do not help their progeny (Curtsinger, 1995b).

Until recently, the evolutionary theory of aging largely rested on theoretically plausible arguments that had not yet been empirically tested; Rose (1991) reviews the limited empirical results. Although there have been some important recent experiments (such as Hughes and Charlesworth, 1994; Charlesworth and

Hughes, 1996), the theory still substantially outpaces available observations. Furthermore, even the theory is based largely on reasoned speculation rather than on well-specified mathematical models with compelling implications.

EMPIRICAL FINDINGS

Demographers have long been interested in the shape of the age-trajectory of human mortality. The general nature of this trajectory from birth to age 80 or so is well known: mortality is high right after birth, falls to a very low level around puberty, and then rises more or less exponentially except for some excess mortality among adolescents and young adults. Due to the painstaking efforts of Kannisto (1994, 1996), Lundström (1995; Vaupel and Lundström, 1994), Thatcher (1992), and others, reliable data on mortality after age 80 are now available for Japan and 13 Western European countries. When these data are pooled, it is possible to accurately estimate the age-trajectory of human mortality up to about age 107 for females and age 105 for males. Reasonable estimates can be made up to about age 110, and shakier "guesstimates" can be boldly ventured up to age 120 (Thatcher et al., 1997). Figure 2-1 clearly shows that human mortality does not increase exponentially after age 80. Mortality decelerates, reaching perhaps a maximum or ceiling around age 110. Whether mortality is slowly increasing, level, slowly decreasing, or rapidly decreasing after age 110 is uncertain.

These results are based on data on some 70 million humans who reached age 80, some 200,000 who celebrated their 100th birthday, and 1 exceptional person, France's Jeanne Calment, who reached age 122 on February 21, 1997.

Humans are animals. Almost all animals show signs of aging; for almost all animals death rates tend to rise after the age of maturity (Finch, 1990). Even researchers who are only interested in people may benefit from biological insights from studies of other species, because these insights may cast light on the biology of humans. The following paragraphs describe some recent findings about age-trajectories of mortality for insects and worms.

The largest nonhuman population followed to natural death consisted of 1.2 million medflies studied in a laboratory near Tapachula, Mexico. These flies were held in cages, each holding several thousand flies. As reported by Carey et al. (1992), the trajectory of mortality rises, peaks, and then falls to a low level around which it hovers until the last fly died at an age of 171 days (compared with an average life span in the experiment of 21 days). The results up to day 100 are shown in Figure 2-2.

Weismann (1889), one of the forerunners of the evolutionary theory of aging, argued that "there is no reason to expect life to be prolonged beyond the reproductive period; so that the end of this period is usually more or less coincident with death" (quoted in Rose, 1991). As noted earlier, Charlesworth (1994) and others who helped develop the evolutionary theory of aging have made

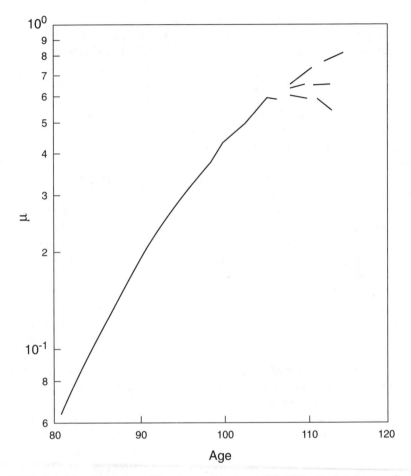

FIGURE 2-1 Mortality at ages 80 and over, females, 1980-1992. Pooled data are from 14 countries (Japan and 13 Western European countries) with the most reliable information. μ = force of mortality. SOURCES: Kannisto (1994, 1996); Lundström (1995); Vaupel and Lundström (1994); and Thatcher (1992).

similar assertions. In the wild there is little egg-laying among medflies after the first month of adult life, so a sharp rise in mortality might be expected around age 30 days. Many of the medflies, however, survived many months after the usual cessation of reproduction.

Following up on this pathbreaking initial study, the Carey laboratory completed life-span analyses on an additional 1.6 million medflies, raised under a variety of conditions. Again, mortality decelerated at older ages. This result was replicated in a study of 1 million *Anastrepha ludens*, the Mexican fruit fly, which is somewhat larger and somewhat longer-lived than the medfly. For this species,

21

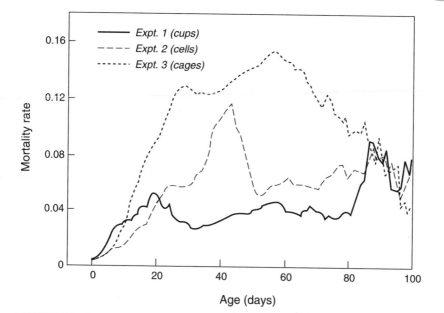

FIGURE 2-2 Smoothed age-specific death rates for three medfly mortality experiments. The total number of individuals remaining alive at age 100 days for experiments 1 (cups), 2 (cells), and 3 (cages) was 307, 31, and 62, respectively. SOURCE: Carey et al. (1992).

mortality peaked around 2 months of age and then roughly leveled off (Boe et al., 1995).

In James Curtsinger's laboratory, the life spans of tens of thousands of *Drosophila melanogaster* have been studied in various controlled experiments. These experiments all involve genetically identical strains of flies. From the earliest reported findings (Curtsinger et al., 1992) on, the experiments have shown a deceleration of mortality at older ages (e.g., Promislow et al., 1996), with strong indications that the mortality rate at older ages is "approximately constant and independent of age" (Curtsinger et al., 1992). Figure 2-3 shows a typical pattern of mortality for one of the isogenetic strains analyzed.

In Thomas Johnson's laboratory, a cohort of 180,000 nematode worms of the species *Caenorhabditis elegans* were followed until the entire population had died (Brooks et al., 1994). The worms were of the same genotype—that is, they were genetically identical, like identical twins. Analysis of these data revealed a definite deceleration in mortality around day 8 or 9, which is the age when reproduction for this genotype falls to very low levels (Vaupel et al., 1994). As shown in Figure 2-4, a two-stage Gompertz model fits the data fairly well. From day 5 to 8 mortality increased at a rate of 0.58, which is more than twice the rate of 0.21 that prevails afterwards. A smooth curve that levels off at the highest ages also fits the data well.

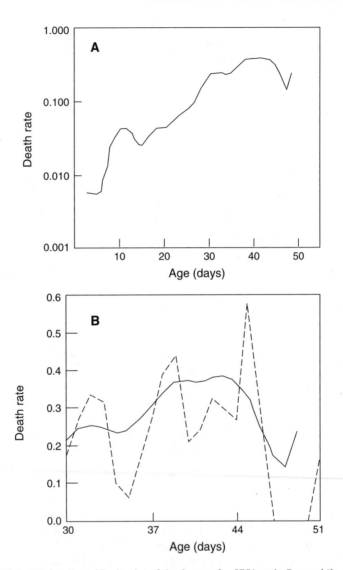

FIGURE 2-3 (A) Semilogarithmic plot of death rates for 5751 male *Drosophila melanogaster* from inbred line. (B) Detail of mortality rate (arithmetic scale) of last 1906 deaths. Dashed line: Observed daily probabilities of death (five final deaths not shown). Solid line: Death rates estimated by smoothing. SOURCE: Curtsinger et al. (1992).

Pamela Larsen directs a nematode laboratory at the University of Southern California. She has compared the mortality trajectory of the so-called wild-type nematode, the genotype usually studied, with mutant strains that differ from the wild type by a point mutation at a single locus known as *DAF2* (Larsen, 1993). As shown in Figure 2-5, her experiments show a sharp rise in mortality in the wild-type strain, but a much slower increase, with signs of a rough leveling off, in the *DAF2* genotypes. What is remarkable is the radical change in the age-trajectory of mortality produced by a point mutation. [Larsen's results look quite different from Johnson's results, as shown in Figure 2-4, but they are not inconsistent. Larsen's experiments involved thousands, rather than hundreds of thousands, of worms. As demonstrated in Carey et al. (1992), the deceleration of mortality may not become apparent until a very large experiment is done. Furthermore, Johnson's experiments were conducted under much harsher conditions than Larsen's experiments, which explains the difference in life expectancy.]

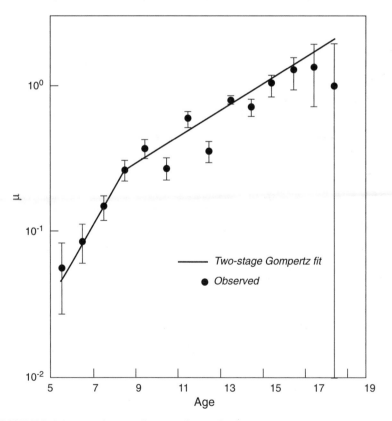

FIGURE 2-4 Nematode mortality. μ = force of mortality. SOURCE: Vaupel, Johnson, and Lithgow (1994).

For all five species for which reliable data are available on large populations—humans, medflies, Mexican fruit flies, *Drosophila*, and nematode worms—mortality tends not to accelerate, but rather to decelerate, at older ages. This finding also appears true in some other species for which smaller populations were studied, including the bruchid beetle *Callosobruchus maculatus* (Tatar et al., 1993) and perhaps the flour beetle *Tribolium confusum* and the common house fly *Musca domestica* (Wilson, 1994). Death rates are such that many individuals in these various species survive well past the ages when reproduction usually ceases or drops to very low levels. Madame Jeanne Calment, who died at age 122, had lived seven decades after menopause. For the flies and worms, which do not care for their progeny, extraordinarily long spans of life have been observed in the "postreproductive" period when fertility is very low. Nematodes, for instance, have very few progeny after the

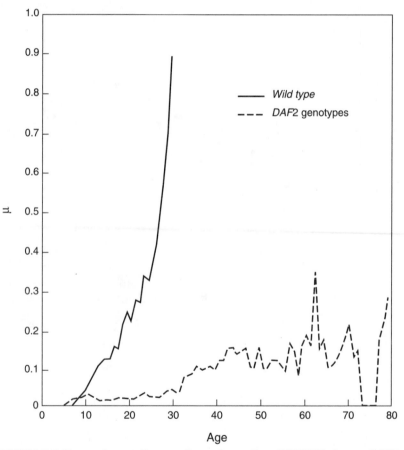

FIGURE 2-5 Nematode mortality. μ = force of mortality. SOURCE: Larsen (1993).

eighth day of their lives, but Pamela Larsen's longest-lived worm wriggled around for some 96 days.

MECHANISMS

Mortality deceleration came as a surprise, indeed as a shock, to many biologists and gerontologists. (Demographers, on the other hand, had long suspected that death rates probably increased more slowly at older ages, although the data available until recently did not permit a definitive conclusion.) A spate of possible explanations were quickly developed. The following paragraphs review the main possibilities.

In most large animal experiments, populations are kept in confined areas of fixed size. As population size declines with age, population density decreases. If lower densities are salubrious, then the observed leveling off and decline in mortality with age might be an artifact of such changes in density (Graves and Mueller, 1993; Nusbaum et al., 1993; Kowald and Kirkwood, 1993). However, populations of medflies raised in solitary confinement in individual cells also showed a deceleration of mortality at older ages (Carey et al., 1992). Further medfly experiments were done in which density were systematically varied and changes in density were statistically controlled (Carey et al., 1995). The level of mortality increased at higher densities, but regardless of density, mortality rose, leveled off, and then fell with age. In addition, *Drosophila* experiments were painstakingly conducted in which density was held constant by replacement of older flies (Khaezeli et al., 1995). These experiments "show a deceleration of mortality at older ages that is not attributable to density effects" (Curtsinger, 1995a).

All populations are heterogeneous. In some of the experiments described above, strong efforts were made to ensure that all individuals in the population were genetically identical and that environmental conditions were highly similar for all individuals. Even in these experiments, however, individuals differed from each other, in size, in weight, and, more generally, in robustness and vitality. Some individuals are frailer than others . . . and the frail tend to die first. This creates a fundamental problem—indeed it seems to me *the* fundamental problem—for demographic analyses in general and for analyses of age-trajectories of mortality in particular. The individuals alive at older ages are systematically different from the individuals alive at younger ages. The age-trajectory of mortality reflects both the underlying age-trajectories of mortality for individuals in the population *and* the effects of compositional change as the frailer individuals drop out of the population.

Some of my colleagues and I have devoted a lot of thought to this problem over the past two decades (e.g., Vaupel et al., 1979; Vaupel and Yashin, 1985; Vaupel and Carey, 1993). Several researchers suggested that deceleration observed in medfly and *Drosophila* mortality might be attributable to heterogeneity

(Olshansky et al., 1993; Kowald and Kirkwood, 1993; Brooks et al., 1994), and this possibility was noted in both the original Carey et al. (1992) report on medfly mortality and the original Curtsinger et al. (1992) report on *Drosophila* mortality. It can be mathematically proven that compositional change (resulting from the higher mortality of the frail) decreases the rate of increase in the age-trajectory of mortality. In fact, even if death rates are increasing with age for every individual in a population, the age-trajectory of mortality can level off or even decline as a result of compositional change. The Gompertz exponential formula could hold for individual medflies, even though death rates for cohorts of medflies fall substantially at older ages.

Vaupel and Carey (1993) show this. They also show, however, that the required degree of heterogeneity is very large. To fit an underlying Gompertz model to the medfly data, they had to divide the population into subgroups that had vastly different chances of death. The frailest subgroup had 5 billion times the chance of death at any age as the most robust subgroup. Although there may be considerable heterogeneity in relative risks of death in a population, it seems unlikely that the degree of heterogeneity is this large. Natural selection will tend to eliminate subgroups with very high mortalities. Such subgroups could, in theory, be blessed with counterbalancing advantages: they could be extremely fertile or they could tend to produce a few very robust individuals. Further research is warranted, but at present it seems implausible that all of the observed deceleration of mortality at older ages is an artifact of heterogeneity.

If the deceleration of mortality is not completely attributable to compositional change, then there has to be some deceleration at the individual level. It seems plausible that some of the observed deceleration is due to behavioral and physiological changes that occur with age and that are associated either with declines in reproductive activity or with repair mechanisms that compensate for damage at younger ages (Finch, 1990; Carey et al., 1992; Kowald and Kirkwood, 1993; Tatar et al., 1993; Carey and Liedo, 1995). More research is required on the importance of these effects and on the extent to which the deceleration of mortality at older ages can be attributable to changes at the individual level.

More generally, research is needed on the mechanisms that produce various details of the pattern of mortality seen in large populations. For instance, what accounts for the prominent hump in medfly mortality around day 30 (as shown in Figure 2-2)? This hump not only appears in the initial population of 1.2 million but also appears in the large populations of several million medflies studied since (Carey and Liedo, 1995; Carey et al., 1995). Mueller et al., (1997) analyze this "mortality surge." Their research shows that careful attention to the details of the bends and bulges of mortality trajectories can lead to deeper understanding of the determinants of survival and longevity. Horiuchi and Wilmoth (e.g., in press) have done some interesting work along these lines for humans.

BIO-RELIABILITY THEORY

Living organisms are complex systems; reliability engineers and systems analysts have learned a great deal about the failure of complex systems. Even the simplest bacterium is vastly more complicated than the most elaborate machinery. Living organisms have repair and homeostatic programs that far excel those in any mechanical device. Nonetheless, it may prove useful to merge perspectives from reliability engineering and evolutionary theory, from systems analysis and biology, from the study of populations of equipment and the study of populations of people and other forms of life.

Reliability engineers often work with stochastic models in which various states represent the "health" of the system, as determined, for instance, by which components are still working and which components are broken. LeBras (1976) and Gavrilov and Gavrilova (1991) provide some examples that they interpret as models of aging. Yashin et al. (1994) show that the LeBras model and a related model presented by the Gavrilovs produce exactly the same age-trajectory of mortality as does the frailty model proposed by Vaupel et al. (1979). In particular, the various models all lead to a deceleration and eventual leveling off of mortality.

Statisticians interested in stochastic models of failure have considerably generalized this line of thinking. Consider a homogeneous Markov chain in continuous time with a single absorbing state, which can be interpreted as failure or death. Such a Markov chain can have many states and many branches from each state; it can include return to healthier states (as the result of recovery or repair). Suppose there is some initial distribution of individuals among the nonabsorbing states. Then time until death is said to follow a phase-type distribution. Under a variety of fairly general conditions, the age-trajectory of mortality for such a system will eventually level off. Under somewhat more restrictive but still fairly general conditions, the age-trajectory of mortality can rise, decelerate, and then level off. Other more restrictive conditions can produce other patterns, including mortality trajectories with bumps and declines such as those observed for medflies (Figure 2-2). Aalen (1995) suggests that such models should find greater application in biostatistics; he provides some examples as well as a lucid review of the basic ideas.

Many biologists seem to believe that it is possible for organisms to approximate the "one-hoss shay" of Oliver Wendell Holmes that ran perfectly until one day when all of its pieces fell apart simultaneously (e.g., Fries and Crapo, 1981; Dawkins, 1995). This is one of the suppositions used to justify the belief in species-specific maximum life spans. Reliability theory, however, strongly suggests that one-hoss shays are impossible to construct—unless there is a built-in time bomb. Empirical data on the failure of equipment is consistent with the theory. Equipment is often designed such that there is a high probability of survival up until some point. The Pioneer space probe, for instance, was designed to reach Mars; consumer durables may be designed to last until the end of the warranty period. Such designs, however, generally result in substantial spans of life after the target age. The Pioneer space probe was still functioning when it escaped the Solar System; some washing machines and refrigerators continue to function years after their warranties have expired. A body design that gives an organism a good chance of surviving long enough to reproduce may be a sufficiently robust design that some of the organisms can survive long thereafter (Hayflick, 1994).

Automobiles are popular pieces of complicated equipment. They are sufficiently standardized that it is meaningfully possible to count their numbers on an age-specific (model-year) basis. Using automobile registration data gathered by the various states of the United States, R.L. Polk and Company did so for July 1, 1941, and then for July 1 of every year from 1947 to the present. These data, which are closely analogous to population count data collected by national statistical offices and census bureaus, have been assembled and analyzed by Vaupel and C.R. Owens (unpublished work). Using standard demographic methods, they estimated, among other summary statistics, the age-trajectory of mortality for automobiles in various cohorts and in various periods, as shown in Figures 2-6 and 2-7. Depending on the period or cohort, it was possible to compute central death rates—the number of deaths in an interval divided by the average number of individuals alive in the interval—from age 1 to an age up to age 17. Several aspects of the age-trajectories of automobile mortality are intriguing and are addressed by Vaupel and C.R. Owens.

What is important here is the deceleration and leveling off of mortality at older ages. If the titles and legends of Figures 2-6 and 2-7 were erased, an unsuspecting observer might think the trajectories pertained to Drosophila or nematode worms or some other living species. The trajectories are also somewhat similar to the human pattern at older ages.

The deceleration and leveling off of automobile mortality is partially due to heterogeneity—the composition of the automobile fleet changes with age because some kinds of cars are built better and last longer than others. As shown in Figure 2-8, however, even if a single make of car were chosen and a single model year were followed, there is still evidence of deceleration and leveling off. Among cars of the same make and model year—roughly analogous to genotype, although there are different models of the same make—there are certainly differences in "phenotype" (i.e., in observable characteristics of individuals), arising from various errors made in constructing particular cars, from the environment in which the car is driven, from the temperament of the car's owner, etc. Lemons driven on dirt roads by careless, impetuous drivers will tend to be selected out.

Beyond the effects of such compositional change, there are almost certainly "physiological and behavioral" changes that contribute to mortality deceleration. Older cars are repaired. Older cars may be driven less frequently and more

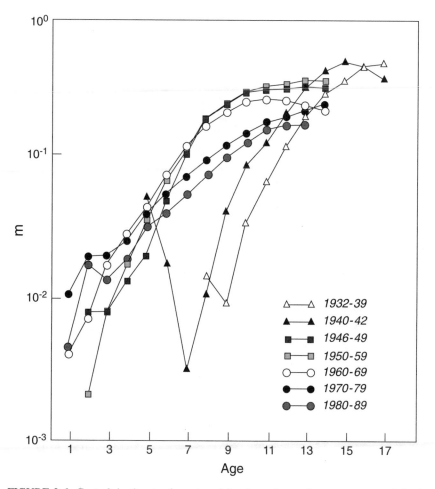

FIGURE 2-6 Central death rates for automobiles in various cohorts. m = central death rate.

carefully. As cars age, their owners may also age and become more stolid and responsible.

On a more general and speculative level, the question arises—is mortality a property of living organisms or a property of complicated systems? When it comes to death, how do people and worms differ from Chevrolets? In particular, is the deceleration and leveling off of mortality a fairly general property of complicated systems (as suggested by phase-type models and by the automobile data)? Better understanding of these questions may lead to new insights into aging and survival. Judicious caution is required, however, because living organ-

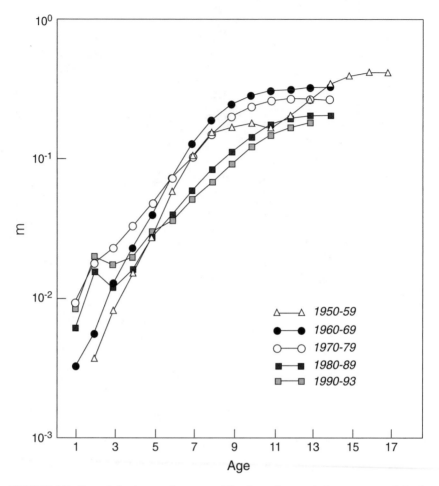

FIGURE 2-7 Central death rates for automobiles in various periods. m = central death rate.

isms are vastly more complicated than equipment and fundamentally different along many key dimensions.

In sum, although living organisms and equipment share only a few common attributes, demographers and biologists may nonetheless be able to learn something from reliability engineers. There is already a splendid example of this—the statistical methods used to analyze survival data were to a considerable extent developed by reliability engineers interested in analyzing failure-time data. Phase-type models, the long postmission life of space probes, and empirical data on the mortality of automobiles suggest the range of potential opportunities for cross-fertilization.

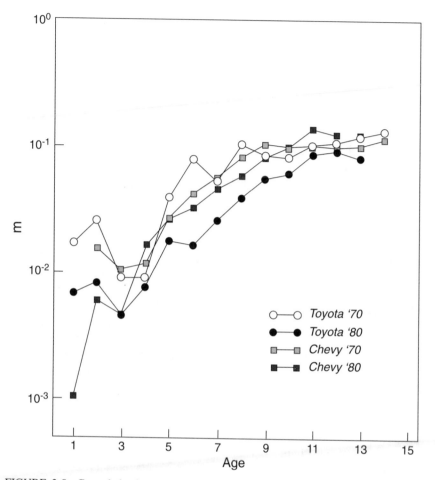

FIGURE 2-8 Central death rates for Chevrolets and Toyotas, 1970 and 1980 model years. m = central death rate.

THE EVOLUTIONARY THEORY OF AGING REVISITED

The discussion so far has addressed a number of explanations for the observed deceleration of mortality in the five species for which large populations have been studied. The deceleration does not appear to be an artifact of declining population densities in the experimental populations. The deceleration is probably partially, but only partially, attributable to compositional change in heterogeneous populations. The deceleration is probably partially attributable to behavioral and physiological changes at the individual level. A deceleration of mortality is also observed in large populations of automobiles—and this deceleration is almost certainly due to a combination of compositional change and changing behavior. It seems clear that various genetic, environmental, behavioral, bio-reliability, and population-heterogeneity mechanisms interact to determine the age-trajectory of mortality in general and its deceleration in particular. The nature of these mechanisms and their relative importance remain to be explored. Specific, testable hypotheses have to be formulated, and appropriate data sets have to be gathered. Experiments with various animal models (and perhaps even with inanimate machines) will almost certainly provide valuable information to supplement observational studies of human populations.

Perhaps the biggest current challenge is to clarify the mystifying puzzle of why the evolutionary theory of aging does not appear consistent with the empirical observation that mortality decelerates at older ages. "Nothing in biology makes sense except in the light of evolution," Dobzhansky (1973) asserted. Evolutionary thinking, however, appears to lead to the prediction that deleterious mutations should accumulate at the age when reproduction falls to low levels. A black hole of bad alleles (i.e., of mutational forms of genes) should preclude survival much past this age. There appear to be at least two ways out of this quandary; neither is, as yet, very well understood, and there may be other solutions as well.

First, it may not be true that the elderly are unimportant from an evolutionary perspective. As Carey and Gruenfelder (in this volume) put it, the elderly may play important roles in nature. For some species this role may consist of helping offspring and other relatives survive. For other species, very rare instances of fertility at older ages may be crucially important and hence of much greater evolutionary significance than simple versions of Lotka's equation imply. In particular, it may be that some species have to make it through bottlenecks, due perhaps to lack of food, cold weather, or drought. Only a very few, exceptionally robust and long-lived individuals may make it through such bottlenecks. These individuals would be the founders of the new populations: all the members of these new populations would have the founder's longevity genes. Even if there are no bottlenecks, there may be considerable stochasticity in a species' environment such that late reproduction is sometimes favored. Tuljapurkar (in this volume) discusses the importance of such stochasticity.

Second, it may be that "mutation-accumulation" alleles are rare. These alleles have bad effects but only at older ages; at younger ages, they are neutral and have no effects. Such alleles may be rare because it is difficult in practice for mutations to occur that produce effects that first start operating at older ages. Nature is constrained by the materials and processes at hand. It is also possible that such alleles are rare because they are knocked-out by subsequent mutations. Most mutations are harmful; many are so harmful that they prevent a gene from properly functioning. Such knock-out mutations can be expected to eventually destroy any allele that does not contribute in some way to an organism's evolutionary fitness. If mutation-accumulation alleles are rare, they may not be of much significance, especially for biological processes that involve many genes in a redundant way that reduces the harmful effects of any particular allele.

"Antagonistic-pleiotropy" alleles (i.e., genes that have multiple effects that pull in different directions) may also be rare. In particular, such alleles are supposed to come in two varieties: some are helpful at younger ages and harmful at middle and older ages, whereas others are harmful at younger ages and helpful at middle and older ages. The older ages in this model do not count for much, if at all, because few individuals survive to older ages, and those that do have low fertility. A tradeoff of good and bad effects between younger and middle ages is, however, theoretically possible. Mutations may arise that lead to the existence of two alleles at the same locus, with opposite age-specific impacts. All species have to make tradeoffs between fertility and survival, between early and late fertility, between early and late survival, etc. Mutations that produce pairs of antagonistic-pleiotropy alleles may be the mechanism that enables alternative choices about such tradeoffs. Both of the two competing alleles may, however, not survive many generations: one may be driven to extinction as the other goes to fixation (Curtsinger et al., 1994). If this were the case, one would observe that species make tradeoffs, but one would only occasionally observe a genetic locus with two or more antagonistic-pleiotropy alleles with different age-specific effects.

The research of Carey, Partridge, Tuljapurkar, and Rose (all of whom have chapters in this volume), as well as Curtsinger (1995a,b), Abrams (1993), and others, is helping clarify the mysterious fact that many individuals survive well past the normal end of reproduction. In addition to the ideas adumbrated above, other possible explanations may prove important. At present, this question appears to be a wide-open, exciting issue on the frontier of knowledge.

CONCLUSION

This chapter was designed to serve two purposes. My charge was to address the question of what demographers, ecologists, and evolutionary biologists can learn from each other. Actually, demographers, ecologists, and evolutionary biologists have learned a lot from each other about the trajectories of mortality at advanced ages. In explaining what they have learned, the potential for this kind of biodemographic collaboration can be conveyed in a concrete, persuasive way. What has been learned—and what could be learned through further collaboration—is fascinating: outlining this was the dual, complementary purpose of this chapter, the other side of the same coin.

Demographers, ecologists, and evolutionary biologists focus on different topics, have memorized different facts and jargon, and have been indoctrinated with different concepts. They share, however, an interest in populations. Although many demographers rigidly restrict demography to the study of human populations, the methods and concepts of demography are useful in studying many kinds of populations, from insects and other forms of life (Carey, 1993) to Chevrolets. If nothing in biology can be understood except in the light of evolution, an equally valid generalization is that nothing in evolution can be understood except in the light of demography. Lotka's demographic equation, which relates survival and fertility to population growth, is the fundamental equation in most evolutionary theorizing in general and in the evolutionary biology of aging in particular.

As Rose (1991) stated, "From these basic features of the demography of populations (i.e., the age-trajectories of survival and fecundity), the crucial evolutionary determinants of aging follow." The research of demographers, ecologists, and evolutionary biologists reviewed in this chapter shows it is still not fully understood how the crucial evolutionary determinants of aging follow from the underlying demography of survival and fertility. Nonetheless, the point is well taken. Deeper understanding of the demography of populations—through research on genetic, environmental, behavioral, bio-reliability, and heterogeneity forces and constraints, including emphasis on the role of the elderly in nature (Carey and Gruenfelder, in this volume)—will almost certainly provide new insights and perhaps the crucial insights into the mechanisms that drive the processes of aging and survival.

REFERENCES

Aalen, O.O.
   1995   Phase type distributions in survival analysis. *Scandinavian Journal of Statistics* 22:447-463.
Abrams, P.
   1993   Does increased mortality favor the evolution of more rapid senescence? *Evolution* 47:877-888.
Boe, C., C. Gruenfelder, P. Liedo, and J.R. Carey
   1995   Mortality Deceleration and Longevity in the Mexican Fruit Fly (*Anastrepha ludens*). Manuscript. Department of Entomology, University of California, Davis, CA 95616.
Brooks, A., G.J. Lithgow, and T.E. Johnson
   1994   Mortality-rates in a genetically heterogeneous population of *Caenorhabditis elegans*. *Science* 263(5147):668-671.
Carey, J.R.
   1993   *Applied Demography for Biologists*. New York: Oxford University Press.
Carey, J.R., and P. Liedo
   1995   Sex mortality differentials and selective survival in large medfly cohorts. *The Gerontologist* 35:588-596.
Carey, J.R., P. Liedo, D. Orozco, and J.W. Vaupel
   1992   Slowing of mortality rates at older ages in large medfly cohorts. *Science* 258:457-461.
Carey, J.R., P. Liedo, and J.W. Vaupel
   1995   Mortality dynamics of density in the Mediterranean fruit fly. *Experimental Gerontology* 30:605-629.
Charlesworth, R.
   1994   *Evolution in Age-Structured Populations*, 2nd ed. New York: Cambridge University Press.

Charlesworth, R., and K.A. Hughes
1996 Age-specific inbreeding depression and components of genetic variance in relation to the evolution of senescence. *Proceedings of the National Academy of Sciences U.S.A.* 93(12):6140-6145.

Curtsinger, J.W.
1995a Density and age-specific mortality [comment]. *Genetica* 96(3):179-182.
1995b Density, mortality, and the narrow view. *Genetica* 96(3):187-189.

Curtsinger, J.W., H.H. Fukui, D.R. Townsend, and J.W. Vaupel
1992 Demography of genotypes: Failure of the limited life-span paradigm in *Drosophila melanogaster*. *Science* 258:461-463.

Curtsinger, J.W., P. Service, and T. Prout
1994 Antagonistic pleiotropy, reversal of dominance, and genetic polymorphism. *American Naturalist* 144:210-228.

Dawkins, R.
1995 God's utility function. *Scientific American* 273:80-85.

Dobzhansky, T.
1973 Nothing in biology makes sense except in the light of evolution. *American Biology Teacher* 35:125-129.

Finch, C.E.
1990 *Longevity, Senescence, and the Genome.* Chicago: University of Chicago Press.

Fries, J.F.
1980 Aging, natural death, and the compression of morbidity. *New England Journal of Medicine* 303:130-135.

Fries, J.F., and L.M. Crapo
1981 *Vitality and Aging: Implications of the Rectangular Curve.* San Francisco, CA: W.H. Freeman.

Gavrilov, L.A., and N.S. Gavrilova
1991 *The Biology of Life Span.* Chur, Switzerland: Harwood Academic Publishers.

Gompertz, B.
1825 On the nature of the function expressive of the law of human mortality. *Philosophical Transactions* 27:510-519.

Graves, J.L., and L.D. Mueller
1993 Population density effects on longevity. *Genetica* 91:99-109.

Hamilton, W.D.
1966 The moulding of senescence by natural selection. *Journal of Theoretical Biology* 12:12-45.

Hayflick, L.
1991 Aging under glass. *Mutation Research* 256(2-6):69-80.
1994 *How and Why We Age.* New York: Balantine Books.

Horiuchi, S., and J.R. Wilmoth
In press Deceleration in the age pattern of mortality at older ages. *Demography.*

Hughes, K.A., and B. Charlesworth
1994 A genetic analysis of senescence in *Drosophila*. *Nature* 367:64-66.

Kannisto, V.
1994 *Development of Oldest-Old Mortality, 1950-1990.* Odense, Denmark: Odense University Press.
1996 *The Advancing Frontier of Survival.* Odense, Denmark: Odense University Press.

Khaezeli, A.A., L. Xiu, and J.W. Curtsinger
1995 Effect of adult cohort density on age-specific mortality in *Drosophila melanogaster*. *Journal of Gerontology* 50(5):B262-269.

Kowald, A., and T.B.L. Kirkwood
1993 Explaining fruit fly longevity. *Science* 260:1664-1665.

Larsen, P.L.
　1993　　Aging and resistance to oxidative damage in Caenorhabditis elegans. *Proceedings of the National Academy of Sciences U.S.A.* 90(19):8905-8909.

LeBras, H.
　1976　　Lois de mortalite a age limite. *Population* 31:655-692.

Lundström, H.
　1995　　Record longevity in Swedish cohorts born since 1700. In B. Jeune and J.W. Vaupel, eds., *Exceptional Longevity: From Prehistory to the Present.* Odense, Denmark: Odense University Press.

Medawar, P.B.
　1952　　*An Unsolved Problem in Biology.* London: H.K. Lewis.

Medvedev, Z.A.
　1990　　An attempt at a rational classification of theories of ageing. *Biological Reviews* 65:375-398.

Mueller, H.G., J.L. Wang, W.B. Capra, P. Liedo, and J.R. Carey
　1997　　Early mortality surge in protein-deprived females causes reversal of sex differential of life expectancy in Mediterranean fruit flies. *Proceedings of the National Academy of Sciences U.S.A.* 94(6):2762-2765.

Nusbaum, T.J., J.L. Graves, L.D. Mueller, and M.R. Rose
　1993　　Fruit fly aging and mortality. Letter to Editor. *Science* 260:1567.

Olshansky, S.J., B.A. Carnes, and C.K. Cassel
　1993　　Fruit fly aging and mortality. Letter to Editor. *Science* 260:1565-1566.

Promislow, D.E.L., M. Tatar, A.A. Khazaeli, and J.W. Curtsinger
　1996　　Age-specific patterns of genetic variance in *Drosophila melanogaster. Genetics* 143(2):839-848.

Rose, M.R.
　1991　　*Evolutionary Biology of Aging.* New York: Oxford University Press.

Tatar, M., J.R. Carey, and J.W. Vaupel
　1993　　Long-term cost of reproduction with and without accelerated senescence in *Callosobruchus maculatus*: Analysis of age-specific mortality. *Evolution* 47:1302-1312.

Thatcher, A.R.
　1992　　Trends in numbers and mortality at high ages in England and Wales. *Population Studies* 46:411-426.

Thatcher, A.R., V. Kannisto, and J.W. Vaupel
　1997　　*The Force of Mortality from Age 80 to 120.* Odense, Denmark: Odense University Press.

Vaupel, J.W., and J. R. Carey
　1993　　Compositional explanations of medfly mortality. *Science* 260:1666-1667.

Vaupel, J.W., T.E. Johnson, and G.J. Lithgow
　1994　　Rates of mortality in populations of *Caenorhabditis elegans. Science* 266:826.

Vaupel, J.W., and H. Lundström
　1994　　The future of mortality at older ages in developed countries. In W. Lutz, ed., *The Future Population of the World.* London: Earthscan.

Vaupel, J.W., K.G. Manton, and E. Stallard
　1979　　The impact of heterogeneity in individual frailty on the dynamics of mortality. *Demography* 16:439-454.

Vaupel, J.W., and A. I. Yashin
　1985　　Heterogeneity's ruses: Some surprising effects of selection on population dynamics. *American Statistician* 39:176-185.

Weismann, A.
　1889　　*Essays upon Heredity and Kindred Biological Problems.* Oxford: Clarendon Press.

Williams, G.C.
 1957 Pleiotropy, natural selection, and the evolution of senescence. *Evolution* 11:398-411.
Wilson, D.L.
 1994 The analysis of survival (mortality) data: Fitting Gompertz, Weibull, and logistic functions. *Mechanisms of Ageing and Development* 74:15-33.
Yashin, A.I., J.W. Vaupel, and I.A. Iachine
 1994 A duality in aging: The equivalence of mortality models based on radically different concepts. *Mechanisms of Aging and Development* 74:1-14.

3

In Search of Limits

John R. Wilmoth

INTRODUCTION

The dramatic rise in life expectancy during the past two or three centuries is arguably the greatest collective human achievement. Fragmentary evidence suggests that early levels of human life expectancy were around 25 years (Acsádi and Nemeskéri, 1970). At the beginning of the twentieth century, many poorer countries still had life expectancies in this range (Preston, 1980; Davis, 1951), although by 1900 the mean life span in the most advantaged countries had already risen to around 50 years (Preston, 1990). According to the latest estimates, life expectancy at birth is still in the low to mid 40s in some African countries but is almost universally above 50 years elsewhere; in Japan and a few other countries, the mean length of life is now around 80 years (Population Reference Bureau, 1995).

As we approach the end of the twentieth century, we are led to question whether this incredible progress has run its course. Is it plausible to believe that these well-documented gains in human longevity can continue? Are limits to the rise in human life expectancy imposed by the structure of the organism itself? Several authors have argued that such limits must exist, based on their understanding of biological mechanisms or a review of demographic evidence. Two common beliefs that have gained an almost mythical status are that human life expectancy is bounded by a limit of around 85 years and that the maximum human life span is around 120 years.

There are numerous means of approaching the question of whether such limits exist. In this chapter, I restrict the discussion to a review of relevant demographic evidence and do not address the many biological arguments related to this issue. My approach is that of a demographer and statistician who attempts to define what limits might look like in terms of aggregate mortality data and then reviews the existing empirical evidence within that framework.

WHAT WOULD LIMITS TO HUMAN LONGEVITY LOOK LIKE?

If limits to human longevity exist, they must have both a mechanism and a manifestation. As noted already, I do not address the issue of mechanisms in this chapter but focus instead on the question of how limits might manifest themselves in aggregate mortality patterns. Based on a review of the literature and my own understanding of this topic, there appear to be three hypotheses about the age distribution of human mortality—and, in particular, about changes in the shape of that distribution over time—which may have a bearing on the issue of limits. In this section, I seek to explain these hypotheses clearly, to review some of the relevant literature, and to examine the most important empirical evidence in light of this theoretical framework. I also discuss briefly the logical connections between the three hypotheses. I conclude by offering a summary view of what a demographic perspective suggests at present about the limits of human longevity.

Notation

The three hypotheses can be stated using the notation of life tables or survival analysis. The former notation is most familiar to demographers and actuaries, while the latter is often used by statisticians, reliability engineers, and many biomedical researchers. To facilitate understanding by a diverse crowd, I will mention both sets of notation whenever convenient. I will favor the notation of survival analysis, however, because it is more general and probably more widely accessible to an interdisciplinary audience.

Mortality distributions can be effectively summarized by any one of several complementary functions. Three functions are particularly useful: the density function, the survival function, and the hazard function. Let X be a (positive) random variable representing the life span of an individual drawn at random from a population of newborns. Following standard statistical practice, let $f(x)$ be the *probability density function* describing the distribution of life spans in this population. The *cumulative density function*, $F(x)$, gives the probability (Pr) that an individual dies before surpassing age x:

$$F(x) = \Pr[X \leq x] = \int_0^x f(a)da. \tag{1}$$

The *survival function*, $S(x)$, gives the complementary probability that an individual is still alive at age x:

$$S(x) = \Pr[X > x] = \int_x^\infty f(a)da = 1 - F(x). \tag{2}$$

The *hazard function, h(x)*, is defined as the ratio of the density and survival functions:

$$h(x) = \frac{f(x)}{S(x)}.$$ (3)

Thus, the hazard function gives the probability density at age x conditional on survival to that age:

$$h(x) = \frac{f(x)}{S(x)} = \frac{\lim\limits_{h \to 0} \dfrac{\Pr[x < X < x + h]}{h}}{\Pr[X > x]}$$ (4)

$$= \lim\limits_{h \to 0} \frac{\Pr[x < X < x + h \mid X > x]}{h} = f(x \mid X > x).$$

In life table notation, the probability of surviving to age x, $S(x)$, would be denoted as lx/l_0 (the *radix* of the life table, l_0, may equal one by definition, although it is usually some large, arbitrary number like 100,000). The continuous density function, $f(x)$, would be replaced by the discrete function, dx (or d_x/l_0), which gives the number (or proportion) of life table deaths in the age interval from x to $x + 1$. Finally, the hazard function, $h(x)$, would be written in the life table as μ_x and is known to demographers and actuaries as the *force of mortality*.

As an illustration, the survival, hazard, and density functions for U.S. females in 1900 and 1992 are shown in Figure 3-1. As the hazard function has fallen across the age range, the area under the survival curve has grown, and the density function has shifted to the right. Three hypotheses about possible limits to human longevity can be described in a similar way. These hypotheses, known as the limited-life-span hypothesis, the compression-rectangularization hypothesis, and the limit-distribution hypothesis, are illustrated in Figures 3-2 to 3-4.

Limited-Life-Span Hypothesis

Perhaps the most common notion of a limit in the study of human longevity is the *limited-life-span hypothesis*, which states that there exists some age ω beyond which there can be no survivors. In the notation of survival analysis, this hypothesis can be expressed by any one of the following three formulas:

$$f(x) = 0 \text{ iff } x \geq \omega$$
$$S(x) = 0 \text{ iff } x \geq \omega$$ (5)
$$\lim\limits_{x \to \omega} h(x) = \infty.$$

Each of these formulas implies the other two. This hypothesis is illustrated in Figure 3-2. These formulas may apply to an individual or to a population; if they

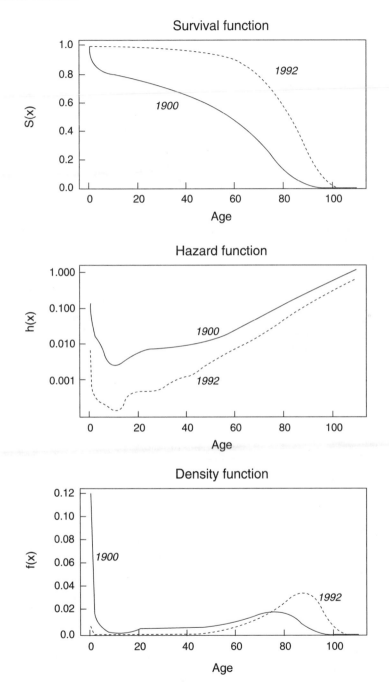

FIGURE 3-1 Mortality curves for U.S. women, 1900 and 1992.

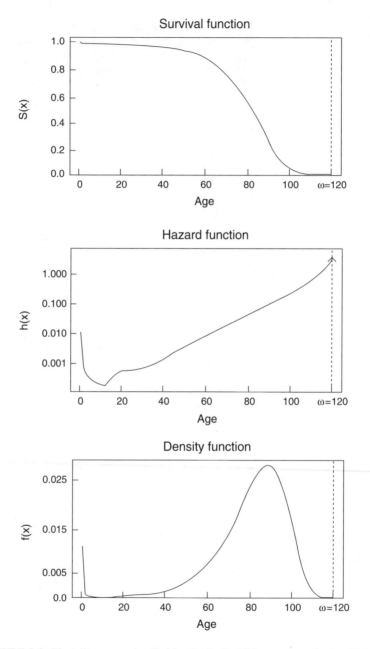

FIGURE 3-2 Mortality curves implied by the limited-life-span hypothesis. Note: The survival function shown here reaches zero at age ω (arbitrarily defined to equal 120 years). Similarly, the density function equals zero above this age. The hazard function becomes infinite as age approaches ω.

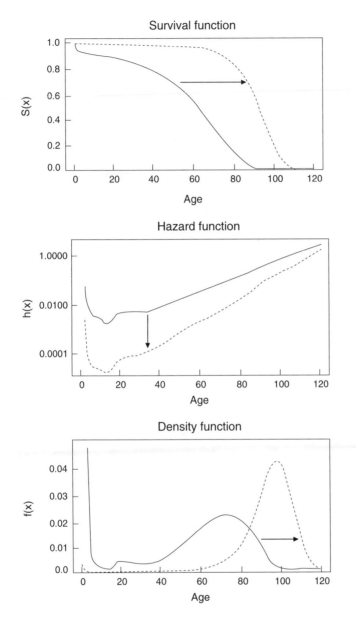

FIGURE 3-3 Mortality curves implied by the compression-rectangularization hypothesis. Note: Changes in these three curves are interrelated: over time the hazard function falls more rapidly at younger than older ages, the area under the survival function grows larger as the curve becomes more rectangular, and the density function shifts to the right and becomes more compressed. The distribution may or may not be truncated at some maximum age. Likewise, the dashed curves may or may not represent ultimate mortality limits.

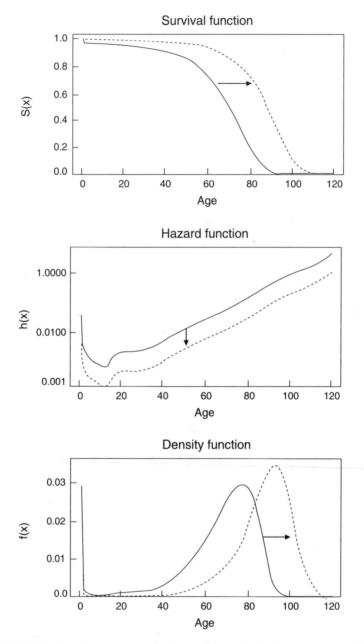

FIGURE 3-4 Mortality curves implied by the limit distribution hypothesis. Note: All three curves are moving toward a limit distribution, which may or may not be more compressed than the original distribution. Likewise, the limit distribution may or may not have a finite right-hand boundary.

refer to a heterogeneous population, then ω is the maximum potential age at death for the most robust individual.

Intuitively, this hypothesis is not very satisfactory. It implies that it is possible to live up to age ω, but that survival to age ω plus 1 day is impossible. The theoretical plausibility of such a truncated mortality distribution was criticized by the eminent probabilist William Feller (1950:8-9). Gavrilov and Gavrilova (1991), who are critical of the idea that there exists a species-specific maximum life span for humans or other animals, devote an entire chapter of their book to this topic.

It is quite clear that a habitual vagueness in the use of the term "life span" has confused the discussion of human mortality limits. According to Webster's dictionary, *life span* is either "the longest period over which the life of any plant or animal organism or species may extend, according to the available biological knowledge concerning it," or "the longevity of an individual." Thus, the life span of an individual refers to his or her age at death; the life span of a species refers to the maximum potential length of life for the most robust member(s) of the species; and the mean life span (of individuals) is equivalent to the familiar concept of *life expectancy*.

Use of this term in the literature has been rather haphazard, however. This confusion has led to some rather remarkable empirical assertions. Economos (1985:110), for example, asserts that "it has long been recognized that the human maximum life span has remained constant, around 100 years, across time, races, and civilizations." I agree with Gavrilov and Gavrilova (1991:119) that this notion appears to have "become established through a long period of mutual citation . . . in the total absence of any convincing proof."

There appear to be two common demographic arguments that are thought to support the limited-life-span hypothesis. One is the assertion that there has been no increase over time in the maximum age at death observed for human populations (Fries, 1980; Olshansky et al., 1990). This assertion is clearly false, however, as illustrated by a recent analysis of trends in the maximum age at death for five countries. Figure 3-5 reproduces a key finding from Wilmoth and Lundström (1996), showing that the maximum age at death for men and women in Sweden has risen steadily for at least 130 years.[1] These authors document a similar trend in three other developed countries (France, England and Wales, and Japan), although only during more limited time periods when the quality of the data appears reliable.[2] Of course, some portion of this upward trend is attributable to population growth, because the extreme values of a sample from any probability distribution are partly a function of sample size (Gumbel, 1937 and 1958). Popu-

---

[1]Data for the earliest decade shown in Figure 3-5, 1851-1860, appear to be contaminated by a handful of exaggerated ages at death. Wilmoth and Lundström (1996) attribute the improvement in data quality around 1860 to the founding of Sweden's National Central Bureau of Statistics.

[2]It is not uncommon to observe a decrease in the maximum reported age at death, although in all known cases this trend can reasonably be attributed to an improvement in data quality rather than a genuine retraction in the tail of the age distribution of deaths.

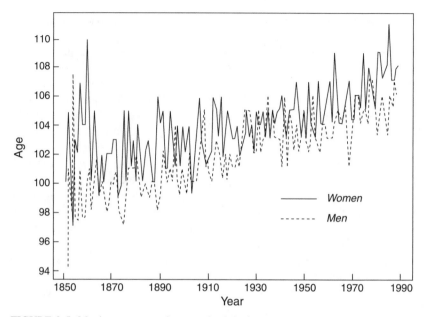

FIGURE 3-5 Maximum reported age at death in Sweden, women and men, 1851-1990.
SOURCE: Wilmoth and Lundström (1996:69).

lation growth, however, is mostly a product of mortality decline, so it is difficult
to separate conceptually the influence of these two factors.

One approach to this problem is to consider the causes of the rapid growth in the
centenarian population of industrialized countries. This "proliferation" of centenarians is due mostly to an increasing probability of surviving into old age (say, until
age 80) and, especially, of surviving from 80 until 100 years of age (Vaupel and
Jeune, 1995). Then, for any underlying mortality function, the age of death of the
oldest individual should rise partly as a function of the increasing number of persons
who become centenarians. A complete analysis of the trend shown in Figure 3-5—
breaking it into components related to the trend in births, the probability of survival
until old age, and the probability of survival within old age—is still lacking. Nevertheless, if the mortality distribution were truncated on the right, this trend would be
subject to an upper limit, regardless of the increasing size of the centenarian population. Therefore, its steady, almost linear rise over time suggests that the tail of the
empirical age distribution has not yet arrived at such a limit. If the theoretical
distribution is bounded on the right, we would expect this trend to level off as it
approaches the limit. The apparent absence of deceleration in this upward trend
suggests that the limit is at least not immediately in sight.[3]

_____

[3]Here, as elsewhere, a more thorough, formal analysis is recommended to answer such questions
as, "How close to the theoretical limit must the observed maximum be before we would observe the
predicted leveling off in the empirical trend?"

The second demographic argument in support of the limited-life-span hypothesis is the assertion that the exponential increase in mortality rates with age, as implied by the Gompertz curve, "ensures a finite life span" (Fries, 1980:131). This argument contains two fallacies. The first fallacy results from the mistaken notion that the Gompertz curve implies a finite life span (Gavrilov and Gavrilova, 1991; Wilmoth, 1992). As noted before, a finite life span results from a hazard function (or force of mortality) that rises abruptly toward infinity as age approaches ω, the species-specific life span. The Gompertz model, on the other hand, implies that there is a non-zero probability of survival even to ages that are well beyond those previously observed (or even imaginable) for humans.[4] Therefore, perhaps contrary to popular belief, the Gompertz mortality curve implies that the limited-life-span hypothesis is false.

A second fallacy in this argument is that the Gompertz curve does not describe human mortality well at old ages. This point is well illustrated in Figure 3-6, which is taken from Gavrilov and Gavrilova (1991). Contrary to the prediction of the limited-life-span hypothesis, observed death rates for humans do not rise abruptly toward infinity at some very high age. In fact, the age-related increase in the hazard rate, or force of mortality, is even less than the exponential rise implied by the Gompertz curve. The data presented in Figure 3-6 are for Swedish men during a limited time period, but all reliable evidence is consistent with the conclusion that the force of mortality continues to rise throughout adult life, but at a decreasing rate after the age of 75 or 80 (Horiuchi and Coale, 1990; Kannisto, 1994; Wilmoth, 1995; Horiuchi and Wilmoth, in press). A similar, or more extreme, finding exists for nonhuman species such as fruit flies (*Drosophila melanogaster*), medflies (*Ceratitis capitata*), and nematodes (*Caenorhabditis elegans*), whose mortality rates appear to level off in old age (Curtsinger et al., 1992; Carey et al., 1992; Fukui et al., 1993; Vaupel et al., 1994).

Of course, it is possible that there exists a maximum human life span at a point that is well beyond current experience. At present, it has been possible to compute reliable death rates for female populations up to a maximum age of around 109 years and for male populations to around 107 years (Kannisto, 1994). The oldest woman whose age has been reliably verified died recently at 122 years old (Robine and Allard, 1995); the oldest man has been verified as 115 years old (Wilmoth et al., 1996). Is it possible that an upper limit to the human life span lies just beyond these ages? We really have no way of denying or affirming this possibility, because verified observations of humans living (or dying) above 110 years of age are so few that we cannot compute reliable death rates in the tail of the distribution. As shown in Figure 3-2, the force of mortality could rise steadily

---

[4]The survival curve (from age 0) for the Gompertz model has the form

$$S(x) = \exp\left[\frac{a}{b}(1 - e^{bx})\right],$$

so that the probability of survival to any age x is above zero.

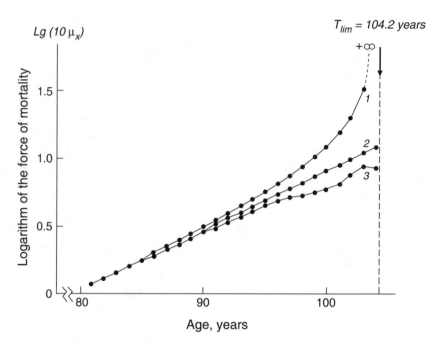

FIGURE 3-6 Force of mortality implied by the limited-life-span hypothesis (1), compared with the Gompertz curve (2), and data for Swedish men during 1945-1967 (3).
SOURCE: Gavrilov and Gavrilova (1991:128). Reprinted with permission from Harwood Academic Publishers.

until just before the upper limit of the life span and only then shoot abruptly
toward infinity. However, such a situation—even if it were the reality—could
never be observed and documented using our present methods.

   In summary, the limited-life-span hypothesis suggests that there exists a
maximum age, ω, beyond which no human being can live. The theoretical
plausibility of such a model is questionable, but the literature on this topic is
confusing due to careless and inconsistent use of terminology. The hypothesis is
not implied by the Gompertz curve or other common models of the age pattern of
human mortality. A review of the empirical evidence also shows that the available demographic data provide no support for this hypothesis. We are led,
therefore, to consider other means of conceptualizing a possible limit to human
longevity.

Compression-Rectangularization Hypothesis

   Another theoretical concept that has been associated with the study of limits
to human longevity is the hypothesis of mortality *compression*, also known as

rectangularization of the survival curve. According to this hypothesis, the variance in life-table ages at death should decrease over time. Recalling that X is a random variable representing the life span of an individual drawn at random from a population of newborns, let $Var(X,t)$ denote the variance of X at time t.[5] In its strictest version, the compression hypothesis states that the following inequality holds for any choice of $t_1 < t_2 < \ldots < t_n$:

$$Var(X,t_1) > Var(X,t_2) > \cdots > Var(X,tn) \tag{6}$$

Alternatively, compression could be defined in terms of the interquartile range of the distribution or some other measure. In general, the compression hypothesis implies that the dispersion in the density function of X, $f(x)$, should diminish over time.

The notion of mortality compression, defined by a successive decrease in the variance of X, seems also to be associated with characteristic changes in the survival function, $S(x)$, and the hazard rate function, $h(x)$ (Wilmoth et al., 1995). Previous empirical analyses indicate that the rectangularity of the survival curve, $S(x)$, is highly correlated with the standard error in the distribution of deaths, $f(x)$. Furthermore, changes in these two characteristics of mortality curves appear to be linked to changes in the hazard function, $h(x)$: a hazard function, $h(x)$, that falls more precipitously at younger than older ages tends to be associated with a compression in the distribution of deaths, $f(x)$, and a rectangularization of the survival curve, $S(x)$, as depicted in Figure 3-3.

Because compression-rectangularization refers to the *variability* in the distribution of deaths, it is not immediately obvious that this hypothesis should be associated with a limit in the *level* of human longevity. It may be instructive to consider, therefore, an argument by Ryder (1975:10-11), which suggests a possible link between these two trends. Although the primary focus of Ryder's discussion was not the question of limits to human mortality, his comments provide some insight. In an article on stationary populations, he noted a strong linear relationship in West model life tables (of the Coale-Demeny system) between life expectancy and the coefficient of variation of ages at death ($r^2 = 0.9882$ for females, and $r^2 = 0.9834$ for males). As life expectancy increases in these model life tables, the coefficient of variation declines. By extrapolation, the variability in age at death should diminish to nothing when $\mathring{e}_0$ equals 85.6 for females or 82.5 for males.

After performing this numerical exercise, Ryder remarks: "The phenomenon of declining coefficient of variation with increasing length of life would be the outcome of a model of survivorship in which one posits, as a species characteristic, a 'normal' life span close to invariant over all populations, with a small

---

[5]Here and elsewhere, "time t" should ideally refer to the birth year of a cohort that is followed from birth until extinction, although in many empirical applications it gives the time reference for a period life table constructed from data for a single year.

but non-zero coefficient of variation; the principal source of variations in observed mean age at death would be the proportion of the population failing to achieve that life span—i.e., experiencing 'preventable' death." Without pushing this view as a prediction of future mortality trends, Ryder anticipated Fries' argument, with both authors suggesting that compression-rectangularization may reflect a process of convergence toward a characteristic human life span of around 85 years (Fries, 1980).

Although compression-rectangularization may be consistent with such a model of mortality change, a decrease in the variability of ages at death is not sufficient proof of the existence of mortality limits. It is certainly possible that the distribution of ages at death could become more and more compressed while also shifting further and further to the right. In such a situation, there might be no fixed life span or maximum life expectancy. Furthermore, there is no reason to believe that an extrapolation of the relationship between level and variability in Coale-Demeny model life tables is an accurate prediction of the course of future mortality change.[6] Alternatively, it is at least theoretically possible that the variability in ages at death could decrease more slowly relative to the increase in life expectancy than predicted by the Coale-Demeny model tables. Thus, Figure 3-3 provides an example of the compression-rectangularization hypothesis in the absence of apparent limits on either the maximum life span or life expectancy.

Because the compression-rectangularization hypothesis suggests a limit in the variability of human longevity, not its level, it is only weakly related to the other two hypotheses considered in this paper. In a situation of mortality decline across the age range, the limited-life-span hypothesis should result in a compression of mortality. Therefore, falling mortality in the absence of compression would suggest that the limited-life-span hypothesis is false.[7] Fries (1980) began by asserting that the limited-life-span hypothesis was true and then concluded that rectangularization of the survival curve must result. In response, some authors have argued that compression-rectangularization has not been observed empirically as a means of countering the limited-life-span hypothesis.

Some of these empirical analyses, however, have offered rather sweeping conclusions based on quite limited evidence. For example, Myers and Manton (1984) conclude that "there is no significant evidence that rectangularization has had a significant effect on the population and mortality dynamics of the elderly, at least through 1979." The empirical basis for this article, and for two other

---

[6]Two characteristics of the Coale-Demeny model life tables make such an extrapolation inappropriate. First, these were constructed using data for populations at relatively higher levels of mortality than implied by the extrapolations. Second, in constructing these tables, relative rates of mortality change at different ages were constrained to be constant across different levels of life expectancy, whereas intuition and recent empirical evidence suggest that the age pattern of mortality change may not be constant over time and mortality level (Horiuchi and Wilmoth, 1995).

[7]Again, it is necessary to add the qualification that we cannot reject the hypothesis of an ultimate life-span limit outside the range of current experience.

papers that also refute the compression-rectangularization hypothesis (Rothenberg et al., 1991; Manton and Singer, 1994), is mortality data for the United States after 1962. Clearly, even a casual inspection of Figure 3-1 demonstrates that the U.S. survival curve has become more rectangular in shape during this century and that the distribution of ages at death has become more compressed.[8] Therefore, Fries was not wrong to observe that human survival curves have become more rectangular over time, although the conclusion that this trend would continue— and any suggestion that it has implications for limits to human longevity—is questionable.

Another analysis of mortality trends in three countries, using up to 130 years of data, has concluded that "rectangularization is by no means a myth" and that "a significant compression of ages at death has clearly occurred over the long-term history of human mortality decline" (Wilmoth et al., 1995). Nevertheless, this study also noted a slowdown and even scattered reversals after 1950 in the compression-rectangularization trend for the countries considered (the United States, Sweden, and Japan). It seems possible and even likely that these trends— so prominent in the past—may not continue indefinitely into the future.

In summary, the compression-rectangularization hypothesis suggests that the variability in the distribution of ages at death should decline as life expectancy increases over time. This compression of the death distribution, $f(x)$, tends to be associated with a progressive rectangularization of the survival curve, $S(x)$, and with a pattern of decrease in the hazard rate, $h(x)$, that is more pronounced at younger ages. An analysis based on model life tables suggests that there exists a consistent negative relationship between the increase in life expectancy and the decline in variability of ages at death; a simple linear extrapolation of this rela-tionship suggests that the current increase in life expectancy at birth may reach a limit around 85 years of age. These calculations are not sufficient proof of limits to human longevity on their own, however, and the empirical evidence demon-strates that compression and rectangularization are by no means universal aspects of mortality decline. Overall, the compression-rectangularization hypothesis seems to have little relevance to questions about the biological limits of human mortality.

Limit-Distribution Hypothesis

A third hypothesis about limits to human longevity asserts that there exists a limiting distribution that mortality curves may approach but not surpass. In terms of the hazard function, this limiting distribution can be written as $h^*(x)$. Thus, $h(x) \geq h*(x) > 0$ for all x in a large, random sample of humans at any point in time. This hazard function has a corresponding density function, $f^*(x)$, and survival

---

[8]Although Figure 3-1 shows mortality curves for U.S. women only, the general pattern for U.S. men is quite similar.

function, $S*(x)$, which have similar interpretations. An example of convergence toward these limiting curves is illustrated in Figure 3-4. In this example, the survival curve may or may not equal zero (exactly) after some age, and the density function may or may not be right-truncated. Similarly, the variance in age at death may or may not decrease in a consistent manner as the distribution converges toward a limit.

Presumably, the limit implied by these curves is the product of some fundamental aspects of human biology in interaction with unavoidable environmental factors. By this argument, all large human populations in all environments should be subject to the same mortality limit. Clearly, the theoretical plausibility of this hypothesis demands some discussion. For example, given what is known about genetic and environmental variability, is it reasonable to suppose that there might be a universal mortality limit that applies to all human populations in all environments? Without this restriction, however, what is the meaning of the limit itself? If we made allowances for subpopulations that possess different mortality limits or environmental conditions that change the limit, it would be necessary to sacrifice the notion of a universal mortality limit.

Consider the issue of genetic variability. There are elements of the human phenotype that show almost no variability (two eyes, two legs, 10 fingers, 46 chromosomes), because in these situations most mutations are deleterious. There are other characteristics that show considerable variability (hair and skin color, height, intelligence), because Darwinian selection does not strongly favor one phenotype over another. In low-mortality populations, longevity probably falls into the latter category, because postreproductive survival can have only limited selective influence.

Empirically, we know from twin studies that roughly one quarter of the variability in individual ages at death may be due to genetic factors (McGue et al., 1993; Herskind et al., 1996). Therefore, it should be possible to find subgroups of the human population that have an unusual genetic endowment for longevity. For a selected subpopulation, we might observe average mortality levels that fall below the theoretical minimum, which applies to a random sample of the total human population. In addition, it is possible that this theoretical minimum could change over time, as a result of Darwinian selection, genetic drift, or conscious manipulation (selective breeding or genetic engineering).

Therefore, for the purpose of discussing ultimate mortality limits, I assume that the forces of Darwinian selection and genetic drift will have only a negligible impact on the genetics of human longevity over the time horizon of interest to demographers and social planners, which is perhaps 50-100 years. Furthermore, although it seems imprudent to speculate about the potential impact that the conscious manipulation of the human genome might have in this area, all statements about ultimate mortality limits must necessarily assume an absence of successful efforts to alter human longevity by this means. Finally, for this discussion, I also neglect the possibility that fundamental changes in the earth's ecosystem (such as the climatic changes associated with geologic eras or human-induced "global warming") might have a significant effect on human mortality levels in the next century.

With these restrictions and qualifications in mind, it is reasonable to consider at least the possibility that some version of the limit-distribution hypothesis might be true. The question associated with the hypothesis might be stated as follows: Given the current genetic composition of the human population and the natural environment as it exists today, does there exist an irreducible mortality level, represented by $h^*(x)$, which thus implies an upper limit to the *mean* life span, or life expectancy (but not necessarily a finite *maximum* life span)?

As with the two hypotheses mentioned previously, there have been several discussions of this topic already in the literature. Bourgeois-Pichat (1952, 1978), Kannisto (1988), and Olshansky et al. (1990) have all used methods for theoretically eliminating certain causes of death as a means of exploring the lower limits of human mortality rates. The justification for such calculations is the belief that certain "exogenous" causes of death could theoretically be eliminated, while other "endogenous" causes may prove intractable.

There are several reasons to criticize the cause-elimination methodology, however. First, the method typically involves an assumption that the various causes operate independently of one another (Keyfitz, 1985), which is not plausible in many situations (Manton et al., 1991). Furthermore, the theoretical distinction between "endogenous" and "exogenous" causes is rather dubious. Mortality rates due to so-called exogenous causes (e.g., infectious disease, accidents, suicide) tend to increase with age, perhaps reflecting an increased propensity to succumb to these causes as a result of internal degeneration. Empirical evidence also demonstrates that mortality rates due to so-called endogenous causes are highly variable, both over time and across populations. Thus, it seems likely that almost all causes of death are both "exogenous" and "endogenous" in nature. Similarly, the notion of death due exclusively to "old age" or "senility," which Fries (1980) referred to as "natural death," has been sharply criticized (Schneider and Brody, 1983).

Nevertheless, cause-elimination models are not the only means of exploring the notion of a mortality limit distribution. Other, mostly ad hoc methods have also been used to estimate one or more parameters of this hypothetical distribution. For example, Fries (1980) derived his estimate of the maximum achievable human life expectancy by extrapolating the total life expectancy at age x, $x + \overset{\circ}{e}x$, at various ages. Because $\overset{\circ}{e}x$ has traditionally been rising much less rapidly at older than at younger ages, the extrapolated curves must eventually intersect. According to Fries, this intersection will occur around the year 2045 for the U.S. population, when an "ideal average life span" of around 85 years should be achieved. This maximum life expectancy corresponds to Fries' "ideally 'rectangular' survival curve" and thus to a limiting mortality distribution.

Fries' argument, however, seems to ignore the problem of a discontinuity at the limit itself. Why would the various values of $x + \mathring{e}x$ follow separate, linear paths until the point of convergence but then merge and remain constant (around 85 years) thereafter? Equally consistent with the empirical evidence—and more plausible theoretically—is a prediction that the values of $x + \mathring{e}x$ may move closer over time along curvilinear paths but never become equal. From this perspective, these curves might or might not be thought to possess an upper limit.

Most evidence from demographic trends seems inconsistent with the notion of a finite mortality limit, but there are some important questions of interpretation. If there exists a non-zero lower bound for age-specific death rates, how would we know if it were approaching? Most authors seem to assume that the approach to a limit would be characterized by a slowdown in the rate of mortality decline over time. The absence of deceleration in the rate of mortality decline, then, is taken as evidence that we are not currently approaching a lower limit in mortality rates.

For example, the reduction in age-specific death rates for most developed countries has been a stable, long-term process. This conclusion is illustrated for the United States in Figure 3-7, which shows age-adjusted death rates for women and men during 1900-1992 based on Social Security data (Bell et al., 1992). This figure is drawn using a semilogarithmic scale to conform with standard practice. Thus, it is the relative, not absolute, rate of mortality decline that has been stable.

If Figure 3-7 showed trends in death rates for separate age groups, the general conclusion (of stable decline) would not change. It would be evident, however, that the rate of decrease has varied enormously by age: although the pattern has changed in recent years, death rates have typically fallen much more rapidly at younger than at older ages. When making mortality projections, it is typical to assume that the differences by age in the pace of mortality decline will continue into the future (Pollard, 1987; Lee and Carter, 1992).

Thus, the trend in Figure 3-7 is influenced by the enormous decline in infant and child mortality, and also by smaller reductions in death rates at older ages. Over the time period shown here, the relative importance to the overall mortality decline of changes in younger and older age groups has reversed itself. As discussed below, the most rapid decreases in mortality are now occurring at older ages, whereas the opposite was true in earlier eras of mortality decline. Thus, it is all the more remarkable that the trend in Figure 3-7, which is a composite of trends across the age range, moves downward with such regularity.

The pace of overall mortality decline has not, however, been constant. From Figure 3-7, it is evident not only that there have been periods of acceleration and deceleration but also death rates have moved steadily downward over the long run. Perhaps the most curious feature of Figure 3-7 is the plateau that appears from around 1954 to 1968, especially for men. A detailed discussion of this phenomenon is given by Crimmins (1981), who analyzes these trends in terms of underlying causes of death. The period around the 1940s was characterized by very rapid mortality decline, owing at least in part to the increased use of drug therapies, primarily antibiotics and sulfa drugs, in the treatment of infectious diseases. By the mid 1950s, however, the potential for further reduction by this means was nearly exhausted, and so the pace of overall mortality decline slowed considerably for women and came to a veritable halt for men.

Crimmins points out that the trend in male mortality around the 1960s was also affected by a mild increase in violent deaths, in particular, deaths due to homicide and suicide. The resumption of rapid mortality decline in the United States after 1968, however, resulted from a new set of changes affecting cardiovascular mortality (i.e., deaths due to heart disease, cerebrovascular disease, and arteriosclerosis). These changes included both life style (exercise, diet, smoking) and medical factors (access to treatment through federal programs, surveillance and treatment of hypertension, pharmaceutical and surgical interventions). Owing to these developments, the relative size of the decline in U.S. mortality rates during 1968-1977 was greater at ages 85 and above than for all other age groups except infants (Crimmins, 1981:230).

What was happening in other developed countries during this time period? A slower pace of mortality decline during the late 1950s and 1960s, especially for men, was characteristic of most developed countries (United Nations, 1982; Spiegelman and Erhardt, 1974; Anderson and Silver, 1994). There is also evidence that the pace of mortality decline in developed countries has quickened in recent decades, especially at older ages (Kannisto et al., 1994). Figure 3-8 shows

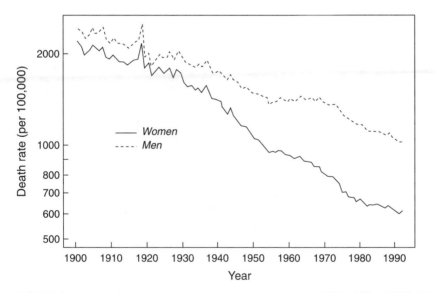

FIGURE 3-7 Age-adjusted death rates, U.S. women and men, 1900-1992. SOURCE: Bell et al. (1992:3-4), updated by the author. Total death rates were standardized using the 1980 census population.

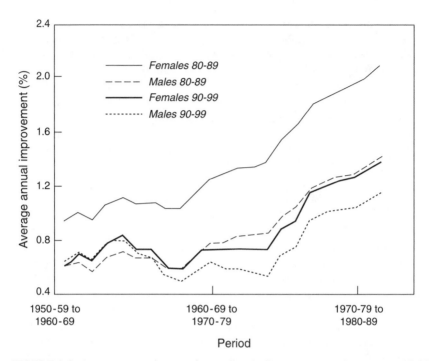

FIGURE 3-8 Average annual rates of mortality decline, women and men, ages 80-89 and 90-99 combined, for an aggregate of nine countries. SOURCE: Kannisto et al. (1994:802). Reprinted with permission. Each observation in this graph gives the annualized rate of mortality improvement over successive 10-year time periods; for example, the last point on the curve gives the improvement between 1972-81 and 1982-91. The nine countries included in the aggregate analysis are Austria, Belgium, England and Wales, France, West Germany, Japan, Scotland, Sweden, and Switzerland.

the average annual reduction in death rates (in percent) for ages 80-89 and 90-99 in an aggregate of eight European countries plus Japan from the 1950s through the 1980s. Rather than slowing down, mortality decline at older ages in industrialized countries seems to have accelerated.

The evidence from the recent study by Kannisto and his colleagues is corroborated by the work of Horiuchi and Wilmoth (1995), who have documented an "aging of mortality decline" for several countries. This trend is illustrated in Figure 3-9 using Swedish data for the period 1861-1990. These graphs demonstrate that the age pattern of mortality decline has evolved over time, with the most recent period characterized by an increase in the age of the most pronounced decline (thus, an "aging of mortality decline"). The more detailed graph in Figure 3-9b shows that this change has continued at least until 1990.

Another empirical result worth mentioning here is the apparent absence of a strong correlation between level of mortality and speed of mortality decline.

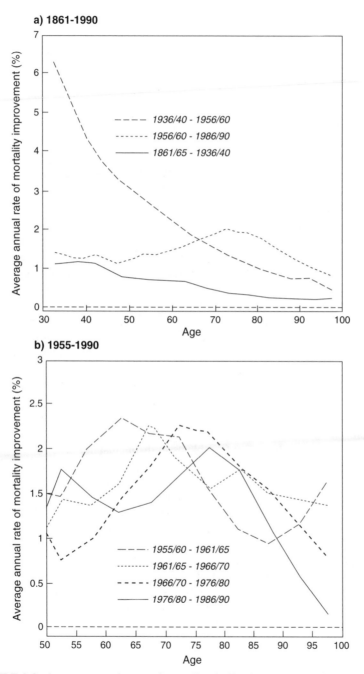

FIGURE 3-9 Average annual rates of mortality decline by age in Sweden for women only in various years during 1861-1990. SOURCE: Horiuchi and Wilmoth (1995).

Figure 3-10 shows a scatter plot of average death rates for ages 80-99 in the 1970s versus the average annual rate of improvement during the 1970s and 1980s, again taken from a study of 27 developed countries (Kannisto et al., 1994). The correlations associated with these graphs are negative: –0.10 for males and –0.35 for females. If the Eastern European countries (shown in darker type) are omitted, these correlations become slightly positive: 0.30 for males and 0.07 for females. In either case, these data do not provide strong evidence of a slowdown in the rate of mortality decline associated with lower mortality levels. Furthermore, it is notable that the values for females lie to the "northwest" of those for males, indicating that women enjoy both lower mortality levels and faster rates of mortality decline.

Kannisto and his colleagues argue (p. 802): "If mortality among the oldest-old were approaching biological or practical limits, then countries that have the lowest death rates would be closer than other countries to such limits. Rates of mortality improvement, however, are only weakly related to levels of mortality . . . ." Thus, the failure to demonstrate a positive correlation between mortality level and rate of improvement is taken as evidence against the limit-distribution hypothesis—but this argument, too, must be qualified by the observation that a limit distribution could still exist but is not currently in sight.

In summary, then, the limit distribution of human mortality is represented by a hazard function, $h^*(x)$, and associated density and survival functions, $f^*(x)$ and $S^*(x)$, which signify the hypothetical level of mortality that would be achieved by a large, random sample of individuals from the present human population if those individuals lived their entire lives under optimal environmental conditions. The most common means of estimating the limit distribution implied by these curves has been some form of cause-elimination, although the validity of this framework is itself questionable, both because of the interdependence between competing causes of death and because of problems in distinguishing between exogenous and endogenous, or between senile and nonsenile, causes of death.

The parameters of a limiting-mortality distribution have also been estimated by extrapolating past trends until some form of convergence is achieved, such that further reductions in mortality may appear improbable, but such arguments are not convincing if they imply a discontinuity at the point of convergence. Empirical studies of trends in total mortality contain no suggestion that human mortality is approaching a lower bound. Contrary to the predictions of the mortality limit hypothesis, mortality decline is accelerating in the oldest age groups in several low-mortality countries, and there is no evidence of a positive correlation between mortality level and the pace of mortality decline.

CONCLUSION

The demographic debate about the limits of human longevity can be expressed in terms of three hypotheses: limited life span, compression-rectangu-

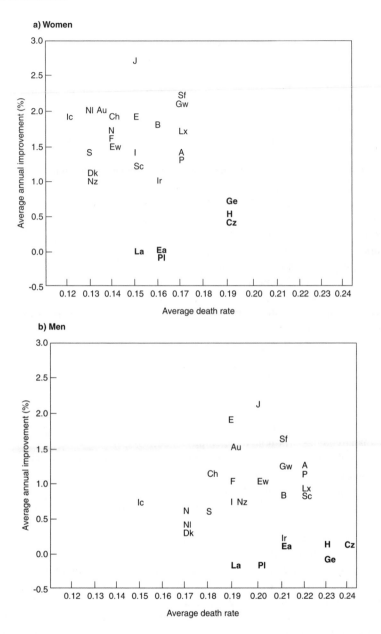

FIGURE 3-10 Average death rate in the 1970s plotted against the average annual rate of mortality decline from the 1970s to 1980s, women and men, ages 80-99 combined, 27 developed countries. SOURCE: Kannisto et al. (1994:803). See source for explanation of country abbreviations. Abbreviations for Eastern European countries are printed in darker type.

larization, and limit distribution. These hypotheses can be stated precisely in the language of statistical survival analysis as limits regarding, respectively, the maximum age attainable by humans, the variability in individual life spans, and the age pattern of human mortality.

Intuitively, the limited-life-span hypothesis is unappealing because it suggests that it is possible to survive to some maximum age, ω, but not to ω plus 1 day. Empirical research provides two pieces of relatively strong evidence that the limited-life-span hypothesis is false (more precisely, that a finite human life-span limit is not presently within sight). First, rather than rising abruptly toward infinity as predicted by the hypothesis, within the measurable range the rise in the human death rate decelerates with age. In some nonhuman species such as fruit flies, medflies, and nematodes, a more extreme pattern is observed, in that death rates seem to level off at advanced ages. It is possible, however, that we simply have not measured the force of mortality at ages near enough to the limit. A second, perhaps more convincing, piece of evidence that humans are not currently approaching an ultimate life-span limit is the observation that the maximum age at death for some national populations has risen and continues to rise in a steady, almost linear fashion. If we were close to observing a biological maximum, intuition suggests that this trend would show some sign of deceleration, although none is evident.

The compression-rectangularization hypothesis describes a trend of decreasing variability in individual life spans that has probably been observed throughout most of the history of human mortality decline. Nevertheless, it is not certain that this trend continues in all low-mortality populations today or that it will be observed there in the future. The failure to observe a continuing pattern of compression-rectangularization seems to deny further the validity of the limited-life-span hypothesis, although the empirical basis for this conclusion is not strong, and its theoretical basis needs more careful consideration as well. Overall, the relevance of the compression-rectangularization hypothesis to the current debate about the limits of human longevity is somewhat dubious.

The most general, and perhaps useful, of these three hypotheses is the limit-distribution hypothesis. It asserts that the age pattern of human mortality possesses an irreducible lower limit (in a large, randomly selected population). This hypothesis implies limits in the mean life span, or life expectancy, and in other parameters of the probability distribution of ages at death, including the median, the variance, and so forth. There have been several attempts to derive this limit distribution by separating causes of death into two mutually exclusive categories—either endogenous versus exogenous or senile versus nonsenile—and then computing the distribution that would result from the hypothetical elimination of exogenous or nonsenile causes. These methods do not appear to be well-grounded in theory, however, and some of their predictions have already been overturned. Attempts to derive a single parameter of the limit distribution—for example, life expectancy—through extrapolation of past trends also lack a firm theoretical justification and are plagued by logical inconsistencies, particularly with regard to discontinuities at the limit.

Three empirical observations provide important evidence in opposition to the limit-distribution hypothesis: (1) the historical stability of rates of mortality decline, (2) the acceleration of mortality decline at older ages, which are now characterized by the fastest age-specific rates of decline currently seen in some populations; and (3) the absence of a strong, positive correlation between levels of mortality and rates of improvement over time. Nevertheless, the link between these patterns and the limit-distribution hypothesis relies on intuition rather than firm theoretical results. Logically, mortality decline might or might not decelerate as the hazard rate approaches an irreducible lower bound.

In any case, demographic evidence can suggest only that we are not close to a limit at present, not that no ultimate limit exists. If the data contain no suggestion of a limit, a facile response is to assert that the limit may still be out there but that we are just not close enough to be able to observe it. In my view, however, proving or disproving the existence of limits that lie far beyond current experience is not a pressing task: the question of interest to policy makers is whether we are now approaching a biological limit to longevity, not whether such a limit exists. Furthermore, any hypothesis about a limit that lies far from current experience would not be falsifiable: anyone could assert or deny that such a limit exists, and there could be no basis for disputing that assertion empirically. Therefore, rather than merely asking, "Are there limits to human longevity?," we should inquire, "Are limits to human longevity presently in sight?" Of course, we should also be asking ourselves, "How good is our eyesight?"

REFERENCES

Acsádi, G., and J. Nemeskéri
   1970   *History of Human Life Span and Mortality*. Budapest: Akadémiai Kiadó.
Anderson, B.A., and B.D. Silver
   1994   A comparison of Soviet mortality in the working ages: 1959-1988. Pp. 295-338 in W. Lutz, S. Scherbov, and A. Volkov, eds., *Demographic Trends and Patterns in the Soviet Union before 1991*. London: Routledge.
Bell, F. C., A.H. Wade, and S.E. Goss
   1992   *Life Tables for the United States Social Security Area 1900-2080*. Actuarial Study No. 107, SSA Publication No. 11-11536.
Bourgeois-Pichat, J.
   1952   Essai sur la mortalité "biologique" de l'homme. *Population* 7(3):381-394.
   1978   Future outlook for mortality decline in the world. *Population Bulletin of the United Nations*, No. 11.
Carey, J.R., P. Liedo, D. Orozco, and J.W. Vaupel
   1992   Slowing of mortality rates at older ages in large medfly cohorts. *Science* 258:457-463.
Crimmins, E.M.
   1981   The changing pattern of American mortality decline, 1940-1977, and its implications for the future. *Population and Development Review* 7(2):229-254.

Curtsinger, J.W., H.H. Fukui, D. Townsend, and J.W. Vaupel
    1992   Demography of genotypes: Failure of the limited lifespan paradigm in *Drosophila melanogaster*. *Science* 258:461-463.
Davis, K.
    1951   *The Population of India and Pakistan*. Princeton, NJ: Princeton University Press.
Economos, A.C.
    1985   Rate of aging, rate of dying and non-Gompertzian mortality—Encore . . . . *Gerontology* 31:106-111.
Feller, W.
    1950   *An Introduction to Probability Theory and its Applications*. New York: John Wiley & Sons.
Fries, J.F.
    1980   Aging, natural death, and the compression of morbidity. *New England Journal of Medicine* 303:130-135.
Fukui, H.H., L. Xiu, and J.W. Curtsinger
    1993   Slowing of age-specific mortality rates in *Drosophila melanogaster*. *Experimental Gerontology* 38:585-599.
Gavrilov, L.A., and N.S. Gavrilova
    1991   *The Biology of Life Span: A Quantitative Approach*. New York: Harwood.
Gumbel, E.J.
    1937   *La Durée Extrême de la Vie Humaine*. Paris: Hermann.
    1958   *Statistics of Extremes*. New York: Columbia University Press.
Herskind, A.M., M. McGue, N.W. Holm, T.I. Sorensen, B. Harvald, and J.W. Vaupel
    1996   The heritability of human longevity: A population-based study of 2872 Danish twin pairs born 1870-1900. *Human Genetics* 97:319-323.
Horiuchi, S., and A.J. Coale
    1990   Age patterns of mortality for older women: An analysis using the age-specific rate of mortality change with age. *Mathematical Population Studies* 2(4):245-267.
Horiuchi, S., and J.R. Wilmoth
    1995   The Aging of Mortality Decline. Presented at the annual meetings of the Population Association of America, San Francisco, April 6-8, and the Gerontological Society of America, November 15-19.
    1995   Deceleration in the age pattern of mortality at older ages. *Demography*.
Kannisto, Väinö
    1988   On the survival of centenarians and the span of life. *Population Studies* 42:389-406.
    1994   *Development of Oldest-old Mortality, 1950-1990: Evidence from 28 Developed Countries*. Odense, Denmark: Odense University Press.
Kannisto, Väinö, J. Lauritsen, A.R. Thatcher, and J.W. Vaupel
    1994   Reduction in mortality at advanced ages. *Population and Development Review* 20:793-810.
Keyfitz, N.
    1985   *Applied Mathematical Demography*. New York: Springer-Verlag.
Lee, R.D., and L.R. Carter
    1992   Modeling and forecasting U.S. mortality. *Journal of the American Statistical Association* 87:659-671.
Manton, K.G., and B. Singer
    1994   What's the fuss about compression of mortality? *Chance* 7(4):21-30.
Manton, K.G., E. Stallard, and H.D. Tolley
    1991   Limits to human life expectancy: Evidence, prospects, and implications. *Population and Development Review* 17(4):603-637.
Manton, K.G., and H.D. Tolley
    1991   Rectangularization of the survival curve: Implications of an ill-posed question. *Journal of Aging and Health* 3(2):172-193.

McGue, M., J.W. Vaupel, N. Holm, and B. Harvald
1993   Longevity is moderately heritable in a sample of Danish twins born 1870-80. *Journal of Gerontology* 48:B237-244.
Myers, G.C., and K.G. Manton
1984   Compression of mortality: Myth or reality? *The Gerontologist* 24(4):346-353.
Olshansky, S. J., B.A. Carnes, and C. Cassel
1990   In search of Methuselah: Estimating the upper limits to human longevity. *Science* 250:634-640.
Pollard, J.H.
1987   Projection of age-specific mortality rates. Pp. 55-69 in *Population Bulletin of the United Nations* No. 21/22.
Population Reference Bureau
1995   *World Population Data Sheet.* Washington, DC: Population Reference Bureau.
Preston, S.H.
1980   Causes and consequences of mortality declines in less developed countries during the twentieth century. Pp. 289-360 in R. A. Easterlin, ed., *Population and Economic Change in Developing Countries.* Chicago: University of Chicago Press.
1990   Sources of variation in vital rates: An overview. Pp. 335-350 in J. Adams, D. Lam, A. Hermalin, and P. Smouse, eds., *Convergent Issues in Genetics and Demography.* Oxford: Oxford University Press.
Robine, J., and M. Allard
1995   Validation of the exceptional longevity case of a 120 year old woman. Pp. 363-367 in B.J. Vellas, J.L. Albarede, and P.J. Garry, eds., *Long-Term Care. Facts and Research in Gerontology.* New York: Springer Publishing Company.
Rothenberg, R., H.R. Lentzner, and R.A. Parker
1991   Population aging patterns: The expansion of mortality. *Journal of Gerontology: Social Sciences* 46(2):S66-S70.
Ryder, N.B.
1975   Notes on stationary populations. *Population Index* 41:3-28.
Schneider, E.L., and J.A. Brody
1983   Aging, natural death, and the compression of morbidity: Another view. *New England Journal of Medicine* 309(14):854-856.
Spiegelman, M., and C.L. Erhardt
1974   International comparisons of mortality and longevity. Pp. 39-64 in C.L. Erhardt and J.E. Berlin, eds., *Mortality and Morbidity in the United States.* Cambridge, MA: Harvard University Press.
United Nations
1982   *Levels and Trends of Mortality since 1950.* New York: United Nations.
Vaupel, J.W., and B. Jeune
1995   The emergence and proliferation of centenarians. In B. Jeune and J.W. Vaupel, eds., *Exceptional Longevity,* Odense, Denmark: Odense University Press.
Vaupel, J.W., T.E. Johnson, and G.J. Lithgow
1994   Rates of mortality in populations of *Caenorhabditis elegans. Science* 266:826.
Wilmoth, J.R.
1992   The Demographer's Crystal Ball: How Long Will We Live During the 21st Century? Presented to the Bay Area Colloquium in Population, October 7.
1995   Are mortality rates falling at extremely high ages? An investigation based on a model proposed by Coale and Kisker. *Population Studies* 49(2):281-295.
Wilmoth, J.R., J.W. Curtsinger, and S. Horiuchi
1995   Rectangularization Revisited: Survival Curves for Humans and Fruit Flies. Presented at the annual meeting of the Population Association of America, San Francisco, April 6-8.

Wilmoth, J.R., and H. Lundström
    1996   Extreme longevity in five countries: Presentation of trends with special attention to
            issues of data quality. *European Journal of Population* 12(1):63-93.
Wilmoth, J.R., A. Skytthe, D. Friou, and B. Jeune
    1996   The oldest man ever?   A case study of exceptional longevity.   *The Gerontologist*
            36(6):783-788.

4

The Evolution of Senescence

Shripad Tuljapurkar

INTRODUCTION

This paper suggests directions for developing an evolutionary theory of senescence with the aim of producing testable predictions or theoretically based tools for data analysis. The evolutionary view of mortality defined by Medawar (1952), Williams (1957), and Hamilton (1966) made the key points that mortality is a fitness component and that the age pattern (which I will call the shape) of mortality is probably under the influence of evolutionary forces (selection, mutation, drift, etc.). These writers also made the important prediction that immortality (or, at least, indefinite extension of life) is unlikely to be the end result of evolution by selection. Recent analyses of experimental data (e.g., Carey et al., 1992, Curtsinger et al., 1992 and 1994; Gaillard et al., 1994) have provided detailed information about the shape of mortality within species and comparisons among species. To understand and analyze this information as well as to predict at an appropriate level of detail will require that we move beyond the classical theories.

Theoretical advance hinges on defining what we wish to understand and how we will proceed. I center my discussion on the concept of an evolutionary equilibrium for a life history, which includes the shape of fertility and mortality and possibly other features such as growth rates. A theory focused on equilibria is limited by the assumption that the forces of evolution have operated long enough that the characters we study are close to their equilibrium states. A nonequilibrium theory is much more difficult, because the characters of interest may be in some transient state that depends on initial conditions unknown to us.

Understanding equilibria is an essential step toward a nonequilibrium theory and should provide greater insights than we now possess. I first discuss different theoretical approaches to the definition of evolutionary equilibria. Next I consider the classical theory and define two special equilibria: the "salmon" limit, and the "bacterium" limit. These equilibria reveal critical issues concerning the assumptions and structure of the theory. The consequences of some specific generalizations of the classical theory will then be reviewed. Finally, I outline a program of theoretical work that should lead to a more useful evolutionary theory of senescence.

EVOLUTIONARY EQUILIBRIA

Consider the dynamics of a population phenotype under the action of selection and mutation. At any time, there is some frequency distribution of the phenotype (among individuals) and an underlying distribution of genotypes. Genotypes map into phenotypes, and phenotypes map into fitness. Fitness differences, mutation, and random drift can lead to a change in the relative numbers of different genotypes and thus to changes in phenotype distribution. Any theoretical analysis makes assumptions about each step in this process. Given such assumptions, an evolutionary equilibrium (EE) is defined as a phenotypic distribution for a population that remains unchanged under the above dynamic process.

For an age-structured population, the individual phenotype of interest is a vector $z = (\mu, m)$. The components $\mu(x)$ and $m(x)$ of the two vectors listed on the right are, respectively, the mortality rate and fertility at age x. For a size-structured population, we would add size-specific growth rate $g(s)$ at size s, and make $\mu(s)$ and $m(s)$ size-dependent to get $z = (\mu, m, g)$. Suppose that time is measured in discrete units (e.g., generations) and that the frequency distribution of the phenotype in the population is given by $f_t(z)$ at time t. The evolutionary dynamic process above changes this distribution, in one time step, into a new one, $f_{t+1}(z)$. An evolutionary equilibrium is a distribution $F(z)$ that remains unchanged under the dynamics. We are mainly interested in stable equilibria: the analysis of stability properties can be difficult, although this paper does consider the stability of some special equilibria. Unstable equilibria can also be interesting, typically in situations where one asks if a newly introduced phenotype can increase in frequency in a population from which it was previously absent. Such invasion analyses are used here to examine the effects of random environments on the evolution of mortality patterns.

There are three ways of modeling the dynamics of a phenotype distribution, and I consider them in turn. In each case, I direct attention to the assumptions and limits of the method. The reader should note that the results of the theory depend not only on the assumptions within each method below but also that different methods can produce different answers.

Evolutionarily Stable Strategy

Evolutionarily stable strategy (ESS) models assume that every genotype maps to a single phenotype and (typically) that the population displays one common phenotype. Instead of a frequency distribution of phenotypes, a single phenotype applies to every individual. An underlying set Z of possible phenotypes is considered, and the dynamics consist of competition between phenotypes. In the usual set-up, a rare (infrequent) phenotype z_R is assumed to compete with a common phenotype z_C. If the rare type can increase in frequency, it is said to invade the population. The object of the theory is to identify a subset Z_E of the best competitors among the possible phenotypes Z. The set Z_E may contain several phenotypes that are equally competitive, or a single "best" phenotype; in either case, the ESS model consists of subset Z_E.

How is competitive success (i.e., fitness) defined here? The definition depends on the population dynamics of competition. The original model of Hamilton (1966) was (implicitly) of this sort and assumed exponential growth in a constant environment, so that fitness equaled the Lotka (intrinsic) rate of increase $r = r(z)$. If we change the model of competition, a different fitness measure may apply. For example, Orzack and Tuljapurkar (1989) assumed exponential growth in a stochastic environment, so their fitness equaled the long-run stochastic growth rate $a = a(z)$. With different fitnesses, the competitive ranking of phenotypes in the same underlying set Z can change.

In this type of model, the ESS depends on the initial set Z of possible phenotypes. Suppose, for example, that the fitness measure is r from classical demography. Then we know that r increases with an increase in fertility at any age. Absent any constraints, the ESS phenotypes would cluster at the point of maximum fertility in the set Z. Absent an upper bound on fertility in the set Z, we would be led to ridiculous conclusions. The set Z of possible phenotypes must contain constraints: one example would be the imposition of correlations between fertility and mortality and another would be the imposition of a maximum fertility (or other measure of reproductive output). I will later discuss a particular model of correlations that has been analyzed in different ways.

A shortcut approach to the ESS is sometimes used, based on the idea that if there is a single fitness for each phenotype z, then the ESS set Z_E is simply that set which yields a maximum of the fitness. This approach works when there is a single maximum but can fail when multiple fitness maxima occur.

Evolutionary Genetic Stability

Evolutionary genetic stability (EGS) is a term coined by Eshel and Feldman (1982) and is a relative of ESS. In this approach, the genetic basis of the phenotypes of interest is taken to be more complex. Eshel and Feldman typically consider two- or three-locus models. As with ESS, there is a set of possible phenotypes, but here competition is described by the dynamics of a rare "modifier" gene at one of the loci. Typically, the modifiers are chosen from a set, and each modifier in the set maps into a phenotypic variant. If a rare modifier gene can invade a given genetic configuration, by increasing in frequency, the genetic configuration is unstable. When a genetic configuration is found such that it cannot be invaded by any modifiers in the set, that configuration is said to be at EGS.

This approach has not been used for life-history characters but rather has been used for characters that are not components of fitness. Examples of the latter are mutation rate and rate of recombination between loci. A virtue of this method is that it forces attention to the genotypic structure. Such attention is conspicuously absent in the literature on the evolution of life-history characters; possible reasons for its absence are the complexity of analysis in EGS theory and the relative dearth of good information on the genetic basis of life-history traits.

Selection-Mutation Equilibrium

The preceding methods do not explicitly invoke mutation. They do implicitly assume that the phenotype set Z is generated by mutational events, but there is no dynamical representation of the mutational process. (This restriction applies to ESS and EGS models for life-history traits; obviously, an EGS model for modifiers of mutation rate will include mutational dynamics, as in Liberman and Feldman, 1986.) However, mutation is central to most arguments about the evolution of mortality rates, and it is clearly important to examine the joint dynamics of mutation and selection.

The first paper to do this, as far as I know, was Charlesworth (1990), following earlier work by Lande (1982). His approach points the way in which, I believe, the theory should go, and I will review it in a little more detail. A central assumption is that the components of the life-history phenotype z are determined by the additive action of many loci that are loosely linked. This, plus an assumption that selection is weak, allows the phenotypic dynamics to be described by the mean and variance of the phenotype distribution (in effect, the phenotype distribution is approximated by a normal distribution). Further, the dynamics of the mean phenotype are independent of the dynamics of the phenotypic variance. Changes in the mean phenotype are driven by selection and mutation.

The selective force acting here is simple competition between phenotypes that differ in mortality, fertility, and so on and is measured in terms of Lotka intrinsic growth rate r and the generation time T. In these models, a selective change in gene frequency first shows up in the youngest age class (new offspring) and then propagates through the population as these offspring, in turn, age and produce further young. As a result, the generation time T is a characteristic time scale for change in the population distribution of genes and phenotypes. The effectiveness of selection also depends on correlations between components of the phenotype; for example, increased fertility may be accompanied by decreased survival.

The Lande-Charlesworth approach summarizes these facts in an equation for the dynamics of the population-average of the life-history phenotype vector. The equation has the form

$$\left\{ \begin{array}{c} \text{Rate of Change} \\ \text{In Mean Phenotype} \end{array} \right\} = \text{Selective Change} + \text{Mutational Change} \qquad (1)$$

Mutational change in the average life-history phenotype is taken to be the result of mutations at each of the many underlying loci that additively determine the phenotype.

Equation 1 provides an equation for the equilibrium mean phenotype that will be maintained under the combined effects of selection and mutation. This is an important feature because it provides an explicit mapping from assumptions about mutation and the phenotype set to the equilibrium state. Such a mapping is essential if we are to make testable predictions. This approach does not, however, resolve the problems of defining the phenotype set; the problems noted above for ESS also occur here, as I will illustrate later.

In contrast to ESS models, this approach yields predictions for equilibrium phenotypes. These predictions can then be confronted with data in an unambiguous way. When mutation is not directly modeled, theory leaves us with no clear guide to possible sources of discrepancy between predictions and observations, because one can always appeal to unspecified mutational effects. Unfortunately, the predictions of a mutationally based theory are also difficult to check because mutational effects are difficult to measure (see Mukai et al., 1972, and Partridge, in this volume).

TWO EVOLUTIONARY EQUILIBRIA

The simplest dynamic process for the evolution of the shape of mortality is based on classical demography, with r as fitness. I now show, in this case, that there are two obvious evolutionary equilibria for life-history phenotypes. These equilibria are derived under the assumptions of the classical theory of senescence—i.e., that there is exponential growth in a constant environment. It is helpful, first, to recall two well-known results from classical demography.

We use discrete ages, survival from age x to $x + 1$ is $p(x)$, survival from birth to age x is $l(x)$, and the stable (Lotka) growth rate is r. Then

$$\left(\frac{\partial r}{\partial p(x)} \right) = \left(\frac{1}{T} \right) \sum_{i>x} m(i)l(e)^{-ri}, \qquad (2)$$

where T is mean length of generation, and

$$\left(\frac{\partial r}{\partial m(x)} \right) = \left(\frac{1}{T} \right) l(x)e^{-rx}. \qquad (3)$$

Note that $\partial r/\partial p(x)$ is constant at the ages before reproduction starts, declines after that until reproduction stops, and is zero postreproduction. However, $\partial r/\partial m(x)$ always decreases with age if $r > 0$.

The Salmon Limit

Assume that there is a fixed age β after which reproduction ceases, so that $m(x) = 0$ for $x > \beta$. Assume also that mutations affecting survival are always deleterious. Then for $x > \beta$ there is no selection to balance the mutational pressures, and it must follow that survival rate will evolve to zero. This is what I will call the salmon limit for mortality, because it corresponds to a catastrophic increase in mortality beyond age β.

It is important to note that this result is unaffected by several changes in the assumptions. First, suppose that we have antagonistic pleiotropy, defined specifically by saying that some mutations have a beneficial effect early in life (i.e., before age β) and also have deleterious effects late in life. Such mutations will be favored, but they will only accelerate the accumulation of postreproductive deleterious effects. Therefore the salmon limit is stable under such mutations.

Second, remove the assumption of a fixed age of last reproduction and allow a tradeoff between mortality and fertility at every age, so that a positive change in $p(x)$ comes at the expense of a negative change in $m(x)$. Such a tradeoff alters the values of the derivatives in Equations 2 and 3 but does not alter the fact that the selective pressure measured by $[\partial r/\partial m(x)]$ declines with age x. Consequently, with deleterious mutations affecting survival there will always be some age β past which the mutation-selection balance will be dominated by mutations and survival will fall catastrophically. This is precisely the pattern observed by Charlesworth (1990).

The Bacterium Limit

For a different limit, let us constrain total reproduction, so that, for example, the total lifetime reproduction is fixed. Now assume that there are both beneficial and deleterious mutations affecting survival and fertility. Because of the age pattern of the selection coefficients, mutations with beneficial effect on early fertility will be most strongly selected. In other words, selection will act to increase early reproduction even at the cost of late reproduction. As long as a supply of some mutations that can increase early reproduction exists, the mortality schedule will be compressed toward earlier ages, leading to a collapse into a one-age-class life cycle. This is what I call the bacterium limit.

Shortcomings of the Classical Theory

Although it is certainly true that we can observe both salmon and bacteria and thus the equilibria described by these limits are observable, most examples that interest us are not described by these limits. Yet these limits are the only equilibrium states possible under the specific assumptions stated, and this fact is rarely discussed. Clearly, theoretical analyses that yield different patterns must make other assumptions. That is the subject of the next section.

OTHER EQUILIBRIA

I now discuss several models that yield ESS patterns or mutation-selection equilibria that depart from the salmon type of mortality pattern, yielding patterns of the kind suggested by Carey et al. (1992).

Tradeoffs: One View

Abrams and Ludwig (1995) have presented an elegant analysis of an ESS model in which the life history is described by the vector $z = (\mu, m)$. They assume that there is a tradeoff at each age between a component of mortality at that age $a(x)$ and fertility at that age. Specifically,

$$\mu(x + 1) = \mu(x) + a(x),$$
$$m(x) = m[a(x)]. \tag{4}$$

The tradeoff is contained in the assumption that fertility is an increasing function of $a(x)$; thus, fertility only increases at the expense of increased mortality. To find the ESS, they maximize reproductive value (equivalent to maximizing r). They then present results of ESS trajectories of $m(x)$ as a function of age x, given different functional relationships between fertility and $a(x)$. Their paper focuses on the conditions under which $\mu(x)$ is or is not of Gompertz form. Here I will point to a different feature of their results. In all the results they present, there is a nonzero trajectory of values of $a(x)$; in some cases $a(x) \rightarrow$ a constant as x increases; in others $a(x)$ increases with increasing x. Notice that Equation 4 implies, in these respective cases, that $m(x) \rightarrow$ a constant as x increases; or $m(x)$ increases with age. Thus in their model there is no prediction of declining reproduction with age, which is surely a correlate of increasing age and/or increasing mortality in most cases. This result is not surprising when we note that they do not include mutation.

Tradeoffs: Another View

Charlesworth (1990) uses a tradeoff model that is similar in spirit to that of Abrams and Ludwig (1995), except that in his model there is no accumulative effect of mortality. He does, however, explicitly include mutation. His model measures the tradeoff at each age x by a reproductive-effort phenotype $e(x)$, and the level of fertility at each age is scaled to a phenotypic value $e(x)$, so that

$$p(x) = a(x) \ b \ [1 - e(x)^k],$$
$$m(x) = a(x) \ e(x). \tag{5}$$

The parameter k is fixed and measures the convexity of the tradeoff. He says (p. 528), "there is directional selection on $[a(x)]$ . . . . There is assumed to be a net negative effect on the means of the $[a(x)]$ values, consistent with the assumption of directional selection." On the other hand, he takes $e(x)$ to be under optimizing selection.

Although this model contains considerably more detail, it is still governed by the sensitivity of classical demography. In agreement with my discussion of the salmon limit, Charlesworth finds in every case that there is a catastrophic onset of high mortality at some age. The age of onset is determined by the mutation rate and other parameters of the model.

Positive Pleiotropy

Curtsinger (1995 and personal communication) has argued that the existence of an equilibrium that displays a high mortality plateau at later ages may be due to positive pleiotropy between mutations affecting early and late ages. This assumption gets past the salmon limit by adducing a positive selection pressure (due to early-age effects) on mutations with pleiotropic beneficial late-age effects. In essence, a catastrophic mortality decline is averted because of the accumulation of mutations that "hitch-hike" on a positive effect of selection early in life.

Variable Environments

A different explanation for the evolution of mortality rates is found in the analysis of life-history evolution in the common situation when vital rates depend on a randomly varying external environment. Tuljapurkar and Boe (1993) examined selection in a environment that affects the age-specific probability of successful reproduction. They model the timing of fertility in two different ways. The first of these is the classical approach in which we specify the age pattern of fertility and examine the impact of shifting the entire schedule of fertility to later ages; the second approach uses the demographic notion of parity progression: individuals make transitions from maturity to states where they have reproduced once, twice, thrice, etc. They assume that a random environment affects the probability of a successful parity transition, so that in severe environments reproduction is very difficult, whereas in favorable environments reproductive success is high.

In the presence of random variation, the relative fitness of phenotypes is measured by a stochastic growth rate a. The value of a is determined by two factors—the growth rate corresponding to the average vital rates and the impact of variability, which is modulated by the generation time. These factors are summarized in an approximate expansion

$$a \approx r - \frac{1}{2T^2} \sum_{(ij),(kl)} S_{i,j} S_{k,l} \sigma_{ij,kl}. \tag{6}$$

Here r is the Lotka growth rate for the time-averaged vital rates, $S_{i,j}$ is the derivative of r with respect to vital rate (i, j), and $\sigma_{ij,kl}$ is the covariance between vital rates (i, j) and (k, l). Therefore fitness depends on the generation length and the age pattern of variability in fertility and mortality.

Results from both formulations of the stochastic model show that phenotypic combinations that differ with respect to the age pattern of fertility can be equally "fit" in a range of stochastic environments. It follows that stochastic selection can produce a range of equally fit phenotypes. This paper concludes that phenotypic polymorphism for the length of reproductive life can be readily maintained by temporally varying selective regimes.

The practical consequence of such polymorphism will be that mortality will not be observed to fall catastrophically but rather will show some kind of plateau at late ages.

Size-Structured Models

An important class of biologically useful models has sensitivity properties that are always very different from the sensitivity properties that underlie age-structured demography. This class of models is based on size and physical growth rate. These models define fitness as do age-based models, but they enforce a correlation between mortality and fertility, because there is usually a positive value to age delays that allow the organism to grow to larger size. Such models have been analyzed by Caswell (1985) and Tuljapurkar and Boe (1993).

In a typical size-structured model, the size s of an individual depends on its age x via a physical growth function,

$$\frac{ds}{dx} = g(x), \tag{7}$$

and mortality $\mu(s)$ and fertility $m(s)$ depend on size. The Lotka equation of classical demography is replaced by a size-structured analog,

$$1 = \int_0^\infty ds\, m(s)\, H(s) \exp^{-rs}, \tag{8}$$

where

$$H(s) = \frac{1}{g(s)} \exp\left[-\int_0^s dz \left(\frac{\mu(z)}{g(z)} \right) \right]. \tag{9}$$

In typical biological situations the physical growth rate $g(s)$ starts at some high value when the organism is at its minimum (birth) size and then decreases until a maximum size is reached. In consequence, $[1/g(s)]$ is an increasing function of size. In Equation 8, then, the exponential factor in $H(s)$ decreases with size s, whereas $[1/g(s)]$ increases with size. The result is that the function H first increases and then decreases with size, typically displaying a maximum at some nonzero size. Hence increases in fertility will have progressively greater positive effect until the organism reaches some size $s*$, beyond which fertility will have progressively smaller effect. The sensitivity to mortality first decreases with size to some minimum value and then increases with size.

These selective pressures on mortality and fertility show a dramatically different qualitative pattern as compared with classical age-structured models. Therefore in size-structured models, different patterns in the timing ("early" versus "late") of reproduction can lead to equivalent fitness, just as in models with temporally varying vital rates. In other words, we have here another mechanism for the existence of equilibrium mortality patterns that are not salmon-like.

DIRECTIONS

The preceding sections suggest the elements of a research program that should yield substantially improved insight into the evolution of equilibrium patterns of life-history phenotypes. I will discuss these below and conclude with some suggestions for work on the analysis of empirical data.

Mutation-Selection Equilibria

It should be clear by now that models must incorporate mutation explicitly if they are to provide unambiguous predictions. The work of Charlesworth (1990) shows how this can be done, at least for some models. An important line of research is the embedding of different dynamical and ESS models in a mutation-selection framework. Such models include models of tradeoffs between different components of the life-history phenotype, models of temporally varying selection, and models of size-structured dynamics.

The assumptions of the mutational dynamics need to be explored carefully, with a clear statement of assumptions. In principle, one can classify all mutations by their age pattern of effects on fertility and mortality. Given such a classification, a mutational variance-covariance matrix will describe any particular assumed pattern of mutational events. It is highly desirable to use such a general framework so that the results of different assumptions can be usefully compared. A careful analysis of the literature on mutations, especially the extensive body of work on fitness-related mutations in *Drosophila*, should help in this regard.

Tradeoffs in Life History

There is growing experimental and theoretical interest in the nature of tradeoffs. Abrams and Ludwig (1995), for example, use a different kind of tradeoff than does Charlesworth (1990), even though there are similarities. It would be useful here to classify tradeoffs in terms of covariances between life-history components. As with mutations, this would provide a systematic framework for comparisons between theoretical studies. Here, too, a careful assessment of the empirical data on plants and animals would be worthwhile.

Temporally Varying Environments

Models of temporal variation predict stable polymorphisms among a range of life-history phenotypes. It would be valuable to extend this theory to a model for quantitative traits using the methods of quantitative genetics and to examine the nature of equilibrium phenotypic distributions that would be predicted by such models.

Size-Structured Models

These models have been relatively little explored in the context of life-history evolution, although considerable work has been done on their application to the modeling of population dynamics. The study of such models is promising because they express ontogenetic correlations between fertility and mortality and may yield new insights into the determinants of evolutionary equilibrium phenotypes. These models, too, need to be extended to incorporate quantitative genetics.

Strong Selection

The quantitative theory of mutation-selection dynamics is based on the assumption of weak selection, under which the demography of the population is always close to equilibrium. It is well known that demographic characters strongly influence dynamics when the population is not in demographic equilibrium. Therefore, it would be very interesting to extend this theory to incorporate the interaction between selection and demographic disequilibrium. Such a theory should reveal similarities with the theory of temporally varying selection, because the latter also deals with demographic disequilibrium.

Empirical Issues

The work of Gaillard et al. (1994) shows that it is possible and necessary to examine field data on populations using careful longitudinal methods where possible. While demographers have the relative luxury of conducting new surveys with more covariates and higher resolutions, ecologists often do not. Demographers could help ecologists by examining the issues that confront the latter when examining field data. In particular, work is needed on the effect of age/size and time resolutions on estimates of mortality, and on practical assessment of senescent patterns (when does senescence occur?). Analyses of comparative data also must to be done with great care and pose interesting statistical questions.

A different direction in comparative analysis is suggested by the work of Sibley and Ahlquist (1990) on bird phylogeny. Using a massive application of DNA-DNA hybridization, they constructed a new phylogeny of birds. Along with the phylogenies, they summarize information on demographic differences between birds. With the increasing accumulation of molecular data leading to phylogenies in many other plants and animals, there is a mine of information on the evolutionary development of demographic differences. This would be a valuable place to look for estimates on the rate at which demographic characters diverge during evolution. Such estimates would add to a broader and more accurate perspective on the evolution of mortality and fertility in humans.

ACKNOWLEDGMENTS

I thank the Morrison Institute for Population and Resource Studies, Marc Feldman, and Jean Doble at Stanford University; the National Institutes of Health for support from HD 16640 and HD 32124; the National Science Foundation for support from DEB 9420153; and Carl Boe, Jim Curtsinger, Ken Wachter, Jim Vaupel, Daniel Promislow, Jim Carey, Mike Rose, and Peter Abrams for useful discussions.

REFERENCES

Abrams, P., and D. Ludwig
  1995   Optimality theory, Gompertz' Law, and the disposable soma theory of senescence. *Evolution* 49:1055-1066.
Carey, J., P. Liedo, D. Orozco, and J. Vaupel
  1992   Slowing down of mortality rates at older ages in large Medfly cohorts. *Science* 258:457-463.
Caswell, H.
  1985   The evolutionary demography of clonal reproduction. Pp. 187-224 in J.B.C. Jackson, L.W. Buss, and R.E. Cook, eds., *Population and Evolution of Clonal Organisms*. New Haven, CT: Yale University Press.
Charlesworth, B.
  1990   Optimization models, quantitative genetics, and mutation. *Evolution* 44:520-538.
Curtsinger, J.W.
  1995   Density, mortality, and the narrow view. *Genetica* 96:187-189.
Curtsinger, J.W., H. Fukui, D. Townsend, and J.W. Vaupel.
  1992   Demography of genotypes: Failure of the limited life-span paradigm in *Drosophila melanogaster. Science* 258:461-463.

Curtsinger, J.W., H. Fukui, A. Khazaeli, L. Xiu, and S. Pletcher
  1994   Rates of mortality in populations of *Caenorhabditis elegans. Science* 266:826.
Eshel, I., and M.W. Feldman
  1982   On the evolutionary genetic stability of the sex-ratio. *Theoretical Population Biology* 21:430-439.
Gaillard, J-M., D. Allaine, D. Pontier, N.G. Yoccoz, and D. Promislow
  1994   Senescence in natural populations of mammals. *Evolution* 48: 509-516.
Hamilton, W.D.
  1966   The moulding of senescence by natural selection. *Journal of Theoretical Biology* 12:12-45.
Lande, R.
  1982   A quantitative genetic theory of life history evolution. *Ecology* 63(3):607-615.
Liberman, U., and M.W. Feldman
  1986   Modifiers of mutation rate: A general reduction principle. *Theoretical Population Biology* 30:125-142.
Medawar, P.B.
  1952   *An Unsolved Problem of Biology.* London: H.K. Lewis.
Mukai, T., S.I. Chigusa, L.E. Mettler, and J.F. Crow
  1972   Mutation rate and dominance of genes affecting viability in *Drosophila melanogaster. Genetics* 72:335-355.
Orzack, S., and S. Tuljapurkar
  1989   Population dynamics in variable environments VII. The demography and evolution of iteroparity. *American Naturalist* 133:901-923.
Sibley, C., and J.E. Ahlquist
  1990   *Phylogeny and Classification of Birds: A Study in Molecular Evolution.* New Haven, CT: Yale University Press.
Tuljapurkar, S., and C. Boe
  1993   No Senescence Before Its Time: Life History and Mortality. Paper presented at the annual meeting of the Population Association of America.
Williams, G.C.
  1957   Pleiotropy, natural selection, and the evolution of senescence. *Evolution* 11:398-411.

5

Evolutionary Biology and Age-Related Mortality

Linda Partridge

INTRODUCTION

Analysis and interpretation of age-specific death rates are of considerable interest to both biodemographers and evolutionary biologists. Of special concern to both groups is the age-related decline in survival probability later in life, characteristic of many organisms including humans. This decline is generally taken to be indicative of a decline in intrinsic state, known as aging or senescence. The exact form of the survival curve differs considerably among human populations living in different areas and at different times (Finch, 1990; Wilmoth, in this volume), and we want to understand these differences and to produce a predictive theory of how mortality rates would change with age in different environments and behave in populations of different composition. Such a theory would be especially useful if it could also help predict patterns of age-related morbidity and cause of death.

Age-specific death rates have three main determinants: age-related changes within individuals, the environment in which they are placed, and qualitative differences between individuals. In addition, these three factors can interact with one another in the determination of mortality. Evolutionary biology has a strong theory for the evolution of age-related changes within individuals (e.g., Cole, 1954; Williams, 1957, 1966; Schaffer, 1974; Pianka and Parker, 1975; Charlesworth, 1980 and 1994; Roff, 1992; Stearns, 1992). Theories for the impact of the environment (Gomulkiewicz and Kirkpatrick, 1992; Scheiner, 1993; de Jong, 1995) and for the effects of individual differences (e.g., McNamara and Houston, 1996) are being increasingly explored. Human populations often inhabit an environment very different from those in which their life history evolved. This

78

considerably weakens the predictive power of evolutionary life-history theory, because interactions between genotypes and environments for life-history traits are pervasive (e.g., Stearns, 1992; Chapman and Partridge, 1996). In addition, much demographic analysis of the impact of aging has relied on various measures of age-specific death rates late in life. The evolutionary theories of aging apply to fertility and survival rates jointly, and from an evolutionary perspective aging is complete when reproduction ceases, unless the old contribute to reproduction by relatives. Deriving any general predictions for death rates alone, especially for postreproductive death rates, is not simple.

The following sections briefly summarize these issues and point to some areas where further work could be profitable. In addition, the broader implications of evolutionary ideas for the aging process are discussed.

AGE-RELATED CHANGES WITHIN INDIVIDUALS

Evolution of Life Histories and of Aging

The intrinsic state of individuals changes with age in humans and other organisms. These changes in state are reflected in changes in vital rates: survival and fertility. Evolutionary life-history theory has been directed at understanding the diverse array of age-related changes seen in different organisms.

From an evolutionary perspective, a life history is the combination of age-specific survival probabilities and fertilities characteristic of a type of organism. These produce the life table of survival probabilities to each age x (l_x) and the fertilities at those ages (m_x). The life history includes traits such as age at first breeding, number of breeding attempts, fecundity at each breeding attempt, and adult life span. The life histories observed in different species and, indeed, populations are extremely diverse, and the forces affecting their evolution are becoming well understood (e.g., Cole, 1954; Schaffer, 1974; Pianka and Parker, 1975; Charlesworth, 1980 and 1994; Stearns, 1992; Roff, 1992; McNamara and Houston, 1996; Tuljapurkar, in this volume). Natural selection is expected to act on the life history so as to incorporate into the population alleles that maximize the intrinsic rate of increase (r), which takes into account changes in the size of the population into which offspring are born or, in a population where numbers do not vary, lifetime reproductive success (R_0). To reach this conclusion requires certain simplifying assumptions such as stable age structure, absence of frequency-dependent selection, and absence of any interaction between the effects of male and female genotype upon the fertility of mating pairs. Other more complex fitness criteria can be used if some of these assumptions are violated (Tuljapurkar, in this volume).

Maximization takes place in the face of two forces. The first is the set of constraints on the combinations of different life-history variables that can be realized. Some of these are internal to the organism, in the form of various physiological constraints such as costs of growth, repair, and reproduction. Others are ecological, in the form of an altered impact of factors such as predation or parasitism in response to an alteration in, for instance, reproductive rate. Life histories evolve by a process of constrained optimization, in which the organism makes tradeoffs between costly competing activities. The environment that the organism inhabits will also affect the evolution of the life history, by imposing characteristic rates of age-specific (or size- or stage-specific) mortality and insults to fertility. These will affect the prospects for future reproduction at each age. In an environment with relatively high, externally imposed adult mortality, for instance, effort expended on reproduction is expected to increase even if survival probability and future fertility are thereby reduced by physiological costs, because prospects for future reproduction are anyway poor for environmental reasons.

The life histories of many organisms include a period of aging or senescence, terms for the deterioration in performance observed later in the adult life span. From an evolutionary point of view, the important manifestations of aging are a drop in survival probability and in fertility. These senescent changes have been very frequently reported, both in nature and in benign environments (Comfort, 1979; Finch, 1990; Rose, 1991; Charlesworth, 1980 and 1994). Aging is a particularly interesting trait from an evolutionary point of view, because taken in isolation it is maladaptive relative to its absence. We have to account for the failure of organisms later in life to achieve the levels of performance of which they were capable in youth. Aging is caused by damage to molecules, cells, organs, and systems. It could therefore be regarded as simply inevitable (Kirkwood, 1977; Kirkwood and Rose, 1991). However, different organisms have very different rates of aging, suggesting that the process is combated to different extents. It is this diversity in resistance to the effects of damage that requires an evolutionary explanation.

The evolution of aging is embedded in the evolution of the life history as a whole. The intensity of natural selection declines over the adult part of the life history because, even in a potentially immortal or indefinitely fecund organism, extrinsic forces such as disease, predation, and accidents impose mortality and damage to fertility. A mutant that is expressed early in adulthood will therefore be subject to strong selection because most of its initial bearers will still be alive and fully fertile. For a mutant expressed later, many initial carriers will already have died or suffered external insults to their fertility at a rate no different from nonbearers of the mutant, so that only the survivors are exposed to selection (Medawar, 1952). For age-specific fertility, selection intensity depends upon the probability of reaching that age, whereas for survival, selection intensity depends both upon survival probability to each age and what is lost by death at different ages, and therefore upon the future prospects for both survival and fertility (Charlesworth, 1980 and 1994).

Aging can therefore evolve as part of the constrained optimization of the life history, because an allele with beneficial effects in the early part of life but with deleterious effects later on will be more strongly selected through the former than through the latter effect (Williams, 1957). Aging can therefore be accounted for as a deleterious side-effect of the evolution of an optimal life history (Partridge and Barton, 1993a). This theory has become known as the pleiotropy theory of aging (Vaupel, Tuljapurkar, in this volume), although the evolutionary processes at work need not include pleiotropy (Partridge and Barton, 1993a; 1996). Although life-history optimization may result in the evolution of aging, it does not follow that a monotonic decline in the intrinsic state of the organism will occur during the adult period. Under some circumstances, a condition is predicted to improve for part of the adult period, for instance as a result of growth or learning, which could lead to gains in future reproductive prospects through improved survival probability and fertility (Hamilton, 1966; Charlesworth, 1980 and 1994).

Aging is not an inevitable feature of life-history optimization and, for it to appear, the age of expression of the beneficial effects of the mutant must precede the age of expression of the deleterious effects. The alternative is an increase in risk (Partridge and Andrews, 1985; Partridge, 1987; Partridge and Barton, 1993a,b). For instance, a mutant individual that reproduced more at a particular age could be more likely to die at that age because it attracted the attentions of predators or became more likely to have a heart attack. When the organism ceased the risky activity, its phenotype would then be no different from that of an otherwise comparable organism that had not taken the risk. Risk contributes to the constraints under which the life history is optimized, but it does not, by definition, in itself induce aging, because it does not alter the phenotype, contrary to a recent claim (Blarer et al., 1995). An example of a beneficial effect with a delayed cost could be a negative effect of increased reproductive rate on various somatic repair processes, which could, in turn, reduce subsequent survival or fecundity (Kirkwood and Rose, 1991; Abrams and Ludwig, 1995), sometimes known as the "disposable soma theory" (Kirkwood, 1977).

Aging can also evolve as a result of depression of the life history below the optimal, through mutation pressure, the "mutation-accumulation theory" of aging (Vaupel, Tuljapurkar, in this volume). Deleterious mutations with effects on the phenotype that become apparent early in life are more strongly selected against than those expressed later in adult life (Medawar, 1952; Hamilton, 1966; Charlesworth, 1980 and 1994). Later-acting mutations are more likely to escape the attention of natural selection because their bearers are more likely to have died or become subfertile from some other cause, at a rate no different from that of nonbearers of the mutation, before the age at which the phenotypic effect of the mutation becomes apparent. Deleterious mutations with a later effect on the phenotype can therefore reach a higher frequency under mutation-selection balance, and their effects would be apparent as an intrinsic decline later in life.

For the mutation-accumulation theory to be important, new mutations should have deleterious effects on the phenotype that are at least partially specific to later ages. This does not mean that the genes should be expressed at these ages. For instance, genes active during development could affect the durability of the soma, while genes affecting levels of activity and reproduction could determine the levels of damage that are incurred. The mutation-accumulation theory does not, therefore, rest on the implausible assumption that the late-life decline in state relies on gene expression of an increasing number of deleterious mutations. Rather, effects of variation between alleles and their patterns of expression at all ages become apparent in the phenotypes of old age.

How Can the Rate of Aging Be Measured?

What do these evolutionary theories allow us to predict about age-related changes in death rate in the later part of life in any population, including human populations? This question raises an important empirical issue, which is how the intrinsic deterioration that causes death rate to increase and fertility to decline at later ages can be detected and compared between different populations. There is considerable current interest in measuring the rate of aging in different natural populations, and in using such measures to deduce the evolutionary mechanisms at work (e.g., Nesse, 1988; Abrams, 1991; Promislow, 1991; Gaillard et al., 1994; Carey et al., 1992; Curtsinger et al., 1992; Abrams and Ludwig, 1995), which has led to lively debate about exactly how aging can be detected and its rate measured.

Most measures of the aging rate used thus far have focused on death rates. If intrinsic deterioration is occurring and death rate alone is used as a measure, then death rate clearly must change with age. Two populations that differ from each another in death rates that remain constant with age within each population do not, by this criterion, differ in their rate of aging (Medawar, 1952; Tatar et al., 1993; Blarer et al., 1995). Various measures of the rate at which death rate increases with age have therefore been proposed (Finch, 1990; Finch et al., 1990; Promislow, 1991; Carey et al., 1992) and have been used, for instance, to examine the occurrence of aging in natural populations (Promislow, 1991; Gaillard et al., 1994), to document the rate of change in death rate with age in humans (Finch et al., 1990), or to show an apparent slowing down in the rate of aging at later ages in insects (Carey et al., 1992; Curtsinger et al., 1992), nematodes (Brooks et al., 1994), and in humans (Vaupel, in this volume). An increase in age-specific death rates in theoretical models has been used to claim that spurious evidence for aging can be found in the absence of any intrinsic decline in the organism (Blarer et al., 1995) or that aging can occur as a direct result of an intrinsic improvement in state (McNamara and Houston, 1996). Superficially, some of these findings might be at variance with evolutionary theories of aging. However, they rest, in part, on the use of an inappropriate measure of aging from the evolutionary point of view, based solely on the way that death rates change with age.

A point that has escaped sufficient emphasis is the inevitability of the joint evolution of death and fecundity rates, rather than the separate evolution of the two traits (Partridge and Barton, 1993b, 1996). Both traits are expected to be affected by aging, and in ways that are not independent. One reason is that aging as a by-product of an optimal life history can occur because of a tradeoff necessitated by the direct physiological connection between survival and fecundity. Another is that the intensity of selection on age-specific fecundity depends upon the survival rate to that age, whereas selection upon age-specific survival depends on the fecundity schedule, because this affects what is lost by death at different ages (Charlesworth, 1980 and 1994). The important issues are to determine (1) how we can combine measures of survival and fertility into a single measure of the rate of aging, and (2) how use of this measure, instead of measures of rates of change in age-specific death rates, would affect conclusions about the pattern of change of intrinsic state in relation to age, and their concordance with evolutionary theories of aging.

Aging, the process we are trying to measure, occurs either because of later-expressed costs of processes beneficial earlier in life or because mutation pressure is depressing the life history below the optimal one. Either of these explanations will lead to an intrinsic decline in state, so that aging alone implies a drop in future prospects for offspring production. How can we detect this decline when it can occur against the backdrop of a state that can, over at least some of the adult life span, increase as part of life-history optimization? During this period of increase, aging may nevertheless be present, because intensity of selection starts to decline at the age of first reproduction (Charlesworth, 1980 and 1994), and its presence will mean that state will not improve as much as it would have in the absence of aging. However, in theory, during this part of such a life history, death rates could increase, decrease, or remain constant, despite the fact that intrinsic state is increasing (Hamilton, 1966; McNamara and Houston, 1996). Furthermore, intrinsic state could not itself be used to indicate the extent of the impact of aging. Only when intrinsic state starts to decline, as it must later on in any life history (Hamilton, 1966), can we start to measure and compare rates of intrinsic deterioration.

As a start in this direction we (Partridge and Barton, 1993b) suggested that the product $l_x m_x$, where l_x is survival from birth to age x and m_x is fecundity at age x could be used as a measure of the extent to which aging has occurred by age x. This product measures the contribution of each age to the total progeny output. However, this measure is taken from birth, and it applies only to age x. No indication therefore is given of the prospects for future reproduction from age x onward, given that age x is reached, which is the real test of intrinsic state at age x. A better measure would be Fisher's "reproductive value":

$$v(x) = \int_x^\infty \frac{l(y)}{l(x)} m(y) e^{r(x-y)} dy.$$

Here, r is the asymptotic rate of population growth, which in many cases could be taken as zero; note that $v(0) = 1$. The "reproductive value" gives the expected number of descendants that will be produced by an individual of age x over the rest of its lifetime, given that it has already survived to that age. It is therefore a measure taken prospectively from each age of the potential of the organism to produce further offspring, which is the evolutionarily relevant indication of the state of the organism (Partridge and Barton, 1996). Note that, as Hamilton (1966) argued, $v(x)$ does *not* give the strength of selection on the life history at age x, since that should also account for the probability of surviving to age x. We also ignore complications from the effects of an individual upon the fitness of its relatives. These effects can be very important in many organisms, including humans (Carey and Gruenfelder; Austad, in this volume), and would require modification of the proposed measure of the rate of aging to account for inclusive fitness effects. The outcome should, nevertheless, be qualitatively similar.

The presence of aging in a population can consequently be detected as a late-life decline in reproductive value, and this is what is predicted by evolutionary theories of aging. The measure can also compare the rate of aging in different populations. Reproductive value is a continuous function of age, which means that any two life histories can differ for it in an infinite number of ways. If the reproductive value is always lower in one life history than another, then one can say that life history involves more rapid aging. If, in contrast, they cross over at one or more points, then the implications become more complex, and the rate of aging can be compared only during late-life decline.

Interpretations of a slowing down in the rate of increase in death rates at later ages (e.g., Carey et al., 1992; Curtsinger et al., 1992; Brooks et al., 1994; Vaupel, in this volume) should be viewed in this light. Because all cases so far reported involve postreproductive individuals and most of them are from species where individuals do not contribute to the survival of relatives, the observed effects are selectively neutral and are, therefore, not at variance with evolutionary theories of aging. Postreproductive survival in the absence of inclusive fitness effects is an epiphenomenon from the evolutionary point of view, and changes in mortality rates at these ages could have a variety of explanations (Charlesworth and Partridge, 1997). One could be the inevitable viability of complex machines after the time for which they are engineered (in this case by natural selection) to guarantee to function (Vaupel, in this volume). Postreproductive survival may be increased in unnaturally benign environments, and cessation of reproduction or an associated reduction in activity levels could both contribute to lowering of the impact of damage. Additional factors could be variation in frailty (Vaupel, in this volume), or a tendency for the elderly to inhabit more benign environments. The important point is that evolutionary theories of aging do not necessarily predict Gompertzian-type increases in postreproductive mortality rates. Nor does the mutation-accumulation theory necessarily predict catastrophic increases in mortality when reproduction ceases, especially as mutations that produce aging also have some small deleterious effect earlier in life (Partridge and Barton, 1993a). The evolutionary theories do predict a monotonic decline to zero in reproductive value at some point in the life history. Re-examination of the reported anomalous cases in which "aging" (measured as mortality rate) appeared in theoretical models where there was either no change (Blarer et al., 1995) or a positive change (McNamara and Houston, 1996) in intrinsic state also shows that use of reproductive value as a measure of aging would have removed the anomaly.

To advance this issue will require the production of explicit theoretical models of the mutation-accumulation and pleiotropy theories that examine outcomes for age-related patterns of mortality in not only the reproductive but also the postreproductive period. Two recent studies (Abrams and Ludwig, 1995; Rose, in this volume) are promising starts in this direction. We also need more data. There is at present a paucity of information about the degree and pattern of age-specificity of fitness effects of new mutations, and of the relevant mutation rates. The timing of the effects of costs of reproduction or of investment in repair processes on future fertility and survival is also poorly known (Partridge and Sibly, 1991). These data are not easy to collect and are a challenge for future work. To understand how postreproductive survival evolves, we need to understand its genetic correlations with survival and mortality patterns during the reproductive period.

Can We Predict Either the Rate of Aging
or the Rate of Change in Death Rate?

What can evolutionary theories of aging predict about its rate in different populations? One of the broadest predictions is that there will be a relationship between the impact of external factors on the survival and fertility of the population, on one hand, and the intrinsic rate of aging that it is expected to evolve, on the other (Medawar, 1952; Williams, 1957; Hamilton, 1966; Charlesworth, 1980 and 1994; Tuljapurkar, Rose, in this volume). For instance, higher externally imposed death rates of adults are expected to cause evolution of higher rates of aging for both survival and fertility. However, the precise nature of this prediction and the nature of the measurements necessary to test it have been the subject of some discussion (Abrams, 1993; Promislow, 1991; Blarer et al., 1995).

Population dynamics are one important consideration. If one vital rate is changed by a change in, for instance, the size-specificity of predators, then for the population to remain regulated in numbers, it must compensate in some way. For an alteration in externally imposed factors to impose a permanent change in selection on the life history, the population must not respond by restoring a pattern of age-specific vital rates that leaves the pattern of selection unaltered (Abrams, 1993). The first thing that must be established, therefore, is that a difference in the impact of external factors results in an altered pattern of age-specific vital rates. This external impact must be separated from any intrinsic changes within the individuals in the study populations. Such studies are extremely difficult in nature. Allocating even differences in natural death rates, in unmanipulated populations, to intrinsic or extrinsic causes is, in general, not possible: are predators catching more great tits in one population because of lack of alternative prey, or because the great tits are distracted by the need to forage for larger broods?

One approach to this problem has been to use differences in life style as an indicator of hazard. For instance, Williams (1957) suggested that the evolution of flight might have resulted in a reduced impact of external hazard. A similar suggestion has been made for bats (Austad and Fischer, 1991). However, information of this kind does not involve any objective measurement of external hazard and does not form the basis for any quantitative statements. The contention about the hazard-reducing effects of flight may well be correct, but there is no direct evidence that it is, and alternative theories for avian longevity have been advanced (Carey and Gruenfelder, in this volume). Another approach has been to use mortality rate in early adulthood as a measure of hazard (Promislow, 1991). However, this mortality rate is affected by intrinsic as well as extrinsic factors. There is therefore a challenge to make the relevant measurements of hazard on natural populations.

The second requirement for a test of the relationship between the impact of environmental hazard and the evolved rate of aging is a measurement of the intrinsic change of state in natural populations and, in particular, its rate of decline in the later part of life. Here, it has been argued that life span under optimal conditions is a suitable measure (e.g., Williams, 1957; Austad and Fisher, 1991; Partridge and Barton, 1993a). There are two objections to this measure. The first comes from the nature of the environments in which such measures are generally made. What is required is an environment with external hazards removed but otherwise similar to the natural one. Typically, measurements of intrinsic change have been made in benign environments, very different from that in which the life history evolved, a problem because life-history traits and the correlations between them are often extremely sensitive to environmental change (e.g., Stearns, 1992; Chapman and Partridge, 1996). The study organism may, through phenotypic plasticity, alter its own intrinsic life history as a proximate response to, for example, changes in nutrition or even the removal of external hazard. The second problem comes from using life span as an indication of the aging rate. Measurement of rate of change of reproductive potential with age is the appropriate measure. Conclusions might be unaltered by its use, but this remains to be seen. Again, these measurements present a challenge for future studies. Although the data from nature are at present equivocal, the results of experimental, laboratory studies support the contention that external hazard is an important determinant of the evolution of both longevity and age-specific fecundity (Rose, 1984; Luckinbill et al., 1984; Partridge and Fowler, 1992; Zwaan et al., 1995).

Predicting the rate of aging for humans is more difficult than for many other organisms because their life history evolved in environments different from those inhabited by most present-day populations. We know rather little about the impact of external hazards on human populations in their evolutionary past, although archaeological, historical, and comparative anthropological data are increasingly being exploited for information on vital rates (Kaplan, in this volume). Disentangling the roles of extrinsic and intrinsic factors in producing these vital rates presents an interesting challenge. Analysis of natural selection on the life histories of humans is complicated by the fact that they can contribute to the care of descendants and other relatives when they themselves have become unable to reproduce (Carey and Gruenfelder, Austad, in this volume). Patterns of personal fecundity do not therefore give an adequate picture of true fitness schedules in the evolutionary past. In any discussion of the implications of evolutionary knowledge for age-related patterns of human death rates, we therefore need to bear in mind that part of the picture is missing, and that this could alter our conclusions. However, the physical frailty of the oldest old may have greatly limited their contribution to the reproductive success of younger kin, so the difficulty may not be too serious.

ENVIRONMENTAL EFFECTS

The environment is an important determinant of the form of life histories. We have already seen that the pattern of hazard that it imposes is expected to determine the way in which natural selection acts on the life history. In addition, environmental change can affect the ways in which life-history traits are expressed and the correlations between them. For instance, *Drosophila melanogaster* reared at lower temperatures develop more slowly and into a larger adult. Environmental effects are not necessarily predictable from evolutionary ones. For instance, *D. melanogaster* that have evolved at lower temperatures, when reared under similar conditions to higher-temperature populations, show more rapid development to larger adult body size. The developmental and evolutionary effects of temperature on rate of development are therefore in opposite directions, while those on body size are in the same direction (for review, see Partridge and French, in press).

An important issue with environmental effects is their timing. Current environment is frequently important. For instance, female fruit flies (*Drosophila*) can switch their egg production on and off almost instantaneously in response to altered food supply (Chapman et al., 1994). Data from large cohorts of medflies (Carey et al., 1992) showed that the way in which adult mortality rate changed with age was affected by the kind of container and social environments in which the flies were kept. Environmental effects can also be persistent. In *Drosophila*, larval density during rearing, to take one of many relevant variables, affects the size, life span, and fertility of adults (e.g., Clark and Feldman, 1981; Zwaan et al., 1991).

Environmental variables can also interact in their effects on the life history. For instance, adult female *Drosophila* that had been reared under standard conditions were exposed to different levels of nutrition, chosen to span the level that the females usually encountered, and to two levels of opportunities for mating. Excess mating can reduce the life span of female *Drosophila* (Fowler and Partridge, 1989; Chapman et al., 1995). Nutrition and opportunity for mating interacted in their effect on female lifetime reproductive success, because the cost of mating reduced lifetime reproductive success only at the highest level of nutrition (Chapman and Partridge, 1996).

Life histories, like any other trait evolving under natural selection, are expected to evolve toward a form optimal only for the environments in which selection occurs. There has been a great deal of theoretical and empirical work on how sensitivity to the environment of life-history traits, their "norm of reaction" or "phenotypic plasticity," is expected to evolve for the range of environments naturally encountered (e.g., Gomulkiewicz and Kirkpatrick, 1992; Scheiner, 1993; de Jong, 1995). The conclusions of such models depend, to some extent, upon their assumptions. For instance, increased plasticity might or might not carry a cost. The trait could be one like insect body size, which is fixed at the onset of adulthood, so that plasticity is expressed only once during the life history, or one like egg-laying rate in female *Drosophila*, which can vary throughout the adult period. Different environments could be encountered equally or unequally frequently. The general theoretical findings are that phenotypic plasticity will evolve under a wide range of circumstances. Further, where different environments are encountered unequally frequently, the pattern of plasticity will produce the most appropriate expression of the trait and minimum additive genetic variance for it in the environment most frequently encountered.

The environments encountered by present-day human populations undoubtedly differ widely from those in which their life history evolved. Factors such as nutrition and disease are probably particularly important. Another peculiarity of human populations is that as their economic status rises, their fecundity declines by design. We are therefore probably dealing with fecundity schedules for both males and females that are very different from those that applied, on average, in the evolutionary past. In humans, changed environment can alter circumstances during development, especially for growth, in a way that is known to affect age at first breeding and adult phenotype. Within the adult period, both fecundity schedule and age-specific death rates are affected by environment. Many peculiarities of modern human populations could be manifestations of adaptive phenotypic plasticity that has evolved in response to the various levels of resources encountered in the past. Some insight into the sorts of plasticity patterns we might expect in response to these variables could, therefore, come from a knowledge of the effects of social and economic structuring in human populations before the demographic transition. The effects on postreproductive survival patterns would be particularly interesting. Whether the effects of the demographic transition on human life histories are so large as to make them difficult to interpret in evolutionary terms remains to be seen.

INDIVIDUAL VARIATION

If individuals differ in either their baseline intrinsic state or how it changes with age, the shape of the aging function for the population will partly reflect these individual differences (Vaupel, in this volume). Individual variation can mean that those individuals that become the oldest old do so because they are a nonrandom sample of their cohort.

Individual variation can be genetic or environmental in origin. Our best method of predicting the form of genetic variation comes from evolutionary theories of aging. The pattern of genetic variation predicted is different for the mutation-accumulation and pleiotropy mechanisms (Charlesworth and Hughes, 1996), with the former predicting an increase in additive genetic variance for survival and fertility with age and the latter not doing so, unless by making some restrictive assumptions. We do not yet know the relative importance of these two processes in determining the rate of aging or whether their contributions vary among different kinds of organisms. With mutation accumulation, we expect individually rare alleles at a large number of loci, but that is about all we can say with confidence. Certainly among the oldest old we should expect to see the effects of these rare mutations, and they must be expected to underlie much of any familial resemblance in age at and cause of death, but we cannot at present predict the pattern of individual variation in age at death that they will produce.

Environmental variation could also cause individual variation, perhaps more than that generated by genotype differences. It would be illuminating to obtain data from one or more of the model organisms on what kinds of individuals, in demographic terms, survive to become the oldest old. For instance, some studies with *Drosophila* have suggested that environmental manipulations that reduce adult fitness (high larval crowding, poor nutrition) can, paradoxically, extend life span (e.g., Luckinbill and Clare, 1986; Chapman and Partridge, 1996). However, at the same time lifetime reproductive success is reduced because of a reduction in fecundity. Furthermore, those individuals with the highest lifetime success produce their offspring, on average, earlier in life and cease reproduction soonest. If these findings generalize to other species, then the oldest old will not include an excess of those individuals that were initially the most robust members of their cohort, but rather of the ones that have been less successful in producing off-spring earlier in life. A fuller exploration of these kinds of environmental effects could be worthwhile.

In the context of the oldest old of the human population, one way to get at the effects of past environmental influences would be to exploit natural reversal experiments, where individuals move to a different environment part way through life. Their subsequent survival and fertility can then be compared with those of individuals who always inhabited the new environment or who always stayed in the old environment. This comparison is analogous to the use of temperature-sensitive mutations to study the effects of mutant gene expression at different ages or of experimental reversal of environmental variables such as reproductive status part way through life. These sorts of experiments raise quite an interesting paradox. In *Drosophila* this type of reversal experiment has been used to examine the timing of the increase in male mortality caused by sexual activity (Partridge and Andrews, 1985). The results suggested that the elevation of mortality is instantaneous and ceases or commences with the end or onset of elevated sexual activity. However, individual differences in frailty, whether genetic or environmental in origin, could complicate the interpretation of these experiments. If mortality rates were higher among the sexually active than among the celibate males before the reversal of reproductive status occurred, then the survivors of sexual activity would presumably be, on average, less frail than the survivors of celibacy. It is therefore possible that in the above experiment sexual activity did have lingering effects on male death rate, but that these were masked by the effects of the variation in frailty (Prowse and Partridge, 1997). We therefore need to apply some caution when studying the timing of environmental effects on death rate. In addition, these experiments failed to account for any possible effects on fertility, which might alter the conclusions about an absence of intrinsic changes in state.

INTERACTIONS

Intrinsic differences between individuals and intrinsic changes caused by aging may interact with the environment, producing a variety of patterns of age-related change in mortality or fertility. Benign environments, defined as those that, on average, improve individual performance, might be expected particularly to favor the frail and the aged, and there are many examples of such changes in relative viability with, for instance, population density. We know rather little about these interaction effects for life histories generally, and they warrant further study.

One of the most important interaction effects for life histories may involve patterns of phenotypic plasticity in relation to individual variation in frailty. There is increasing interest in theoretical analysis of life-history optimization in individuals that differ in state. The issue first became clearly apparent in work on optimization of clutch size in birds, where experimental work with field populations revealed that individual optima varied (e.g., Gustaffson and Sutherland, 1988; Pettifor et al., 1988). The basic finding was that, if brood size was experimentally manipulated, those individuals that laid larger clutches were also more capable of rearing those clutches successfully to fledging. These findings have helped to encourage the development of theoretical analysis of state-dependent life-history optimization (e.g., McNamara and Houston, 1996). Individual variation in human populations may reflect this type of plasticity and could have a major bearing on individual variation in the aging process. These findings underline the need to understand what kinds of individuals survive to later ages.

BROADER IMPLICATIONS OF AN EVOLUTIONARY APPROACH FOR HUMAN AGING

An evolutionary approach to aging has a number of messages in addition to any for age-specific death rates. Any gene that does not have an effect on fertility or survival would be lost by mutation pressure, so all genes must influence one or both of these traits at some ages (Partridge and Barton, 1993a). The deduction is that genetic variation for the rate of aging will be polygenic, making aging a quantitative genetic trait, as has been frequently demonstrated (Hutchinson and Rose, 1991; Hutchinson et al., 1991; Hughes, 1995a,b). We are also not expecting most genes that influence the aging rate to be specialists, in that they did not evolve to their present form to cause aging, which, is, in fact, a deleterious trait. Aging is not like development (Partridge and Harvey, 1993; Martin et al., 1996), which is an orchestrated process under the control of a highly specialized gene hierarchy. Rather, genes active during development will affect the eventual resistance of the adult soma and reproductive processes to damage, while others that determine, for instance, levels of reproduction and activity will affect the rate at which damage is accumulated. Some genes, to be sure, will determine the extent to which damage is repaired, but they may well be the minority.

Another prediction is that, because the rate of aging evolves in response to the external hazards, we would expect the different systems underlying continuing survival and fertility to wear out in parallel, because of the common pattern of natural selection maintaining them in the face of damage. In consequence, we would not expect to find major genes that reduce the aging rate, unless they also had a deleterious effect on some other life-history aspect. Even if a genetic or other kind of intervention ameliorated one aspect of the aging process, we would expect the recipients to become infertile or die as a result of failure of other systems at a time very little later than the controls. The same argument does not apply to single genetic lesions that accelerate the aging process; they can and do cause early death and infertility (e.g., Yu et al., 1996). There have been reports of reduction in the rate of aging through single gene mutations or transgenes (see Johnson, in this volume), which contrasts interestingly with the predictions of evolutionary theory. There could be several explanations. (1) If the whole life history is not measured, perhaps because only survival is examined, there may well be negative, compensatory effects on fertility, preadult survival, or rate of development to adulthood. (2) If the effect of the genetic change is measured in an environment other than that where the life history evolved, complications from gene-environment interaction could result. (3) Particularly where the effects of transgenes are measured, the possibility of mutagenic effects of the insert, over and above any effects of transgene expression, must be considered. It is essential to control for the insert size, the position of the transgene in the genome, and the genetic background into which it is placed (Kaiser et al., 1997), controls rarely found in published studies.

CONCLUSIONS

An evolutionary approach does allow some strong predictions about aging patterns but does not, at present, have strong predictive power for patterns of mortality and morbidity in the elderly members of human populations. However, refinement of theory and data should greatly improve our understanding of these issues, and there may be other ways in which evolutionary thinking can inform future work on these issues. For instance, it would be helpful, at a physiological level, to know what the main tradeoffs are in mammalian life histories. It would be useful to know the cost of repair processes in any organism and how the level of different repair processes interacts with various environmental variables to determine rate of intrinsic deterioration. To this end, it would be extremely illuminating to know whether there are any major "public mechanisms" of aging (Martin et al., 1996), common to all species, in which case work on detailed mechanisms in model species could be directly relevant to humans. It would be useful to look for biomarkers of intrinsic state in natural populations and to learn more about evolution of norms of reaction for life-history traits, to predict the impact of changed environment.

Perhaps one of the most useful contributions of evolutionary thinking in this area is cautionary. We are interested in human senescence because we wish to maintain healthy life as long as possible. Because the rate of aging is affected by genetic variation, it is tempting to apply the kind of thinking to it that is applied to genetic disorders, including exploration of the possibility of genetic intervention. However, everything that we know about the evolution of aging suggests that it is probably the most polygenic of all traits. Fertility and viability are affected by all genes in the genome. The prospects for genetic intervention, therefore, must be explored with some circumspection.

REFERENCES

Abrams, P.A.
    1991   Fitness costs of senescence: The evolutionary importance of events in early adult life. *Evolutionary Ecology* 5:343-360.
    1993   Does increased mortality favor the evolution of more rapid senescence? *Evolution* 47:877-887.
Abrams, P.A., and D. Ludwig
    1995   Optimality theory, Gompertz law, and the disposable soma theory of senescence. *Evolution* 49:1055-1066.
Austad, S.N., and K.E. Fischer
    1991   Mammalian aging, metabolism, and ecology: Evidence from the bats and marsupials. *Journal of Gerontology* 46:B47-53.

Blarer, A., M. Doebeli, and S.C. Stearns
1995   Diagnosing senescence: Inferring evolutionary causes from phenotypic patterns can be misleading. *Proceedings of the Royal Society of London, Series B. Biological Sciences* 262:305-312.

Brooks, A., G.L. Lithgow, and T.E. Johnson
1994   Mortality rates in genetically heterogeneous populations of *Caenorhabditis elegans*. *Science* 263:668-671.

Carey, J.R., P. Liedo, D. Orozco, and J.W. Vaupel
1992   Slowing of mortality rates at older ages in large medfly cohorts. *Science* 258:457-461.

Chapman, T., L.F. Liddle, J.M. Kalb, M.F. Wolfner, and L. Partridge
1995   Cost of mating in *Drosophila melanogaster* females is mediated by male accessory gland products. *Nature* 373:241-244.

Chapman, T., and L. Partridge
1996   Female fitness in *Drosophila melanogaster*: An interaction between the effects of nutrition and encounter rates with males. *Proceedings of the Royal Society of London, Series B. Biological Sciences* 263(1371):755-759.

Chapman, T., S. Trevitt, and L. Partridge
1994   Remating and male-derived nutrients in *Drosophila melanogaster*. *Journal of Evolutionary Biology* 7:51-69.

Charlesworth, B.
1980   *Evolution in Age-Structured Populations*. 1st ed. New York: Cambridge University Press.
1994   *Evolution in Age-Structured Populations*. 2nd ed. New York: Cambridge University Press.

Charlesworth, B., and K.A. Hughes
1996   Age-specific inbreeding depression and components of genetic variance in relation to the evolution of senescence. *Proceedings of the National Academy of Sciences U.S.A* 93(12):6140-6145.

Charlesworth, B., and L. Partridge
1997   Ageing: Levelling of the grim reaper. *Current Biology* 7:R440-R442.

Clark, A.G., and M.W. Feldman
1981   Density dependent fertility selection in experimental populations of *Drosophila melanogaster*. *Genetics* 98:849-869.

Cole, L.C.
1954   The population consequences of life history phenomena. *Quarterly Review of Biology* 29:103-137.

Comfort, A.
1979   *The Biology of Senescence*, 3rd ed. Edinburgh: Churchill Livingstone.

Curtsinger, J.W., H. Fukui, D. Townsend, and J. Vaupel
1992   Failure of the limited-lifespan paradigm in genetically homogeneous populations of *Drosophila melanogaster*. *Science* 258:461-463.

de Jong, G.
1995   Phenotypic plasticity as a product of selection in a variable environment. *American Naturalist* 145:493-512.

Finch, C.E.
1990   *Longevity, Senescence and the Genome*. Chicago: University of Chicago Press.

Finch, C.E., M.C. Pike, and M. Whitten
1990   Slow mortality rate accelerations during aging in some animals approximate that of humans. *Science* 249:902-905.

Fowler, K., and L. Partridge
1989   A cost of mating in female fruitflies. *Nature* 338:760-761.

Gaillard, J-M., D. Allaine, D. Pontier, N.G. Yoccoz, and D.E.L. Promislow
1994   Senescence in mammals: A reanalysis. *Evolution* 48:509-516.

Gomulkiewicz, R., and M. Kirkpatrick
1992   Quantitative genetics and the evolution of reaction norms. *Evolution* 46:390-411.
Gustaffson, L., and W.J. Sutherland
1988   The costs of reproduction in the collared flycatcher *Ficedula albicollis. Nature* 335:813-815.
Hamilton, W.D.
1966   The molding of senescence by natural selection. *Journal of Theoretical Biology* 12:12-45.
Hughes, K.A.
1995a   Evolutionary genetics of male life history characters in *Drosophila melanogaster. Evolution* 49:521-537.
1995b   The inbreeding decline and average dominance of genes affecting male life-history characters in *Drosophila melanogaster. Genetical Research* 65(1):41-52.
Hutchinson, E.W., and M.R. Rose
1991   Quantitative genetics of postponed aging in *Drosophila melanogaster.* I. Analysis of outbred populations. *Genetics* 127:719-727.
Hutchinson, E.W., A.J. Shaw, and M.R. Rose
1991   Quantitative genetics of postponed aging in *Drosophila melanogaster.* II. Analysis of selected lines. *Genetics* 127:729-737.
Kaiser, M., M. Gasser, R. Ackermann, and S.C. Stearns
1997   P-element inserts in transgenic flies: a cautionary tale. *Heredity* 78(1):1-11.
Kirkwood, T.B.
1977   Evolution of ageing. *Nature* 270(5635):301-304.
Kirkwood, T.B.L., and M.R. Rose
1991   Evolution of senescence: Late survival sacrificed for reproduction. *Philosophical Translations of the Royal Society of London, Series B. Biological Sciences* 332:15-24.
Luckinbill, L.S., R. Arking, M.J. Clare, W.C. Cirocco, and S.A. Buck
1984   Selection for delayed senescence in *Drosophila melanogaster. Evolution* 38:996-1003.
Luckinbill, L.S., and M.J. Clare
1986   A density threshold for the expression of longevity in *Drosophila melanogaster. Heredity* 56:329-335.
Martin, G.M., S.N. Austad, and T.E. Johnson
1996   Genetic analysis of aging: Role of oxidative damage and environmental stresses. *Nature Genetics* 13:25-34.
McNamara, J.M., and A.I. Houston
1996   State-dependent life histories. *Nature* 380:215-221.
Medawar, P.B.
1952   *An Unsolved Problem of Biology.* London: H.K. Lewis.
Nesse, R.M.
1988   Life table tests of evolutionary theories of senescence. *Experimental Gerontology* 23:445-453.
Partridge, L.
1987   Is accelerated senescence a cost of reproduction? *Functional Ecology* 1:317-320.
Partridge, L., and R. Andrews
1985   The effect of reproductive activity on the lifespan of male *Drosophila melanogaster* is not due to an acceleration of senescence. *Journal of Insect Physiology* 31:393-395.
Partridge, L., and N.H. Barton
1993a   Optimality, mutation and the evolution of ageing. *Nature* 362:305-311.
1993b   Evolution of aging: Testing the theory using *Drosophila. Genetica* 91:89-98.
1996   On measuring the rate of ageing. *Proceedings of the Royal Society of London, Series B. Biological Sciences* 263(1375):1365-1371.

Partridge, L., and K. Fowler
1992   Direct and correlated responses to selection on age at reproduction in *Drosophila melanogaster. Evolution* 46:76-91.
Partridge, L., and V. French
1996   Why get big in the cold? Pp. 265-292 in *Animals and Temperature*, L.A. Johnston and A.B. Bennett, eds. Cambridge: Cambridge University Press.
Partridge, L., and P.H. Harvey
1993   Methuselah among nematodes. *Nature* (News and Views) 366:404-405.
Partridge, L., and R. Sibly
1991   Constraints in the evolution of life histories. *Philosophical Transactions of the Royal Society of London, Series B. Biological Sciences* 332:3-13.
Pettifor, R.A., C.M. Perrins, and R.H. McCleery
1988   Individual optimization of clutch size in great tits. *Nature* 336:160-162.
Pianka, E.R., and W.S. Parker
1975   Age-specific reproductive tactics. *American Naturalist* 109:453-464.
Promislow, D.E.L.
1991   Senescence in natural populations of mammals: A comparative study. *Evolution* 45:1869-1887.
Prowse, N., and L. Partridge
1997   The effects of reproduction on longevity and fertility in male *Drosophila melanogaster. Journal of Insect Physiology* 43(6):501-512.
Roff, D.A.
1992   *The Evolution of Life Histories: Data and Analysis.* New York: Chapman and Hall.
Rose, M.R.
1982   Antagonistic pleiotropy, dominance, and genetic variation. *Heredity* 48:63-78.
1984   Laboratory evolution of postponed senescence in *Drosophila melanogaster. Evolution* 38:1004-1010.
1991   *Evolutionary Biology of Aging.* Oxford: Oxford University Press.
Schaffer, W.M.
1974   Selection for optimal life histories: the effects of age structure. *Ecology* 5:291-303.
Scheiner, S.M.
1993   Genetics and evolution of phenotypic plasticity. *Annual Review of Ecology and Systematics* 24:35-68.
Stearns, S.C.
1992   *The evolution of life histories.* Oxford: Oxford University Press.
Tatar, M., J.R. Carey, and J.W. Vaupel
1993   Long-term cost of reproduction with and without accelerated senescence in *Callosobruchus maculatus*: Analysis of age-specific mortality. *Evolution* 47:1302-1312.
Yu, C-E, J. Oshima, Y.H. Fu, E.M. Wijsman, F. Hisama, R. Alisch, S. Mathews, J. Nakura, T. Miki, S. Ouasis, G.M. Martin, J. Mulligan, and G.D. Schellenberg
1996   Positional cloning of the Werner's Syndrome gene. *Science* 272:258-262.
Williams, G.C.
1957   Pleiotropy, natural selection, and the evolution of senescence. *Evolution* 11:398-411.
1966   Natural selection, the cost of reproduction and a refinement of Lack's principle. *American Naturalist* 100:687-690.
Zwaan, B., R. Bijlsma, and R.F. Hoekstra
1991   On the developmental theory of aging. I. Starvation resistance and longevity in *Drosophila melanogaster* in relation to pre-adult breeding conditions. *Heredity* 66:29-39.
Zwaan, B., R. Bijlsma, and R.F. Hoekstra
1995   Direct selection on life span in *Drosophila melanogaster. Evolution* 49:649-659.

6

Toward an Evolutionary Demography

Michael R. Rose

INTRODUCTION

Our quantitative understanding of the actuarial features of human populations has been dominated by ad hoc models from the field of demography, from Benjamin Gompertz in 1825 to the present day (e.g., Finch, 1990; Easton, 1995). This situation has continued despite the parallel development of an evolutionary theory for life history, including aging, from the 1930s to the present (see Charlesworth, 1994). On the one hand, we have the ad hoc models of demography, and on the other we have the a priori models of evolutionary theory. An obvious goal, then, would be to seek a synthesis of these two fields, a synthesis here termed "evolutionary demography."

Naturally, there is resistance to the wholesale introduction of evolutionary theory into research on demography and aging. It is often supposed that demographic and aging patterns are fixed species properties, analogous to chromosome number or breeding system. This definition removes the topic from the reach of normal evolutionary theory. A hardy perennial is that aging is somehow good for the species, a theory that underemployed physicists seem to rediscover every decade. One side effect of this theoretical confusion is the displacement of evolutionary and demographic theories of aging by hypotheses from the realm of molecular or cellular biology. It has been argued that because aging is due to free radicals, the evolutionary history of the organism is irrelevant. Likewise, limited cell replication in vitro or a hypothalamic clock may be offered as the ultimate determinant of aging patterns. Elsewhere, I have published a lengthy critique of this type of reasoning (Rose, 1991) and will not repeat it here. My conclusion, in any case, is that the proper ground for building theories of demography, aging, life history, and the like is evolutionary theory.

BASIC THEORY OF EVOLUTIONARY DEMOGRAPHY

The fundamental starting point for evolutionary analysis is an ecologically determined demography: particular age-specific survival probabilities and fecundities, varying also with time, organismal size, population density, and a range of other factors (Charlesworth, 1994). Frequently, however, factors other than age are neglected in the theory, and I will follow this practice for the sake of convenience and clarity. Some of the literature on the other characters (e.g., size) is discussed in Stearns (1992) and Roff (1992). For the present purposes, however, evolutionary demography starts from a simplified evolutionary situation defined by a set of age-dependent survival probabilities, $P(x)$ and fecundities, $m(x)$.

When density-dependence can be neglected (cf. Charlesworth, 1994), population growth rate is given by the largest real-valued root, r, of

$$\sum e^{-rx} \, l(x)m(x) = 1, \tag{1}$$

where $l(x) = \prod_{y=0} P(y)$ and x is age as well as the upper limit of multiplication. This ecological situation, in turn, determines the evolution of $P(x)$ and $m(x)$, where the equations for gene frequency change have terms weighted by

$$s(a) = \sum_{x-a+1} e^{-rx} l(x)m(x) \text{ and } s'(a) = e^{-ra} l(a) \tag{2}$$

for selection coefficients involving $ln \, P(a)$ and $m(a)$, with genetic effects at age a, respectively (Hamilton, 1966; Charlesworth, 1980; Rose, 1985). The s and s' functions play a *scaling* role. When the scaling functions are large, selection is more powerful, and conversely, when these values are small, selection is weak.

The forms of the s and s' scaling functions reveal the most important features of evolutionary demography in its crudest form. The form of $s(a)$ is such that it remains at 1.0 for ages below the start of reproduction. But for ages *after* the start of reproduction, $s(a)$ falls with age until it approaches zero. In terms of selection equations, this makes allelic effects on early survival of large impact on the evolutionary outcome, but allelic effects on late survival have little or no impact. Except for populations declining rapidly to extinction, similar patterns apply for $s'(a)$, which will usually be large at early ages and small at late ages. Put simply, this situation is summarized as "the force of natural selection tends to fall with adult age" (Medawar, 1952). This basic idea is hinted at in the classic writings of R.A. Fisher and J.B.S. Haldane and then broadly sketched by P.B. Medawar (e.g., 1952). However, it wasn't adequately developed mathematically until the work of Hamilton (1966) and Charlesworth (e.g., 1980), as outlined above. The most obvious corollary derivable from this situation is that components of fitness should deteriorate at later adult ages, due to the weakness of natural selection, and thus aging occurs (Rose, 1991). No decline in the force of natural selection acting on age-specific mortality is expected until the onset of reproduction in a cohort of same-aged organisms. Once at ages having reproductive individuals, the force of natural selection acting on survival begins to decline, as indicated by the equation for $s(a)$. There are analogous results for selection acting on age-specific fecundity, although they do not necessarily take the same form (Hamilton, 1966; Charlesworth, 1994). Overall, this might be described as the "basic" or "general" evolutionary theory for demography, aging, life history, and the like. There are many important special cases that depend on adding particular assumptions to this theory, some of which are discussed below. The foregoing should not be taken as a complete presentation of the theory of selection on age-structured populations, for which the best summary remains that of Charlesworth (1994).

EMPIRICAL EVIDENCE CONCERNING THE FORCE OF NATURAL SELECTION

Unlike many other global theories in population biology, the basic evolutionary theory of demography leads to some directly testable theoretical predications. It is categorically not the case that evolutionary theory provides a mere backdrop for reductionist research on the real "causes" of aging. Indeed, some of the most elegant and powerful experimental designs in life-history research are derivable from this basic evolutionary theory. Edney and Gill (1968) were among the first to point out that altering imposed demographic regimes in the laboratory should lead to corresponding shifts in the organism's demographic pattern. Wattiaux (1968a, b) inadvertently performed two tests of this kind in *Drosophila*, and Mertz (1975) performed some *Tribolium* experiments along these lines. But the most important work has used laboratory populations of *Drosophila melanogaster* since the late 1970s (Rose and Charlesworth, 1980; Luckinbill et al., 1984; Rose, 1984a; Luckinbill and Clare, 1985; Partridge and Fowler, 1992; Leroi et al., 1994; and Fukui et al., 1995).

Most of the *Drosophila* selection experiments have taken a broadly similar form and can be described generically. Normal fruit fly culture involves the production of a cohort of eggs from adults of similar age, where these eggs are typically laid on fresh fly medium. The adults are then discarded, and the eggs become larvae, pupae, and then young adults as a same-aged cohort. Typically, at 25 °C, the young adults are used to lay eggs for the next generation about 2 weeks after they were eggs themselves. With demographic manipulation, the period between emergence from pupa and egg laying to start the next generation is stretched—often to 8 weeks or more. Note that this procedure does not require the denial of copulation or egg laying in general. But any such eggs are discarded before they can contribute to the next generation. The typical experiment, then, combines these regimes: (*i*) controls in which reproduction is early, typically at

2 weeks, and later reproduction is denied; and (*ii*) selected lines in which reproduction is later, typically at 10 weeks, and early reproduction is denied. In terms of the force of natural selection, these two regimes define two rectangular patterns for *s*(*x*), one truncated at 2 weeks and one truncated at 10 weeks. It should also be emphasized that these experiments often involve replication of the selected and control lines, up to five of these lines for each treatment. When such lines are created from a common ancestral stock, it can take as little as 10 generations for the late reproduced lines to evolve significantly increased longevity. After 50 or more generations of late reproduction, these lines may have 60-80 percent greater mean longevity, compared to the controls, and maximum longevity may be increased more than that. The general conclusion from this work has been that the laboratory evolution of aging broadly follows the expectations of basic evolutionary theory: when the force of natural selection at later ages is artificially prolonged by denying early reproductive opportunities, evolution progressively postpones aging (e.g., Rose, 1984a; Luckinbill et al., 1984; Partridge and Fowler, 1992).

The force of natural selection can also be returned to its initial pattern by the simple expedient of returning late-reproduced lines, or derivatives of them, to early reproduction. Evolution then returns the population to its ancestral demography, with longevity falling back to its original value over subsequent generations (Graves et al., 1992). Other characters also tend to return to their original values, sometimes after considerable delay, sometimes not (Service et al., 1988; Graves et al., 1992). In any case, this is yet another case where demography effectively determines evolutionary destiny.

By the standards of evolutionary biology, there is now a wide spectrum of experimental results of this kind, where the force of natural selection determines the pattern of evolution, only some of which is reviewed in Rose (1991). Broadly, this is the well-corroborated core of evolutionary demography: as predicted by theory, experimentally imposed demography determines the subsequent evolution of demography by changing the age-specific forces of natural selection. Indeed, this is one of the best instances of the application of the experimental method within evolutionary biology, a field that normally has to rely on very indirect inferences. At the same time, these results are also the best warrant for the introduction of evolutionary ideas into biodemography, in that these experimental systems dramatically reveal the interplay between selection and demography.

One exemplary field study also deserves mention. Austad (1993) has studied natural populations of opossums in Virginia, one on the continental land mass, the other on islands that have been separated from the mainland for thousands of years. Island populations are exposed to less natural predation and suffer lower adult mortality rates, compared to mainland populations. Evolutionary theory predicts that the island populations should show slower aging. Austad's data corroborate this expectation: island populations show improved adult survivorship and later fertility, as well as ameliorated pathophysiology. In effect, the Virginia opossums have been a reasonable "natural experiment," like those in the laboratory with *Drosophila*.

THEORETICAL POPULATION GENETICS OF LIFE-HISTORY EVOLUTION

But the force of natural selection does not entirely determine the pattern of demographic evolution. An additional determinant is the nature of the genetic mechanisms that affect particular life-history characters. These genetic mechanisms can be grouped under two broad headings: nonpleiotropic genetic effects and pleiotropic genetic effects. I discuss each further in turn.

The most elegant possibility for the genetic mechanisms of demographic evolution is for each age-specific life-history character to evolve on its own, with the alleles that affect it lacking in effects on any other such character. It should be noted that this is a severe assumption, which is being offered here primarily for its simplicity. In particular, I do not wish to convey the impression that I think that this is the normal evolutionary situation where aging is concerned. At the same time, this severe constraint on allele action makes the mathematical specification of the evolutionary dynamics of life history, demography, etc. extremely elegant. Essentially, the entire evolutionary process reduces to two components: age-specific mutation and age-specific selection. In particular, because few beneficial alleles will be segregating at high frequencies at any one time, the evolutionary dynamics become mutation-selection balance, where there would typically be one favored allele and one or more deleterious alleles. For simplicity, the favored and deleterious alleles can be grouped into two allelic classes, and the frequency of the deleterious allele, when it is of minor effect and not fully recessive, can be approximated as

$$u/\{[\ln P_{11}(x) - \ln P_{12}(x)]s_{11}(x)\}, \tag{3}$$

where u is mutation rate from beneficial to deleterious alleles and the ij subscripts refer to genotypes having alleles i and j at the locus in question (Charlesworth, 1994). The beneficial allele is indicated by the numeral 1, and the deleterious allele is indicated by 2. Note that since the demography of the population will be determined largely by the homozygote of the fitter allele, the scaling function is specified by that demography. As discussed above, the scaling function is going to fall with age after the onset of reproduction. And because the scaling function is in the denominator of the allele-frequency formula, the frequency of deleterious alleles will theoretically increase enormously at later ages, producing a deterioration in survival probability. At early ages, of course, selection mutation should keep the frequency of deleterious alleles low, and thus age-specific survival would be high. An additional expectation, with this population genetic mechanism, is that the additive genetic variance for life-history characters should increase substantially at later ages, subject to comparability in the number of loci affecting each age class, as well as showing roughly uniform mutation rates over age classes and similar magnitude effects of the individual alleles over age classes. Of course, if these ceteris paribus conditions are violated, the additive genetic variance may not increase with age. But that is a typical caveat for population genetics theory.

Essentially all other possible population mechanisms fall under the pleiotropic heading. When pleiotropic effects are in the same direction, such that one allele is beneficial for all affected life-history characters, then evolution is somewhat analogous to that in the case with nonpleiotropy. The balance between selection and mutation will be determined primarily by genetic effects at early ages, and the form of the equation determining allele frequency will be much more complicated, but qualitatively the results will be similar. One complication, however, might be a reduction in the genetic variance at later ages, if early, stronger, selective forces are determining allele-frequency equilibria. If allelic effects are opposed among life-history characters, then antagonistic pleiotropy arises. Under these conditions, selection will often be the dominating factor in the evolutionary outcome, favoring alleles that are beneficial at early ages but deleterious later (Williams, 1957; Charlesworth, 1980; Rose, 1985).

Overall, both mutation-selection balance and pleiotropy can act so that aging evolves. They can also maintain genetic variability for demographic characters. However, these two mechanisms have different implications for the nature of that genetic variability. With mutation-selection balance, genetic variance should increase with age (Charlesworth, 1990, 1994), all other things being equal, while with pleiotropy it may or may not. Antagonistic-pleiotropy models also require that there be antagonistic genetic effects between some life-history characters, which may (Rose, 1985) or may not (Houle, 1991) be manifest as negative genetic correlations between some life-history characters. Fortunately, these corollaries are testable in experimental systems.

EXPERIMENTAL POPULATION GENETICS
OF LIFE-HISTORY EVOLUTION

The first thing to be said about the experimental population genetics of life history is that additive genetic variation is maintained for a variety of demographic characters in a variety of species (Rose, 1991; Roff, 1992). This is a corollary of both of the theoretical population genetic mechanisms described above. Beyond this point most of our experimental information comes from *Drosophila*. In that genus, at least, there are some cases in which genetic variances increase with age (e.g., Hughes and Charlesworth, 1994), and other cases where it does not (Rose and Charlesworth, 1981; Promislow et al., 1996). There are some cases where negative genetic correlations between life-history characters have been inferred (Rose and Charlesworth, 1981; Rose, 1984a; Luckinbill et al., 1984; Luckinbill and Clare, 1985) and other cases where they have not been (Partridge and Fowler, 1992). Still other studies find evidence both for and against antagonistic pleiotropy, as well as for and against mutation accumulation (Service et al., 1988; Leroi et al., 1994; Promislow et al., 1996; Tatar et al., 1996). The question is, then, how these results reflect on the validity of the two mechanisms of demographic evolution.

Many of the aforementioned studies have been plagued by artifacts. Indeed, it may be that almost all experiments of this kind are afflicted to at least some degree by problems like inbreeding depression, inadequate replication, genotype-by-environment interaction, and so on (Rose and Service, 1985). Nonetheless, it is sometimes possible for further experimentation to sort out many of these problems (e.g., Rose, 1984b; Service and Rose, 1985; Leroi et al., 1994; Chippindale et al., 1994).

Another point to make is that the experimental evidence can't plausibly be viewed as an either-or competition between mutation and pleiotropy models. There is some empirical support for both, some of it coming from the same experiments (e.g., Service et al., 1988; Tatar et al., 1996). Therefore, the only balanced point of view is that both of these genetic mechanisms are somewhat supported. They may both be involved in the evolution of demography, but neither is necessarily involved. Either is, in any case, sufficient for the evolution of demography to be dominated by the force of natural selection.

GOMPERTZ MODELS: PHENOMENOLOGICAL THEORY

From age 15 years or so, the rate of mortality accelerates exponentially in long-industrialized human populations, and this has been a commonplace of both demography and gerontology (e.g., Comfort, 1964). The Gompertz equation

$$\mu(x) = R \exp(\alpha x) \tag{4}$$

attempts to summarize this pattern using what amounts to a linear regression of the logarithm of the mortality rate (μ) on age, x, where α gives the slope of that regression and R is the initial rate of mortality. It has been argued that this ad hoc demographic model is key to understanding aging (e.g., Finch et al., 1990; Finch, 1990), and it certainly has much to recommend it, particularly in comparison with alternative indices, like mean or maximum life span, when the data are collected under dubious conditions.

My colleagues at the University of California, Irvine, and I have recently explored the extent to which the Gompertz model can be used to predict accurately the demography of experimental *Drosophila* populations (Mueller et al., 1995; Nusbaum et al., 1996). We did so because we do not regard human data as a particularly good way to test any general population-level theory; there is too much complexity introduced by culture and history. We also have reservations concerning the uncritical use of field data. We began with considerable doubts about the robustness of the Gompertz model. However, when the model is fitted using maximum-likelihood or nonlinear-regression methods, as opposed to conventional numerical approaches, we find that Gompertz parameters can be used to predict the mortality patterns of experimental populations of *Drosophila* after just 20-30 percent of the deaths of an observed cohort. The fit of these predictions can achieve respectable levels of accuracy, placing such parameters as mean longevity and 95 percent mortality within tight 95 percent confidence intervals. In effect, once the two Gompertz parameters have been fit to the data, there is usually only a little residual pattern to be modeled in the age-specific mortality data. Moreover, there is a high degree of correlation between the *a* parameter of the Gompertz model and other measures of aging, like maximum life span (Nusbaum et al., 1996), over diverse replicated populations. Having started as skeptics, we became convinced of the practical value of the Gompertz model in uncomplicated demographic situations. (However, as will be discussed, we remain concerned about the model's failures.)

Results like these, as well as those of many other investigators, show that the Gompertz model and its comparable first-order demographic equivalents (e.g., the Weibull model) are accurate representations of the demography of some experimental populations. In effect, Gompertz models are outstanding phenomenological models for some biodemographic situations.

THE OLDEST OLD

However, this situation may break down in human populations at extremely advanced ages (Comfort, 1964; Finch, 1990; Gavrilov and Gavrilova, 1991; Vaupel, in this volume, among others). Among these "oldest old," the probability of dying may not increase with age. This phenomenon has recently been demonstrated dramatically in various diptera, as well (e.g., Carey et al., 1992; Curtsinger et al., 1992). This problem of the oldest-old survival rates clearly merits serious attention. In particular, it makes continued reliance on the Gompertz model uncertain. Somehow, demographic theory needs to be refashioned.

Note, however, that the cases where the oldest old break from Gompertzian patterns may involve the latest-age classes only, when few individuals are still alive. For this reason, there is no necessary incongruence between the many cases in which the Gompertz model works to within reasonable limits of accuracy and the few cases where the model breaks down. Most cases where the model seems to work involve too few organisms to detect a late-life deviation from Gompertz expectations. In other words, the violations of the Gompertz model have usually arisen in unusual circumstances, in which the detailed data are either much more extensive or extensive and of very high quality.

The analogy that suggests itself is that of relativistic mechanics, which is based on cases that are usually not important in physical systems, most obviously cases where velocities approach the speed of light or very high masses are involved. Normally, Newtonian theory "works." But we know now that this is because it is only a first-order approximation to the truth, which is better approached by relativistic mechanics.

The strategy that Laurence D. Mueller and I have adopted is to look for a theory that can naturally, without forcing, generate phenomena like plateaus in mortality rates among the oldest old. This theory is thus the analog of relativistic mechanics in physics. We feel that we have taken the first significant steps toward developing such theory, but I do not have the opportunity to introduce this theory for evolutionary demography here.

Abrams and Ludwig (1995) have recently published an optimality approach to the kind of the theory that Mueller and I have tried to develop using population genetics. As a population geneticist, I have long had grave reservations about the use of optimality models for biological situations that are not defined by "free choices," such as those of sex allocation (Charnov, 1982), for example, in which there seems little reason to doubt that an optimal phenotype can evolve. Life-history evolution, instead, involves material resources and genetic constraints that may entirely prevent the attainment of any optimal phenotype (cf. Gould and Lewontin, 1979), and it is at least arguable that the evolution of actual life histories does not proceed toward optimal outcomes (Rose et al., 1987). For example, is it likely that the later life history will evolve toward optimal values if the allelic variation that shapes it is subject to very weak natural selection or none at all, given recurrent mutation pressure? For these reasons, we have proceeded instead to develop a population genetics theory for demography.

CONCLUSION

Recent work on age-specific mortality rates strongly suggests that conventional demographic models are in need of repair. Rather than resorting to yet another ad hoc tuning up of the same mathematical tools, consider the alternative approach provided by the population genetics theory of age-structured populations. This theory has been well-characterized mathematically and has been extensively supported in experimental genetic systems, although neither theory nor experiment are complete or perfect. Results obtained from evolutionary theory offer the best prospects for the development of demographic models, in general. In this way, demography could leave its ad hoc traditions behind and join together with evolutionary biology to forge a much stronger theoretical foundation. While the Gompertz model is an excellent approximation to mortality rates for most individuals from some iteroparous populations, it appears inadequate for the description of even the qualitative pattern of the full life history of most organisms, granting that such full life histories are not usually adequately observed. Biodemography should now move on to the task of developing proper evolutionary foundations.

ACKNOWLEDGMENTS

I am grateful to the other members of the National Research Council Bio-demography of Aging group for their helpful comments. In particular, I thank C.E. Finch for his editorial advice. The aging research of the author has recently been supported by U.S. Public Health Service PO1 Grant AG0-9970.

REFERENCES

Abrams, P.A., and D. Ludwig
    1995   Optimality theory, Gompertz' Law, and the disposable soma theory of senescence. *Evolution* 49:1055-1066.
Austad, S.A.
    1993   Retarded senescence in an insular population of Virginia opossums *Didelphis virginiana. Journal of Zoology* 229:695-708.
Carey, J.R., P. Liedo, D. Orozco, and J.W. Vaupel
    1992   Slowing of mortality rates at older ages in large medfly cohorts. *Science* 258:457-461.
Charlesworth, B.
    1980   *Evolution in Age-Structured Populations.* London: Cambridge University Press.
    1990   Optimization models, quantitative genetics, and mutation. *Evolution* 44:520-538.
    1994   *Evolution in Age-Structured Populations*, 2nd ed. London: Cambridge University Press.
Charnov, E.L.
    1982   *The Theory of Sex Allocation.* Princeton, NJ: Princeton University Press.
Chippindale, A.K., D.T. Hoang, P.M. Service, and M.R. Rose
    1994   The evolution of development in *Drosophila melanogaster* selected for postponed senescence. *Evolution* 48:1880-1899.
Comfort, A.
    1964   *Ageing, The Biology of Senescence*, 2nd ed. London: Routledge.
Curtsinger, J.W., H.H. Fukui, D.R. Townsend, and J.W. Vaupel
    1992   Demography of genotypes: Failure of the limited life-span paradigm in *Drosophila melanogaster. Science* 258:461-463.
Easton, D.M.
    1995   Gompertz survival kinetics: Fall in number alive or growth in number dead? *Theoretical Population Biology* 48:1-6.
Edney, E.B., and R.W. Gill
    1968   Evolution of senescence and specific longevity. *Nature* 220:281-282.
Finch, C.E.
    1990   *Longevity, Senescence, and the Genome.* Chicago: University of Chicago Press.
Finch, C.E., M.C. Pike, and M. Witten
    1990   Slow increases of the Gompertz mortality rate during aging in certain animals approximate that of humans. *Science* 249:902-905.
Fukui, H.H., S.D. Pletcher, and J.W. Curtsinger
    1995   Selection for increased longevity in *Drosophila melanogaster:* A response to Baret and Lints. *Gerontology* 41:65-68.
Gavrilov, L.A., and N.S. Gavrilova
    1991   *The Biology of Lifespan, A Quantitative Approach.* Chur, Switzerland: Harwood Academic Publishers.
Gould, S.J., and R.C. Lewontin
    1979   The sprandrels of San Marco and the Panglossian Paradigm: A critique of the adaptationist programme. *Proceedings of the Royal Society of London Series B, Biological Sciences* 205:581-598.

Graves, J.L., E.C. Toolson, C. Jeong, L.N. Vu, and M.R. Rose
  1992   Desiccation, flight, glycogen, and postponed senescence in *Drosophila melanogaster*.
          Physiological Zoology 65:268-286.
Hamilton, W.D.
  1966   The moulding of senescence by natural selection. *Journal of Theoretical Biology* 12: 12-
          45.
Houle, D.A.
  1991   What genetic correlations are made of, and why it matters. *Evolution* 45:630-648.
Hughes, K.A., and B. Charlesworth
  1994   A genetic analysis of senescence in *Drosophila*. *Nature* 367:64-66.
Leroi, A.M., A.K. Chippindale, and M.R. Rose
  1994   Long-term laboratory evolution of a genetic trade-off in *Drosophila melanogaster*. I. The
          role of genotype x environment interaction. *Evolution* 48:244-257.
Luckinbill, L.S., R. Arking, M.J. Clare, W.C. Cirocco, and S.A. Buck
  1984   Selection for delayed senescence in *Drosophila melanogaster*. *Evolution* 38:996-1003.
Luckinbill, L.S., and M.J. Clare
  1985   Selection for lifespan in *Drosophila melanogaster*. *Heredity* 55: 9-18.
Medawar, P.B.
  1952   *An Unsolved Problem in Biology*. London: H.K. Lewis.
Mertz, D.B.
  1975   Senescent decline in flour beetle strains selected for early adult fitness. *Physiological
          Zoology* 48:1-23.
Mueller, L.D., T.J. Nusbaum, and M.R. Rose
  1995   The Gompertz equation as a predictive tool in demography. *Experimental Gerontology*
          30:553-569.
Nusbaum, T.J., L.D. Mueller, and M.R. Rose
  1996   Evolutionary patterns among measures of aging. *Experimental Gerontology* 31:507-516.
Partridge, L., and K. Fowler
  1992   Direct and correlated responses to selection on age at reproduction in *Drosophila
          melanogaster*. *Evolution* 46: 76-91.
Promislow, D.E.L., M. Tatar, A. A. Khazaeli, and J.W. Curtsinger
  1996   Age-specific patterns of genetic variance in *Drosophila melanogaster*. I. Mortality. *Ge-
          netics* 143:839-848.
Roff, D.A.
  1992   *The Evolution of Life-Histories: Data and Analysis*. London: Chapman and Hall.
Rose, M.R.
  1984a   Laboratory evolution of postponed senescence in *Drosophila melanogaster*. *Evolution*
          38:1004-1010.
  1984b   Genetic covariation in *Drosophila* life history: Untangling the data. *American Naturalist*
          123:565-569.
  1985   Life history evolution with antagonistic pleiotropy and overlapping generations. *Theo-
          retical Population Biology* 28:342-358.
  1991   *Evolutionary Biology of Aging*. New York: Oxford University Press.
Rose, M., and B. Charlesworth
  1980   A test of evolutionary theories of senescence. *Nature* 287:141-142.
  1981   Genetics of life-history in *Drosophila melanogaster*. I. Sib analysis of adult females.
          Genetics 97:173-185.
Rose, M.R., and P.M. Service
  1985   Evolution of aging. *Review of Biological Research in Aging* 2:85-98.
Rose, M.R., P.M. Service, and E.W. Hutchinson
  1987   Three approaches to constraints in life-history evolution. In V. Loescheke, ed., *Genetic
          Constraints on Adaptive Evolution*. Berlin: Springer-Verlag.

Service, P.M., and M.R. Rose
   1985   Genetic covariation among life-history components: The effect of novel environments. *Evolution* 39:943-945.
Service, P.M., E.W. Hutchinson, and M.R. Rose
   1988   Multiple genetic mechanisms for the evolution of senescence in *Drosophila melanogaster. Evolution* 42:708-716.
Stearns, S.C.
   1992   *The Evolution of Life Histories.* London: Oxford University Press.
Tatar, M., D.E.L. Promislow, A.A. Khazaeli, and J.W. Curtsinger
   1996   Age-specific patterns of genetic variance in *Drosophila melanogaster.* II. Fecundity and its genetic covariance with age-specific mortality. *Genetics* 143:849-858.
Wattiaux, J.M.
   1968a Cumulative parental effects in *Drosophila subobscura. Evolution* 22:406-421.
   1968b Parental age effects in *Drosophila pseudoobscura. Experimental Gerontology* 3:55-61.
Williams, G.C.
   1957   Pleiotropy, natural selection, and the evolution of senescence. *Evolution* 11:398-411.

7

Identification and Mapping of Genes Determining Longevity

Thomas E. Johnson and David R. Shook

INTRODUCTION

The world of modern biology is unified by genetics. Genetic approaches have the ability to transcend species and provide cross-links between fields for several reasons. First, is the fact that all species are evolutionarily related. Thus, distinct species have similar gene function, and DNA sequence homology can be found between even distantly related species. Indeed, DNA sequence homology is used as a metric to determine evolutionary relationships among species. Second, molecular genetic manipulation changes both the genotype and the phenotype of an organism. Such manipulations represent an extremely fine-scale tool for dissection of the underlying biochemistry, physiology, anatomy, and development of an individual species. Because virtually any gene can be manipulated at will in many species, a dedicated approach can lead to an unraveling of the relationship between genotype and phenotype for almost any gene in these species. In the study of longevity, genetic approaches can play a key role because the phenotype of longevity can be studied only at the whole-organism level; nevertheless, understanding at the molecular level could lead to accurate predictions of the dynamics of life-expectancy change. The unraveling of this genotype/phenotype relationship in determining organismic life span has only just begun. Third, and most important, is the fact that genetics has the power to reveal causality by factors that are not dependent upon investigator prejudice. Unlike a biochemical approach, which by its very nature must focus on one physiological system and on even one molecule or one part of that molecule (for example), a genetic approach can survey and identify alterations in any subsystem in the species in which the genetic alteration is detected (Botstein and Mauer, 1982). It should be noted, however, that genetics alone has little hope of unraveling molecular mechanisms and that the strongest analysis results from the combined use of biochemistry, cell biology, and genetics.

I will first review the concept of genetic determination of life span and life expectancy and the concept of longevity-determining genes that we call "gerontogenes." Next, we will review relevant literature and experiments done in an effort to identify such gerontogenes. This review will focus mostly on invertebrates because few experiments in vertebrates, notably the mouse, have tried to identify gerontogenes. We will speculate as to how these gerontogenes might be identified in other species, paying careful attention to the mapping of quantitative trait loci (QTLs). This discussion will focus on identifying gerontogenes in nematodes and mice; much of the material has been selected from ongoing experiments in our own laboratory. Their subsequent extension to humans and/or the identification of gerontogenes directly in humans is the subject of another author. Finally, we will review work from our laboratory on the genetic determination of mortality rates. Many recent reviews are available on the genetics of aging (Johnson et al., 1996; Fleming and Rose, 1996; Jazwinski, 1996; Lithgow, 1996; Martin et al., 1996; Nooden and Guiamét, 1996).

CONCEPT OF GERONTOGENES

The gene is the basic unit of inheritance; typically a gene makes a protein. A gerontogene, then, makes a protein involved in aging and, more precisely, a protein involved in determining life span. Gerontogenes are defined functionally: they can be altered by mutation such that animals carrying them have a longer-than-normal life span. Vijg and Papaconstantinou (1990) suggested that gerontogenes might be separated into four distinct categories based upon their effects on life span and their evolutionary origin. "*Deleterious*" and "*pleiotropic*" genes are predicted by the evolutionary theory of aging (Charlesworth, 1980; Rose, 1991) and have evolved as a result of mutation accumulation or pleiotropic gene action, respectively. "*Aging*" genes that actively kill the organism are thought not to operate in organism senescence by evolutionary criteria; "*longevity*" genes promote survival, and presumably most genes that are fixed in an organism are of this type. "Longevity assurance gene," a term used by Sacher (1978) and by D'mello et al. (1994), means essentially the same as the term gerontogene.

METHODS FOR IDENTIFYING GERONTOGENES

Five methods have been used to identify genes involved in aging, with variable success. These approaches mirror the approaches used to identify genes involved in other biological processes. These approaches are: (1) gene association, (2) selective breeding, (3) quantitative trait locus (QTL) mapping, (4) induc-

TABLE 7-1 Approaches Used to Identify Gerontogenes

Allelic association
Mapping quantitative trait loci
Selective breeding
Induction of new mutations
Construction of transgenic stocks

tion of new mutations, and (5) construction of transgenic stocks (Table 7-1). The first three approaches use genetic variation latent in the species studied. In the first approach, these genes are studied as found; this is the only approach useful for studying genes in humans because of constraints inherent in human studies. The second approach involves selective breeding using the phenotype [or more recently the genotype, as in marker-assisted selection (Tanksley, 1993)] of interest to establish a strain in which genes leading to the desired phenotypic alterations (in this case increased longevity) have been differentially accumulated in one line as compared with another. Selected lines differing in traits of interest have been used by humans since the beginning of the agricultural era. The third approach, QTL mapping, is a method for separating the overall polygenic effects of a selected line, for example, into individual components, providing estimated map positions and effect sizes for each QTL (Tanksley, 1993). Approaches 4 and 5 differ from the former two approaches in that they do not rely on preexisting genetic variation and instead involve the creation of new mutations that then become the object of study. Approach 4 involves the identification of mutants induced by mutagens; these mutants are identified solely on the basis of their effect on the phenotype of interest—i.e., longevity. The last approach targets genes of interest to test a specific hypothesis and to determine whether that gene is actually causally involved in aging.

Gene Association

In humans and in other vertebrates the length of the life span and other problems (ethical, technical, and budgetary) have prevented the analysis of longevity by methods other than the study of naturally occurring variation. Studies of human longevity genes have involved either the identification of syndromes leading to reduced life expectancy that in many cases are mimics of the aging process (Martin, 1978; Brown, 1987; Van Broeckhoven, 1995; Yu et al., 1996) or on gene association (Schächter et al., 1994; Takata et al., 1987). The former approach involves the identification of genetic diseases of potential relevance to aging, while the latter has most often involved the study of candidate genes for association between allelic variants in that candidate and life expectancy. In mice, a few studies have attempted to go beyond the use of candidate genes by using genetic markers spanning the whole genome (Gelman et al., 1988; Puel et al., 1995). These studies are difficult both because of problems with maintaining strains of mice in a "clean" environment uncontaminated with pathogens for their entire life span and because of statistical problems in conducting whole-genome scans. Thus, most associations that have been discovered to date are of doubtful significance. [See Lander and Kruglyak (1995) for a discussion of the statistical problems associated with whole-genome scans and see the section on QTL mapping for a more complete description of this approach.]

Selective Breeding

In this approach the breeder chooses animals showing the desired character-istics and mates them; the same breeding scheme is followed for successive generations of their offspring, which leads eventually to an alteration in the trait being assessed or "selected for." This method can be as simple as "mate the best with the best and hope for the best" or can involve very sophisticated strategies wherein phenotype assessment is based on a variety of test matings and progeny testing (Falconer, 1989). Selective breeding has been conducted in *Drosophila*, selecting either on age of reproduction (Luckinbill et al., 1984; Rose, 1984; Partridge and Fowler, 1992) or directly on life expectancy (Zwaan et al., 1995). Most selection studies have identified a negative interaction between longevity and reproductive effort.

QTL Mapping

Overview

When many genes are coordinately involved in the specification of a genetic trait, we can refer to the individual genes contributing to the overall phenotype as QTLs (Table 7-2). We intend to first describe how QTLs are "mapped" (local-ized to specific regions of the genome). Next we will address some issues in evolutionary theory and demography to which QTL mapping may be relevant. We will then describe our work on QTL mapping of life-history traits in the nematode *Caenorhabditis elegans* and some early work on mapping QTLs in-volved in specifying adult demographic characters. Finally, we will speculate as to how these studies may be extended to other demographic parameters not yet assessed in *C. elegans* or other species. Refer to Table 7-2 for definitions; for more background on QTL mapping see Tanksley (1993).

The Basis of QTL Mapping

All genetic mapping is based on the fact that genetic loci, whether QTLs or genetic markers, close together on the chromosome remain together (cosegregate) in crosses, except where recombination occurs. Genes that are close are said to

TABLE 7-2 A Lexicon of QTL Terminology

Term	Definition
Allele	A variant of a gene or genetic marker
Effect size	The amount of genetic variation explained by a particular QTL
Genetic marker	An easily-assessed DNA segment with a known genetic map position and many alleles. It should have no effect on the phenotype
Interval mapping	A method for QTL mapping in which one takes into account genotype information from markers on either side of the region being studied; this allows the detection of recombination events within the interval that can be used to position the QTL within the interval
Quantitative trait	A trait whose phenotypic variation is continuous (rather than discrete) and is determined by the segregation of many genes or QTLs
QTL	Quantitative trait locus; one of a suite of genes specifying any particular phenotype
QTL mapping	The process of determining probable sites and probable effect sizes of a QTL or QTLs
RI	Recombinant inbred; an inbred strain generated by 20 generations of sibling mating from the F_2 of two inbred strains or by 10 generations of self-fertilization (hermaphroditic species)
SDP	Strain distribution pattern; the pattern of alleles at a locus across a series of RI strains derived from crosses between the same initial inbred parents

be genetically linked. For 75 years, single-gene traits have been "mapped" by taking advantage of such cosegregation and the fact that the frequency of recombination events that separate linked genes is proportional to the physical distance between genes on the chromosome. The mapping of quantitative traits, especially demographic traits, is more difficult because these traits are influenced by more than one gene. However, the basis of QTL mapping has been apparent for some time. If a QTL for mean life span, for example, is genetically close (linked) to a genetic marker, then, on average, progeny that carry the marker allele from the "low" parent will have a shorter life span than progeny carrying the marker allele from the "high" parent. The Human Genome Project has provided "dense" genetic maps of the human and mouse with highly polymorphic marker loci; as a result, the mapping of QTLs over practically the entire human genome has become possible. Nevertheless, QTL mapping in humans is difficult and involves large population sizes. Several other animal model systems are also under intense study and are of more immediate relevance for our discussion. These include other mammalian models, particularly the mouse and rat, and invertebrate models such as fruit flies and the nematode *C. elegans*.

Mapping of QTLs involves (1) assaying the phenotype of interest in each offspring, (2) characterizing the pattern of genetic markers in each offspring, and (3) a statistical assessment of whether any part of the phenotypic variation is significantly associated with any marker. For example, a marker allele tightly linked to a QTL involved with the determination of longevity will be overrepresented in the most long-lived individuals in a population in which alleles of this QTL are segregating. Exactly this method was used by Ebert et al. (1993) in mapping genes that contributed to longevity in *C. elegans*. Similarly, the shortest-lived individuals in the population will carry a higher proportion of the marker allele associated with the short-life-span allele of the QTL. Of course, this mapping assumes a significant genetic component to the determination of life span in the particular population being studied.

The degree of correlation between the marker and the phenotype is based on two things: the effect size of the QTL and the genetic distance between the QTL and the marker. If the QTL is close to the marker, then detection and mapping of the QTL can be performed easily and accurately. If the QTL is far from the marker gene, then recombination between marker and QTL will lead to a lower frequency of association, resulting in a lower observed "effect size" attributed to the QTL linked to that marker. This problem can be partially alleviated by using allelic information from markers on both sides of the QTL; this results in the determination of linkage using an "interval-mapping approach." Interval mapping is more mathematically sophisticated and more biologically precise because algorithms have been developed that can account for recombination events in the interval. Interval mapping uses these detected recombination events to suggest most probable locations and effect sizes for the QTL within the interval. Interval mapping can be done by using either regression approaches (Haley and Knott, 1992) or maximum-likelihood procedures, such as those developed by Lander and Botstein (1989) or by Zeng (1994). The interval-mapping procedure involves fitting an additive model for a putative QTL, Q, at a series of positions in the interval, d, between two markers A and B.

Induced Mutants

In this approach, genomes are mutagenized, and the offspring are subsequently screened for phenotypic alterations. This is the most powerful approach in that any gene in the genome can potentially be identified, even those that are essentially fixed in natural populations. A second major advantage of this approach is that it can reveal genes that were not logical candidates. This element of surprise and lack of being tied in with specific hypotheses makes mutant induction the method of choice. This approach has the major disadvantage of being time consuming and expensive and consequently unpopular in the study of aging and senescence. Only in *Neurospora* (Munkres and Furtek, 1984), in the nematode (Klass, 1983; Duhon et al., 1996), and in yeast (Kennedy et al., 1995) has the approach really been successfully employed. However, there is at least one reported example of an increased-longevity mutant in *Drosophila* (Maynard Smith, 1958).

Identification of Gerontogenes in Yeast

D'Mello et al. (1994) isolated the *LAG1* gerontogene based on differential times of expression by screening gene libraries for young-expressed genes and late-expressed genes. *LAG1* appears to be a 411-amino acid protein that is predicted to be an integral membrane protein. Further analysis of *LAG1* revealed that both null mutants, as well as dominant, C-terminal-deletion mutants in *LAG1*, lead to extension of yeast life span.

Kennedy et al. (1995) selected for gerontogene mutants by using prolonged survival under starvation conditions. Their results offer evidence that two phenotypes, extended survival under nongrowing conditions and extended replicative life span, cosegregate. Their finding that eight mutants in four genes (*UTH1-UTH4*) selected on the basis of extended vegetative survival under nongrowing conditions also had increased replicative life spans argues for considerable coordinate control. One gene was studied in detail and shown to be a mutation in *SIR4*, a gene involved in transcriptional silencing. A number of other intriguing studies were described, including a requirement for *SIR3* but not for *SIR1* and evidence that a dominant negative construct of *SIR4* can extend the replicative life span.

Identification of Gerontogenes in *C. elegans*

Eight gerontogenes have been identified in nematodes, and mutants in all of those tested have increased resistance to a variety of stresses (see also Lithgow et al., 1995; Murakami and Johnson, 1996; Martin et al., 1996). (1) Klass (1983) isolated the first mutant, which we subsequently called *age-1* (Friedman and Johnson, 1988). (2) Mutants in *spe-26* show an 80 percent increase in life expectancy of the hermaphrodite (VanVoorhies, 1992). (3) Mutants in *daf-2* have consistently extended adult life expectancy under some conditions (Kenyon et al., 1993). (4) Larsen et al. (1995) demonstrated that *daf-23* mutants also have a prolonged life under some conditions, and she also demonstrated that a double mutant (*daf-12 daf-2*) has a 4-fold life extension (*daf-12* is a dauer-defective mutant, see below). (5) Wong et al. (1995) isolated a new class of mutants, and the first of these, *clk-1*, showed a longer adult life for several alleles. In a subsequent study, Lakowski and Hekimi (1996) showed that *clk-1*, *clk-2*, *clk-3*, and *gro-1* are gerontogenes as well. *rad-8* mutants have extended life at 16°C (Ishii et al., 1994), but this is mostly due to an extended developmental period, and thus *rad-8* is not a true gerontogene.

Only *age-1* was identified by screening for increased longevity. All the other mutants have defects other than the altered life expectancy. *spe-26* is a gene involved primarily in sperm activation and isolated on the basis of its male-specific sterility; *rad-8* was isolated based on its increased sensitivity to radiation; *daf-2* and *daf-23* are temperature-sensitive, dauer-constitutive mutations that cause dauer formation even in the presence of food at 25°C, *clk-1* mutants show a variety of alterations in the timing of cell division and development. In addition, the dauer-defective mutant (*daf-16*) interacts to block the effects of *daf-2*, *daf-23* as well as all of the other mutants tested (Murakami and Johnson, 1996; Kenyon et al., 1993; Larsen et al., 1995). The extended life span of these mutants was detected in a search for extended life expectancy in some cases and serendipitously in others.

Mapping Induced Mutants

The fact that genes located close together on the chromosome remain together during crosses allows the construction of genetic maps and ultimately even the identification of genes by "positional cloning." There is only one example of "mapping" a gerontogene using assessment of life expectancy as the character that is being mapped, and that is the mapping of *age-1* (Friedman and Johnson, 1988; Johnson et al., 1993). More recent studies have relied on the mapping of other traits associated with the gerontogene mutant, such as resistance to stress (Duhon et al., 1996). Problems with directly mapping life expectancy include the lengthy period of time it takes to assess the phenotype and the influence of other genes and environmental effects, such that the mapping can become very problematic. Additional attempts to localize QTLs specifying longevity are described below.

Transgenic Strategies

A final approach for identifying gerontogenes has been successful in only a few instances. This involves the construction of transgenic lines carrying additional copies or altered copies of the genes of interest. Chen et al. (1990) and Sun et al. (1994) used a candidate-gene approach in that they identified genes probably involved in the determination of replicative life span based not on direct screens for longevity but on other evidence. They subsequently showed that disruption of either of two yeast candidate genes, *RAS1* or *RAS2* alters the replicative life span. *RAS1* deletions prolong replicative life about 40 percent, while *RAS2* deletions shorten it. Overexpression of *RAS2* led to an increased longevity, but overexpression of *RAS1* had no effect.

In two cases this approach has been used in *Drosophila*: with EF-1α (a protein elongation factor; Shepherd et al., 1989) and superoxide dismutase/catalase, double transgenics, which both help to detoxify free radicals (Orr and Sohal, 1994). Both studies reported life extension. Subsequent studies on additional EF-1α transgenics (Shikama et al., 1994) failed to replicate the earlier findings. Although the studies on the superoxide dismutase/catalase double mutants are not without problems, they were widely replicated initially and are consistent with a large additional body of evidence showing that reactive oxidant species are involved in many aspects of aging and senescence.

REVIEW OF QTL MAPPING OF LONGEVITY

The most extensive genetic analysis of longevity ever conducted in a mammal was that of Gelman et al. (1988), who used the B × D (C57BL/6J × DBA/2J) series of recombinant inbred strains of mice to identify QTLs for life expectancy. They found six significant associations; however, the statistical significance of these findings is in some doubt because their stringency levels were not sufficiently high (Lander and Kruglyak, 1995); however, see Yunis and Salazar (1993). Lines of mice that have been selected for different immune response have quite different life expectancies (Covelli et al., 1989). Unfortunately, most of the variance between the lines was for decreased life span, since the lines selected for decreased immune function were very short lived. Puel et al. (1995) mapped QTLs that were associated with the different immune response and found that five QTLs explained much of the variance in immune response in the F_2 population but have no data on life expectancy.

Besides our work described below and those in mice just described, we are aware of only three other studies mapping or attempting to find the genes specifying longevity in animals. Ebert et al. (1993) used F_2 populations of *C. elegans* to localize QTLs for longevity by genotyping the longest-lived members of the populations. They were not able to distinguish various aspects of life history, because these aspects were not studied independent of survival—but they were able to apply a novel approach to studying increased longevity. Using two different approaches, they found QTLs for increased survival on chromosomes II and IV and the X chromosome. These QTLs are not the same as those found by Shook et al. (1996, see below). Ebert et al. (1996) also positioned a QTL for H_2O_2-resistance to a site on chromosome V (*stP6*) near the site previously identified that is involved in longevity determination.

In *Drosophila*, Fleming et al. (1993) used two-dimensional gel electrophoresis in a direct approach to identifying the proteins leading to long life in selected lines. These strategies identified genetic regions or gene products that were associated with increased survival, but neither study critically examined life-history traits other than survival, and neither could examine more sophisticated interactions among loci. Luckinbill et al. (1988) showed that most of the effect of life extension in their selected *Drosophila* lines mapped to chromosome 3 with chromosome 2 negatively affecting life span. The findings were corroborated by Arking et al. (1993) on an independent population originally selected at the same time under the same conditions. Several laboratories are currently attempting to generate QTL maps for *Drosophila* longevity, and several studies are under way in mice.

Use of Recombinant Inbred Strains (RIs) in Mapping QTLs for Longevity and Other Life-History Traits

C. elegans, a nematode worm, is a prime candidate for QTL mapping and the study of coadapted gene complexes, since it is normally inbreeding but can also out-cross. Shook et al. (1996, unpublished work) used QTL mapping strategies to localize genetic regions influencing life-history traits in *C. elegans*. These investigators mapped QTLs for mean and maximum survival, mean and maximum fertility, temperature-sensitive fertility, and internal hatching of progeny (bagging). QTLs for mean life span were identified on linkage groups (LGs) II, IV, and the X chromosome, and QTLs for fertility were identified on LGs II, III, and IV. The QTLs for mean life span accounted for 23 percent of observed phenotypic variance (comparable to total genetic variance of 26 percent). The loci for mean fertility accounted for 46 percent of the observed phenotypic variance (genetic component of variance: 52 percent). Additional QTLs for temperature-sensitive fertility (LGs II and V) and internal hatching (LG IV) were also mapped in these crosses.

The two sets of studies (Shook et al., 1996; Ebert et al., 1993) did not replicate each other. Essentially none of the markers associated in the two studies were the same. In the only marker associated in both studies (*spP5* on chromosome V), the association was in the opposite direction in the two studies. There were many differences between the two studies in conduction of the experiments, and the reasons for the lack of replication are unclear. RI-based QTL mapping allows an analysis of the effects of individual genes on different traits and of interactions among genes in specifying individual traits not possible in F_2 populations. We found several instances where genes do not act independently and instead interact to determine mean life span and mean fertility. Negatively correlated effects between mean life expectancy and internal hatching were found linked to the *stP5* genetic marker.

These QTLs were mapped using RI strains described previously (Johnson and Wood, 1982; Johnson, 1987; Brooks and Johnson, 1991). The study was facilitated by a polymerase-chain-reaction method for marker assessment (Williams et al., 1992) based on the assessment of a repeated genetic sequence element (Tc1) found with different frequencies in the two wild-type parental strains that were crossed to generate the RIs; the Bergerac strain has several hundred Tc1s not found in the N2 strain. The use of RIs has a tremendous advantage for the study of demographic parameters—stable unchanging genotypes that can be examined for multiple distinct phenotypes over a period of months or years. In addition to our analysis of demographic parameters, studies on behavior and sensitivity to anesthetic action in these strains are already under way. This study provides a first step toward determining the particular genes involved in specifying life-history traits and in elucidating the mechanisms underlying the interrelationships among these traits. This type of study will contribute to our understanding of the coordinated evolution of life-history traits and the genetic constraints that are placed on evolution.

TABLE 7-3 Basic Theoretical Questions to Be Addressed

Number of genes specifying various aspects of the life course
Location of genes specifying various aspects of the life course
Size of effects specified by each gene
Interactions between genes
Effects of individual genes on more than one aspect of the life course
Identification of and characterization of genes involved in these events

Issues in Evolutionary Theory and in Demography That Can Be Addressed by QTL Mapping

Gene interactions have been postulated to be important in many aspects of evolution and speciation. It is a general assumption in much evolutionary theory that most genes affect many different traits (pleiotropy). Antagonistic pleiotropy has been suggested as a mechanism for maintaining genetic variation and as a mechanism for the evolution of genes that limit life span, trading off survival with some early fitness trait.

In summary, the value of QTL mapping is that it allows the assessment of effects resulting from individual loci rather than the genome as a whole. More specifically, there are a number of questions that QTL mapping can answer (Table 7-3). The genes, their location, and the amount of genetic variation explained by each can be determined by QTL mapping. Most importantly, it is possible to gain some insight into the interactions between and among these QTLs in specifying their respective phenotypes. It is also possible to identify QTLs that are pleiotropic in their action, affecting more than one stage or aspect of life history or demography.

CLONING THE GENES

There is an "ultimate question" which one hopes to eventually answer in these mapping studies: "What is the nature of the genes responsible for these life extensions?" This same ultimate question was asked almost 50 years ago when quantitative genetics and Mendelian genetics made their great rapprochement. It is still not clear if the "mutations" identified and used to such good measure by *Drosophila* and nematode geneticists are stronger alleles of the same genes underlying quantitative traits. The cloning of the gerontogenes themselves should allow us to answer this question directly.

The only successful cloning of gerontogenes based primarily on their extended survival has been in yeast. These studies have focused on the limited proliferative life span of individual yeast cells (Jazwinski, 1996), as well as on the limited length of viability of these cells in stationary phase (Kennedy et al., 1995). The mutants (*UTH1-UTH4*) isolated by Kennedy et al. (1995) had increased life expectancy in stationary culture. One mutant gene was cloned by complementation of its associated sterility phenotype and shown to be a mutation in *SIR4*, a gene involved in transcriptional silencing.

Positional Cloning of Induced Mutants

Only in the nematode has positional cloning been successfully used to identify a gerontogene. The *spe-26* gerontogene was cloned last year and encodes an actin-associated protein (Varkey et al., 1995). How life extension results from the altered gene is not obvious, although increased stress resistance of *spe-26* has been observed for both temperature (Lithgow et al., 1995) and ultraviolet light (Murakami and Johnson, 1996). Our laboratory has been attempting to clone *age-1* for several years, and that effort resulted in a narrow map assignment to the center of chromosome II (Johnson et al., 1993). Recently, it was proposed that *daf-23* and *age-1* are the same gene based on noncomplementation for an unusual phenotype, dauer formation at 27°C (Malone et al., 1996) and the fact that *daf-23* also maps to the center of chromosome II. We have confirmed these results and shown noncomplementation between *age-1* and *daf-23* alleles for several other traits as well. *daf-23* has been recently cloned and shown to have homology to the phosphatidylinositol 3-kinase family (Morris et al., 1996) and thus could play a role in transducing signals of environmental stress to the worm genome. No mutations previously assigned to the *age-1* gene have been found, as yet, in the *daf-23* sequence, leaving open the definitive answer whether *daf-23* and *age-1* are the same gene.

Positional Cloning of QTLs

Unfortunately, cloning QTLs specifying gerontogenes will be even more problematic than cloning induced mutants leading to increased life span. For positional-cloning approaches to work, the site of the mutation must be localized to a small area of the genome. Unlike a single-gene mutant, in which a single recombination event can indicate whether the mutant is to the left or right of the recombination site, a QTL cannot be localized based on the results of any single recombinant chromosome. Instead, QTLs must be localized by making congenic strains carrying the QTL region and subsequent analysis of inbred strains carrying these regions. This approach can lead to localizing the region in which the QTL could be located to as small a region as desired but could be quite expensive; perhaps as much as $100,000 could be spent localizing the QTL to a region less than 1 map unit (2.1 Mb) in size, if these experiments are done in mice. This region may contain 100 or more genes.

An approach successfully used in mice in my laboratory is to identify a QTL based on the effect of an additional gene added to the genome by transgenic manipulations. Both in the nematode (Murakami and Johnson, unpublished work) and in the mouse (Rikke et al., unpublished work), the construction of transgenic animals carrying additional DNA, derived from yeast artificial chromosomes (YACs) has been successfully used to show that a QTL is carried in a candidate region. Subsequent cloning of the genes involved in life expectancy and drug sensitivity, respectively, are still under way.

GENETICS OF AGE-SPECIFIC MORTALITY IN *C. ELEGANS*

Mortality increases with chronological age in *C. elegans* just as in many other species. The standard laboratory wild-type strain, N2, shows age-specific mortality rates (the fraction of worms that die in a 24-hour period) that are highly correlated with age. The normal mortality doubling time is about 4-6 days (Johnson, 1987 and 1990; Brooks et al., 1994).

Mortality of Gerontogene Mutants

The mortality doubling time of strains carrying mutations in *age-1* (a gene that can be mutated to increase mean life span 70 percent) has been increased about 3-fold, and this increase is recessive to the normal allele in that individuals with one normal and one mutant allele have mortality doubling times no different from wild type (Johnson, 1990). Males have shorter life spans and a more rapid rate of mortality increase than hermaphrodites (Johnson, 1990). Males carrying *age-1* mutations also show a lengthening of life and a slowing of the acceleration rate of mortality, although not as much as hermaphrodites, and *age-1* mutant males still have significantly shorter life spans than do hermaphrodites of the same genotype. A major limitation of almost all studies on age-specific mortality rate is the lack of analysis of large populations of nematodes. Only small numbers (200) of worms have been studied, and these results may be modified after larger populations are analyzed.

RI Strains

Both long-lived mutants and RI strains also have been analyzed to see how age-specific mortality rate is altered. Long-lived RI strains, some having mean and maximum life spans up to 70 percent longer than wild type, still showed exponential rates of increase of mortality with chronological age, as did both wild-type progenitor strains (Johnson, 1987). Longer life results from a slowing of the characteristic increase in mortality rate that had been thought typical of aging populations in most, if not all, species. The lengths of the developmental and reproductive period were unrelated to increased life span but instead were under independent genetic control. Lengthened life resulted entirely from an increase in postreproductive life span. General motor activity decayed linearly with chronological age in all genotypes. The loss of general motor activity was both correlated with and a predictor of life expectancy, suggesting that both share at least one common, rate-determining component (Johnson, 1987).

Mortality of Pure Strains

Because increased mean life expectancy could result from lower initial mortality rate, or from a slower rate of increase in mortality (or to alterations in both), we asked how these components varied in the various RI strains. The slopes of the age-specific mortality rates vary among the RI strains (Johnson, 1987; Brooks et al., 1994). The longest-lived strain had a consistent increase in both mean and maximum life span and a highly significant, 1.5-fold decrease in the rate of change of age-specific mortality rate. Another short-lived strain had a significant increase in the rate of change of age-specific mortality rate. No significant change in initial vulnerability was seen for either (Johnson, 1987).

Mortality of Quartiles, Clustered by Life Expectancy

When the combined survival data from these 79 RIs were assessed (Brooks et al., 1994), we found mortality kinetics of the combined population to be similar to that observed in the medfly (Carey et al., 1992) and in *Drosophila* (Curtsinger et al., 1992). In other words, the survival curve had a long tail, and mortality rates approached 5 percent daily mortality by 17 days of age and remained at that level for several weeks. The experiment was replicated with essentially the same observations. In contrast, when we then divided the set of RIs into quartiles based on life expectancy (Brooks et al., 1994), we observed quite distinct mean survival times and survival curves for each quartile. Not surprisingly, each had significantly different life expectancies ($p < .001$) from the other. Now, within each quartile, age-specific mortality rate increased almost exponentially with chronological age until considerably later in life. The differences among quartiles was modeled using a Gompertz model and was due almost entirely to differences in the rate of increase of the exponent with essentially no significant difference in initial mortality rate. There still was evidence of a linear period late in life when mortality rates stopped increasing exponentially with increasing age, as demonstrated by a model-comparison approach (Brooks et al., 1994). However, the detailed interpretation of the exact kinetics await analyses of larger populations.

Survival and mortality kinetics of the combined RI populations closely approximate that previously observed by Carey et al. (1992) and Curtsinger et al. (1992). We also observed periods of several weeks at the end of life when the mortality rate did not increase with chronological age. We conclude that heterogeneity within populations (genetic or environmental) will lead to a deceleration of the age-specific mortality curve as soon as the most at-risk population has expired. Exploration of the effects of this genetic heterogeneity on age-specific mortalities is a primary focus of our future studies in which we characterize and genetically map QTLs specifying various aspects of the demography of mortality, and it is also being explored by Curtsinger and his colleagues.

Although it is clear that genetic and phenotypic heterogeneity can produce mortality deceleration, there may also be some inherent slowing of mortality with age. Even when both environment and genotype have been kept constant, variability in life span or in other quantitative variables are still observed (Brooks et al., 1994). In this study, variability was a function of average life span, as shown by the constancy of the coefficient of variation, consistent with the hypothesis that those inbred populations that die late in life do not fundamentally differ from those that die early. The biphasic mortality rate seen in the genetically heterogeneous populations of nematodes results from the genetic heterogeneity in the population. Genetic heterogeneity could explain similar mortality kinetics in human populations (Vaupel et al., 1979) in which, beyond 85 years, the mortality rate stops increasing exponentially and becomes constant, or actually decreases. Genetic heterogeneity could play a large role in the long period of "flat" mortality rate increases separated by Carey et al. (1992).

Mortality Rates in Large Populations

The relationship between age-specific mortality rate and chronological age on a population of 180,000 worms has been modeled using an exponential function of chronological age (Brooks et al., 1994). Vaupel et al. (1994) used a two-stage Gompertz model and showed that two curves (each with exponential rates of increase) provided a significantly better fit. The break in the curves occurred at day 8, about the time the wild type stops reproducing. Clearly the "best" model for mortality in large populations of *C. elegans* does not fit a two-parameter Gompertz model.

CONCLUSIONS

It is clear that gerontogenes exist. Identification of these genes has been achieved in lower eukaryotes and in one metazoan, *C. elegans*. The most powerful approach, inducing single-gene mutants, may be too expensive to ever be pursued in mammals. QTL mapping offers a useful alternative to localizing genes, but cloning of the genes underlying these QTLs will be problematic. Mortality alterations that result from changes in these genes can be studied, and results from the Johnson laboratory suggest that much of the flattening of mortality rates at later ages in humans could result from genetic heterogeneity among individuals. Clearly such heterogeneity leads to an extended period of nonexponentially increases in age-specific mortality at the end of life.

REFERENCES

Arking, R., S.P. Dudas, and G.T. Baker III
  1993   Genetic and environmental factors regulating the expression of an extended longevity phenotype in a long-lived strain of *Drosophila*. *Genetica* 91:127-142.
Botstein, D., and R. Mauer
  1982   Genetic approaches to the analysis of microbial development. *Annual Review of Genetics* 16:61-83.
Brooks, A., and T.E. Johnson
  1991   Genetic specification of life span and self-fertility in recombinant-inbred strains of *Caenorhabditis elegans*. *Heredity* 67:19-28.

Brooks, A., G.J. Lithgow, and T.E. Johnson
1994   Mortality rates in a genetically heterogeneous population of *Caenorhabditis elegans*. *Science* 263:668-671.

Brown, W.T.
1987   Genetic aspects of aging in humans. *Review of Biological Research in Aging* 3:77-91.

Carey, J.R., P. Liedo, D. Orozco, and J.W. Vaupel
1992   Slowing of mortality rates at older ages in large medfly cohorts. *Science* 258:457-461.

Charlesworth, B.
1980   *Evolution in Age-Structured Populations*. London: Cambridge University Press.

Chen, J.B., J. Sun, and S.M. Jazwinski
1990   Prolongation of the yeast life span by the v-HA-RAS oncogene. *Molecular Microbiology* 4:2081-2086.

Covelli, V., D. Mouton, V. Di Majo, Y. Bouthillier, C. Bangrazi, J.-C. Mevel, S. Rebessi, G. Doria, and G. Biozzi
1989   Inheritance of immune responsiveness, life span, and disease incidence in interline crosses of mice selected for high or low multispecific antibody production. *Journal of Immunology* 142:1224-1234.

Curtsinger, J.W., H.H. Fukui, D.R. Townsend, and J.W. Vaupel
1992   Demography of genotypes: Failure of the limited life-span paradigm in *Drosophila melanogaster*. *Science* 258:461-463.

D'mello, N.P., A.M. Childress, D.S. Franklin, S.P. Kale, C. Pinswasdi, and S.M. Jazwinski
1994   Cloning and characterization of *LAG1*, a longevity-assurance gene in yeast. *Journal of Biological Chemistry* 269:15451-15459.

Duhon, S.A., S. Murakami, and T.E. Johnson
1996   Direct isolation of longevity mutants in the nematode *Caenorhabditis elegans*. *Developmental Genetics* 18:144-153.

Ebert, R.H., V.A. Cherkasova, R.A. Dennis, J.H. Wu, S. Ruggles, T.E. Perrin, and R.J.S. Reis
1993   Longevity-determining genes in *Caenorhabditis elegans*: Chromosomal mapping of multiple noninteractive loci. *Genetics* 135:1003-1010.

Ebert, R.H., M.A. Shammas, B.H. Sohal, R.S. Sohal, N.K. Egilmez, S. Ruggles, and R.J.S. Reis
1996   Defining genes that govern longevity in *Caenorhabditis elegans*. *Developmental Genetics* 18:131-143.

Falconer, D.S.
1989   *Introduction to Quantitative Genetics*, 2nd ed. London: Longman.

Fleming, J.E., and M.R. Rose
1996   Genetics of aging in *Drosophila*. Pp. 74-93 in J.W. Rowe and E.L. Schneider, eds., *Handbook of the Biology of Aging*, 4th ed. New York: Academic Press.

Fleming, J.E., G.S. Spicer, R.C. Garrison, and M.R. Rose
1993   Two-dimensional protein electrophoretic analysis of postponed aging in *Drosophila*. *Genetica* 91:183-195.

Friedman, D.B., and T.E. Johnson
1988   A mutation in the *age-1* gene in *Caenorhabditis elegans* lengthens life and reduces hermaphrodite fertility. *Genetics* 118:75-86.

Gelman, R., A. Watson, R. Bronson, and E. Yunis
1988   Murine chromosomal regions correlated with longevity. *Genetics* 118:693-704.

Haley, C.S., and S.A. Knott
1992   A simple regression methods for mapping quantitative trait loci in line crosses using flanking markers. *Heredity* 69:315-324.

Ishii, N., N. Suzuki, P.S. Hartman, and K. Suzuki
1994   The effects of temperature on the longevity of a radiation-sensitive mutant *rad-8* of the nematode *Caenorhabditis elegans*. *Journal of Gerontology and Biological Science*, 49:B117-B120.

Jazwinski, S.M.
   1996   Longevity-assurance genes and mitochondrial DNA alterations: Yeast and filamentous
          fungi. Pp. 39-54 in J.W. Rowe and E.L. Schneider, eds., *Handbook of the Biology of
          Aging*, 4th ed. New York: Academic Press.
Johnson, T.E.
   1987   Aging can be genetically dissected into component processes using long-lived lines of
          Caenorhabditis elegans. *Proceedings of the National Academy of Sciences U.S.A.*
          84:3777-3781.
   1990   The increased life span of *age-1* mutants in *Caenorhabditis elegans* results from lowering
          the Gompertz rate of aging. *Science* 249:908-912.
Johnson, T.E., G.J. Lithgow, S. Murakami, S.A. Duhon, and D.R. Shook
   1996   Genetics of aging and longevity in lower organisms. Pp. 1-17 in N. Holbrook, G.R.
          Martin, and R.A. Lockshin, eds., *Cellular Aging and Cell Death*. New York: John Wiley
          and Sons.
Johnson, T.E., P.M. Tedesco, and G.J. Lithgow
   1993   Comparing mutants, selective breeding, and transgenics in the dissection of aging pro-
          cesses of *Caenorhabditis elegans*. *Genetica* 91:65-77.
Johnson, T.E., and W.B. Wood
   1982   Genetic analysis of the life-span of *Caenorhabditis elegans*. *Proceedings of the National
          Academy of Sciences U.S.A.* 79:6603-6607.
Kennedy, B.K., N.R. Austriaco, Jr., J. Zhang, and L. Guarante
   1995   Mutation in the silencing gene *SIR4* can delay aging in *C. cerevisiae*. *Cell* 80:485-496.
Kenyon, C., J. Chang, E. Gensch, A. Rudner, and R. Tabtiang
   1993   A *C. elegans* mutant that lives twice as long as wild type. *Nature* 366:461-464.
Klass, M.R.
   1983   A method for the isolation of longevity mutants in the nematode *Caenorhabditis elegans*
          and initial results. *Mechanisms of Ageing and Development* 22:279-286.
Lakowski, B., and S. Hekimi
   1996   Determination of life-span in *Caenorhabditis elegans* by four clock genes. *Nature Genet-
          ics* 272:1010-1013.
Lander, E.S., and D. Botstein
   1989   Mapping Mendelian factors underlying quantitative traits using RFLP linkage maps. *Ge-
          netics* 121:185-99.
Lander, E.S., and L. Kruglyak
   1995   Genetic dissection of complex traits: Guidelines for interpreting and reporting linkage
          results. *Nature Genetics* 11:241-247.
Larsen, P.L., P.S. Albert, and D.L. Riddle
   1995   Genes that regulate both development and longevity in *Caenorhabditis elegans*. *Genetics*
          139:1567-1583.
Lithgow, G.J.
   1996   The molecular genetics of *Caenorhabditis elegans* aging. Pp. 55-73 in J.W. Rowe and
          E.L. Schneider, eds., *Handbook of the Biology of Aging*, 4th ed. New York: Academic
          Press.
Lithgow, G.J., T.M. White, S. Melov, and T.E. Johnson
   1995   Thermotolerance and extended life-span conferred by single-gene mutations and induced
          by thermal stress. *Proceedings of the National Academy of Sciences U.S.A.* 92:7540-
          7544.
Luckinbill, L.S., R. Arking, M.J. Clare, W.C. Cirocco, and S.A. Muck
   1984   Selection for delayed senescence in *Drosophila melanogaster*. *Evolution* 38:996-1003.
Luckinbill, L.S., J.L. Graves, A.H. Reed, and S. Koetsawang
   1988   Localizing genes that defer senescence in *Drosophila melanogaster*. *Heredity* 60: 367-
          374.

Malone, E.A., T. Inoue, and J.H. Thomas
1996   Analysis of the roles of *daf-28* and *age-1* in regulating *Caenorhabditis elegans* dauer formation. *Genetics* 143:1193-1205.
Martin, G.M.
1978   Genetic syndromes in man with potential relevance to the pathobiology of aging. Pp. 5-39 in D. Bergsma and D.E. Harrison, eds., *Genetic Effects on Aging*. The National Foundation March of Dimes Birth Defects: Original Article series Vol. 15. New York: Alan R. Liss.
Martin, G.M., S.N. Austad, and T.E. Johnson
1996   Genetic analysis of aging: Role of oxidative damage and environmental stresses. *Nature Genetics* 13:25-34.
Maynard Smith, J.
1958   The effects of temperature and of egg-laying on the longevity of *Drosophila subobscura*. *Journal of Experimental Biology* 35:832-842.
Morris, J.Z., H.A. Tissenbaum, and G. Ruvkun
1996   A phosphatidylinositol-3-OH kinase family member regulating longevity and diapause in *Caenorhabditis elegans*. *Nature* 382:536-539.
Munkres, K.D., and C.A. Furtek
1984   Selection of conidial longevity mutants of *Neurospora crassa*, *Mechanisms of Ageing and Development* 25:47-62.
Murakami, S., and T.E. Johnson
1996   A genetic pathway conferring life extension and resistance to UV stress in *Caenorhabditis elegans*. *Genetics* 143:1207-1218.
Nooden, L.D., and J.J. Guiamét
1996   Genetic control of senescence and aging in plants. Pp. 94-118 in J.W. Rowe and E.L. Schneider, eds., *Handbook of the Biology of Aging*, 4th ed. New York: Academic Press.
Orr, W.C., and R.S. Sohal
1994   Extension of life-span by overexpression of superoxide dismutase and catalase in *Drosophila melanogaster*. *Science* 263:1128-1130.
Partridge, L., and K. Fowler
1992   Direct and correlated responses to selection on age at reproduction in *Drosophila melanogaster*. *Evolution* 46:76-91.
Puel, A., P.C. Groot, M.G. Lathrop, P. Demant, and D. Mouton
1995   Mapping of genes controlling quantitative antibody production in Biozzi mice. *Journal of Immunology* 154:5799-5805.
Rose, M.R.
1984   Laboratory evolution of postponed senescence in *Drosophila melanogaster*. *Evolution* 38:1004-1010.
1991   *Evolutionary Biology of Aging*. New York: Oxford University Press.
Sacher, G.A.
1978   Evolution of longevity and survival characteristics in mammals. Pp. 151-168 in E.L. Schneider, ed., *The Genetics of Aging*. New York: Plenum Press.
Schächter, F., L. Faure-Delanef, F, Guénot, H. Rouger, P. Froguel, L. Lesueur-Ginot, and D. Cohen
1994   Genetic associations with human longevity at the APOE and ACE loci. *Nature Genetics* 6:29-32.
Shepherd, J.C.W., U. Walldorf, P. Hug, and W. J. Gehring
1989   Fruit flies with additional expression of the elongation factor EF-1α live longer. *Proceedings of the National Academy of Sciences U.S.A.* 86:7520-7521.
Shikama, N., R. Ackermann, and C. Brack
1994   Protein synthesis elongation factor EF-1α expression and longevity in *Drosophila melanogaster*. *Proceedings of the National Academy of Sciences U.S.A.* 91:4199-4203.

Shook, D., A. Brooks, and T.E. Johnson
  1996   Mapping quantitative trait loci specifying hermaphrodite survival or self fertility in the nematode Caenorhabditis elegans. Genetics 142:801-817.

Sun, J.Y., S.P. Kale, A.M. Childress, C. Pinswasdi, and S.M. Jazwinski
  1994   Divergent roles of RAS1 and RAS2 in yeast longevity. Journal of Biological Chemistry 269(28):18638-18645.

Takata, H., M. Susuki, T. Ishii, S. Sekiguchi, and H. Iri
  1987   Influence of major histocompatability complex region genes on human longevity among Okinawan-Japanese centenarians and nonagenarians. Lancet 2:824-826.

Tanksley, S.A.
  1993   Mapping polygenes. Annual Review of Genetics 27:205-233.

Van Broeckhoven, C.
  1995   Presenilins and Alzheimer disease. Nature Genetics 11:230-232.

VanVoorhies, W.A.
  1992   Production of sperm reduces nematode lifespan. Nature 360:456-458.

Varkey, J.P., P.J. Muhlrad, A.N. Minniti, B. Do, and S. Ward
  1995   The Caenorhabditis elegans spe26 gene is necessary to form spermatids and encodes a protein similar to the actin-associated proteins kelsh and scruin. Genes and Development 9:1074-1086.

Vaupel, J.W., K.G. Manton, and E. Stallard
  1979   The impact of heterogeneity in individual frailty on the dynamics of mortality. Demography 16:439-454.

Vaupel, J.W., T.E. Johnson, and G.J. Lithgow
  1994   Rates of mortality in populations of Caenorhabditis elegans (Technical Comment). Science 266:826.

Vijg, J., and J. Papaconstantinou
  1990   EURAGE workshop report: Aging and longevity genes: Strategies for identifying DNA sequences controlling life span. Journal of Gerontology 45:B179-B182.

Williams, B.D., B. Schrank, C. Huynh, R. Shownkeen, R.H. Waterston, and A.P. Wong
  1992   A genetic mapping system in Caenorhabditis elegans based on polymorphic sequence-tagged-sites. Genetics 131:609-624.

Wong, A., P. Boutis, and S. Hekimi
  1995   Mutations in the clk-1 gene of Caenorhabditis elegans affect developmental and behavioral timing. Genetics 139:1247-1259.

Yu, C.-E., J. Oshima, Y.-H. Fu, E. M. Wijsman, F. Hisama, R. Alisch, S. Matthews, J. Nakura, T. Miki, S. Ouais, G. M. Martin, J. Mulligan, and G. D.Schellenberg
  1996   Positional cloning of the Werner's Syndrome gene. Science 272:258-262.

Yunis, E.J., and M. Salazar
  1993   Genetics of life span in mice. Genetica 91:211-223.

Zeng, Z.-B.
  1994   Precision mapping of quantitative trait loci. Genetics 136:1457-1468.

Zwaan, B., R. Bulsma, and R.F. Hoekstra
  1995   Direct selection for life span in Drosophila melanogaster. Evolution 49:649-659.

8

Population Biology of the Elderly

James R. Carey and Catherine Gruenfelder

INTRODUCTION

An important, yet widely overlooked incongruity in ecological and evolutionary literature concerns the gap between the emphasis on understanding age-structured populations (Caswell, 1989; Charlesworth, 1994) and the elderly as a subgroup of the population. This disparity implies that age structure is important, but only within a restricted subset of younger age classes. Indeed, the elderly are often viewed as expendable and thus as possessing little real or potential ability to contribute to the fitness of the population (Williams, 1957).

There are several likely reasons for historical neglect of the elderly in behavioral ecology literature. First, it is widely known from field life tables that most individuals in the wild die young and even fewer survive to older ages (Deevey, 1947). Thus, it is argued that their role is negligible, since the elderly subgroup of animals in the wild is not only frail but also is only a small minority of the total population.

Second, the evolutionary theory of aging (Williams, 1957) suggests that older individuals contribute little to fitness of populations because, according to the Lotka model (Lotka, 1907), the force of selection decreases with age (Rose, 1991; Kirkwood, 1985). One of the problems with the use of the Lotka model to define fitness is that it does not consider some situations where the elderly may contribute substantially to the fitness of the population. For example, it does not consider circumstances in which only older adults, particularly females, overwinter and regenerate the population in the spring (Izquierdo, 1991), in which the elderly provide infant care, or in which the older matriarchs or patriarchs provide critical leadership and cohesion.

Third, senility is often used as the physical and behavioral criterion for defining and identifying the elderly in the wild—i.e., those individuals that are decrepit, moribund, and near death. Unfortunately, this anecdotal "aging" of wild individuals is subject to substantial error. Only in the last several decades have detailed longitudinal data been systematically gathered on individuals of known ages and greater emphasis been placed on understanding age structure of populations (Finch and Ricklefs, 1991). Researchers have found that the variability in the rate of aging in wild animals is as great as that in humans, and in most species, it is virtually impossible to determine the exact age of an individual by its appearance or a biomarker. This is particularly true at older ages. Indeed, "physiologic heterogeneity" is a consistent characteristic of the elderly population (Timiras, 1994).

The broad objective of this paper is to extract important facts about aging and social and community structure in nonhumans and to reassemble them on a foundation of ecology and population biology. Just as certain morphological traits in animals, such as antler type, leg length, wing shape, visual acuity, gut length, and ear design, have been successfully related to the ecology and life histories of different animal species, we expect longevity and mortality patterns to be interpretable in the same context. We believe that this approach will provide insight into questions such as: What aspects of natural history favor the evolution of greater longevity? To what extent is life span a function of ecology and social structure? Is slowing of mortality at older ages a consequence of selection for certain adaptive traits at younger ages?

We organized this paper into three broad sections and a discussion. In the first section we introduce foundational principles we believe are important for understanding the relationship between longevity and life history of animals. These include biodemographic concepts and behavioral characteristics, such as altruism, dominance, territoriality, learning, and culture. In the second section we present a synopsis of roles and life histories of the elderly in three selected animal groups, including elephants, cetaceans, and primates, to provide specific biological context. In the third section we explore the concept of extended longevity as a preadaptation for the evolution of eusociality in wasps. This concept is important because it broadens the evolutionary scope from microevolution, as is discussed by Rose (1991) and Kirkwood (1985), to macroevolution concerned with speciation and the evolution of broad taxonomic groups (Strickberger, 1996). In the discussion we attempt to synthesize the general findings of the natural history and roles of the elderly, discuss some common life-history patterns associated with extended life span, and suggest future directions.

FOUNDATIONAL CONCEPTS

The Elderly: An Integration of Biodemographic Concepts

Defining the Elderly

Life span of animals is not an orderly unfolding of precisely timed events from fertilization to death, with the elderly as a distinct, definitive stage. There exists no objective physiological landmark for aging, such as occurs with sexual

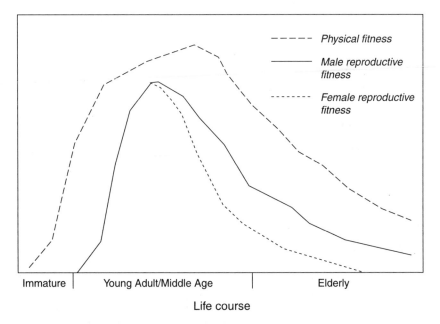

FIGURE 8-1 Physical and reproductive fitness generally peak during middle age and tend to steadily decline throughout the elderly stage (shown here to be the last third of the life course).

maturation in most animals. Its onset occurs at some indeterminate point following maturity, and its progression follows timetables that differ with each individual (Timiras, 1994). Consequently, a consistent characteristic of the elderly in nature is the wide range of frailty and robustness; therefore, it is impossible to specify for any species the age at which the elderly stage begins. However, as an operational definition, we consider the elderly in nature as those individuals who survive to the later half to third of the life span (Figure 8-1). Perhaps a more realistic framework, but one that would not serve the current purposes, would be to consider functional, rather than chronological, markers to define old age (Silverstone, 1996).

Life-Course Premises

Many of the premises outlined by Riley (1979) for the life course and demography of older humans are general and thus relevant for understanding the life course, population dynamics, and aging of populations for any species. These premises are as follows: (1) Aging for all animals is a continual process of development, maturation, and growing old. Thus, no single stage of an individual's life can be understood apart from its antecedents and consequences. (2) Aging consists of several sets of processes, including biological, social, and experiential processes, all of which are systematically interactive over the life course. (3) The life-course pattern of any particular individual is affected by changes in the group and in the environment. (4) Not all individuals survive to old age. However, the importance of the elderly to the overall dynamics and welfare of the population may be disproportionately greater than their numbers.

Consequences of Long Life

Long life has several consequences for individuals in animal populations (Riley and Riley, 1986). First, long life prolongs opportunity to accumulate social and biological experiences. For example, long-lived individuals in social species may possess unique knowledge, such as the location of water during a drought or how to manufacture and use tools. Second, long life maximizes an individual's opportunities to complete or to change role "assignments." For example, a long-lived animal can ascend, lose, and re-attain alpha status within a troop, serve as a grandparent "caregiver"; become a forager after having been a colony "nurse"; become a breeder, by inheriting breeding territory, rather than remain a nest helper. Third, greater longevity prolongs an individual's relationships to others, including mates, parents, offspring, and associates. This feature increases the structural complexity of an individual's social networks, such as kinships, alliances, and communities. For example, when a monogamous pair of birds survives over multiple years, the relationship can become highly complex, leading to large clutch sizes and increased breeding success not seen in short-lived species (Coulson, 1966). In general, these consequences demonstrate that longer-lived individuals can significantly influence change within their group.

Relevant Behavioral Principles

The elderly often exhibit behaviors fundamental to behavioral ecology. This section provides background on several of these concepts that frequently appear in literature on the elderly and thus are basic to understanding the broader nature of the roles of elderly individuals.

Altruism

Altruism, defined by Wilson (1975) as "self-destructive behavior performed for the benefit of others," is relevant to understanding the role of the elderly in nature in several social contexts, including care-giving, allomothering, group defense, and nest care. Altruism is also apparent among the elderly in some nonsocial species. For example, altruism is demonstrated by older, foul-tasting Saturnid moths that sacrifice themselves to "teach" predators that younger counterparts are repugnant (Blest, 1963).

Hamilton (1964) proposed the primary theoretical background for explaining the evolution of altruistic behavior. Hamilton's theory based altruism on the fundamental kinship relations of donor and recipient (Rosenberg, 1992). Altruism has since been generalized to include any form of nonselfish behavior and serves as the cornerstone for much of sociobiology (Wilson, 1975). In this sense, altruistic behavior includes care-giving to kin other than an individual's direct offspring. Feeding, protecting, warning, defending, and teaching kin, in proportion to their consanguinity, emerges as an adaptationally optimal strategy for older individuals.

Many forms of altruism are evident within social species. Maxim (1979) lists four altruistic roles of aging in primates: (1) defense of territory, (2) defense against predation, (3) control of troop movement, and (4) aunt behavior. These activities are of little or no direct benefit to the elderly individuals but do serve to directly benefit the kinship community. Further, Medawar (1957) comments that altruistic behavior of grandparents should be indirectly selected for because, although grandparents are infertile and their behavior is of no benefit to themselves, "grandmotherly indulgence" does benefit the community. Hamilton (1966) also proposed that postreproductive life spans may have evolved when the older animal benefits its younger kin. For example, old postreproductive female langurs ardently defend their troops and protect troop infants to a much greater degree than younger females (Hrdy, 1981). Also, Norris and Pryor (1991) suggest that many postreproductive, yet still lactating, females in dolphin societies may be present as a source of nourishment to offspring of younger mothers while those mothers dive to great depths for prey. Diamond (1996) supports the occurrence of altruistic postreproductive females by stating that aging human females can, evidently, "do more to increase the number of people bearing her genes by devoting herself to her existing children, her potential grandchildren, and her other relatives than by producing yet another child."

An example of altruism in a nonsocial species is given by Blest (1963). Blest found that cryptic New World Saturnid moths, which rely on camouflage to escape detection but are quite palatable to predators, die shortly after completing reproduction. The aposematic subgroup of New World Saturnid moths, which rely on their terrible taste to discourage predators, exhibit a long postreproductive period. Postreproductive survival of the tasty moths is detrimental to conspecifics because a predator can establish a search image of the cryptic species by feeding on palatable individuals. However, a predator's unpleasant experience with an aposematic individual would benefit its kin and other conspecifics. Thus, Blest argued that the sustained physical fitness of postreproductive aposematic moths contributes to the survival of the younger reproductives.

Dominance and Leadership

To dominate is to possess priority of access to the necessities of life and reproduction (Wilson, 1975). Understanding the governance of animal societies by dominance hierarchies provides the fundamental basis for studying the behavioral dynamics of social groups. Because social groups are often headed by older individuals, such as in primate societies, it follows that understanding dominance relations is basic to understanding the role of the elderly in nature.

Allee (1931) addressed the issue of stable hierarchies and argued that dominance hierarchies created cooperative groups that were better able to compete with other groups. One of the classic studies on chickens, from which the concept of "pecking order" was derived, was by Guhl and Allee (1945), who found that chickens with stable hierarchies had individuals that consumed more food and laid more eggs than chickens without hierarchies. Dugatkin (1995) provides further support to this study by demonstrating that subordinate chickens do not challenge superiors but often prefer to wait their turn. Dugatkin shows that this complacency occurs not because subordinates fear damage and retribution but that group selection has "chosen" genotypes that will not contest authority. Closely related to dominance is leadership, which is initiative and control of an activity, usually by one individual. Whereas dominance alone suggests suppression of group activity, even though it may stabilize the social interactions, an individual who is also a leader can contribute to group survival by synchronizing and stimulating group activity (Greenberg, 1947).

Wilson (1975) lists several "special properties" of dominance order that have important bearing on understanding the role of the elderly in social species. First, "the peace of strong leadership" refers to how dominant animals of some primate societies, including those of gorillas, chimpanzees, macaques, spider monkeys, and squirrel monkeys, use their power to terminate fighting among subordinates. Species organized by despotisms also live in peace due to the universally acknowledged power of the tyrant (e.g., the queen bumblebee). Second, "social inertia" refers to the intrinsic stability of a dominance hierarchy. An animal that attempts to change its position in a fixed dominance hierarchy is less likely to succeed than if it made the exertion during the formative, fluid stages of the hierarchy (Guhl, 1968). Third, societies structured as "nested hierarchies" are partitioned into units and exhibit dominance both within and between components. For example, in some primate societies, hierarchies exist both within and between family lines.

Territoriality

A territory is an area occupied either directly by overt defense or indirectly through advertisement (Wilson, 1975). This area usually contains a scarce resource (e.g., steady food supply, shelter, space for sexual display, a site for laying eggs or bearing offspring, etc.). The adaptive advantage of territorial behavior is that successful defense of a territory increases the chances of an individual to secure its necessary share of environmental resources, to mate, and to increase survival of offspring (Kluijver and Tinbergen, 1953). Individuals resident in an area have more to gain from retaining the territory than do intruders from taking it. This is true because residents invest a great deal of energy and time into mastering their area and resources and may well have dependent young. A challenger is devoid of these properties and thus has nothing to lose (Gosling, 1982).

Age is virtually never the sole criterion for achieving dominance or acquiring territory. However, there is likely to be a strong association with age because of two factors. First, the territory holder almost always triumphs in one-on-one encounters. Therefore, territory holders often have held their territories for a long time and thus tend to be older. Second, there is a positive relationship between age and dominance of subordinates, who are continually competing for "next-in-line" status.

Learning and Culture

Learning, defined as any change of behavior of individuals due to experience (Cavalli-Sforza and Feldman, 1981; Alcock, 1993), is found in virtually all animal species from the simplest bacteria and protozoa to complex mammals, such as cetaceans, primates, and elephants. The mechanisms of learning can occur at different levels. Self-teaching occurs when a young individual eats a food that tastes bad and subsequently avoids it. Birds acquire songs and repertoires through imitation. Teaching occurs when inexperienced young of predator species accompany their parents on a hunt to acquire skill. The cumulative learning experiences of groups constitute unique cultures that can often be transmitted from one generation to the next (Alcock, 1993). It is widely believed that selection favors specific learning abilities as solutions to specific ecological problems (Alcock, 1993). For example, solitary animals gain useful flexibility by adjusting their diets to whatever nourishment is available. Also, many animals that hoard food must remember where their food cache is located. The ability of social animals to adjust to the behavior of others (e.g., who is dominant to whom, what one individual did to another individual, etc.) may greatly affect their reproductive success (Alcock, 1993). Information that can only be transmitted through learning includes home range, migratory pathways, location of food sources, tool construction and use, acceptability of food items, parental-care skills, and social relationships, such as pair bonding and alliances (Bonner, 1980).

THE ELDERLY IN NATURE: SELECTED CASE STUDIES

Although there are few papers published on the elderly in nature, the biological literature contains a surprising amount of information on nonhuman elderly that has never been compiled and synthesized. The life history and field biology of a large number of endangered or economically important species in all major taxonomic groups has been studied and documented in meticulous detail. This includes longitudinal studies of marked individuals or monitoring, for decades, individuals in laboratories and in zoos. The purpose of this section is to introduce the concept of the role of the elderly in nature, using information extracted from the biological literature on elephants, cetaceans, and primates. We begin each subsection with background information on the biology and social structure of each group to provide ecological context for the information on aging and the roles of the elderly.

Elephants

Ecological Background

Elephants belong to the order Proboscidea, which includes the extinct mastodon and mammoth. There are only two extant species, the African elephant and the Asian elephant, although there are a number of subspecies within each group (Estes, 1991). The African forest elephant lives in the West African rain forest, whereas the savanna race inhabits lowland forests, low-lying swamps, flood plains, and woodland. Elephants also live in subdesert terrain where gallery forest or neighboring mountains provide shade, browse, and water. These animals must frequently move large distances for food and water due to seasonal variations in food distribution and abundance. Elephants are mixed feeders, concentrating on grasses in the rainy season and on woody plants in the dry season (Buss, 1961, 1990). Thus, they wander widely across the savanna during the rains, yet remain near forest and water sources at other times.

Both African and Asian elephants appear to have identical social structures, of which the family is the core unit (Figure 8-2). The family consists of closely related females, including the matriarch, several younger, yet mature, females, and their calves (Eltringham, 1982). Juvenile males remain with their group until they reach sexual maturity, at which time they are driven away by the matriarch (Buss, 1990). Adult males are either solitary or remain on the distant periphery of the herd. Elephant populations are migratory within large home ranges. Activity, direction, and rate of movement are determined by the matriarch, which is typically the largest (and oldest) cow. Typically, the matriarch leads the group, while another large (and old) female brings up the rear (Douglas-Hamilton, 1987). If disturbed, the group clusters around the matriarch awaiting instruction and protection. If the matriarch is shot, the family becomes a frantic, disorganized mob and, most often, falls prey to the same fate as their leader (Eltringham, 1982). Female leadership and experience play a crucial role in elephant social organization, and thus, female life span extends well past the reproductive years (Laws, 1970).

Elephants do not exhibit seasonal breeding (Poole and Moss, 1989). A female elephant is in estrus for only 3 to 6 days at a time and may conceive only once every 3 to 9 years (Poole and Moss, 1989). Thus, given the short female receptive period and the high investment in each offspring, it is crucial for a

Bachelor Group

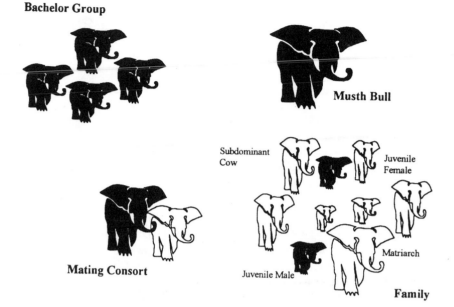

FIGURE 8-2 The social organization of elephants includes a central family core consisting of the matriarch, other adult females, sexually mature and immature female offspring, and sexually immature juvenile males. The sexually mature juvenile males roam in isolated bachelor groups. Adult males will form mating consorts with adult females. Old musth bulls remain solitary and away from the family unit.

female to find a high-quality mate. Usually a female will prefer to mate with an old male that will chase away the younger males and allow the female to rest, a necessity for successful elephant reproduction (DiSilvestro, 1991).

Reproduction, Life Span, and Aging

Females are sexually mature at 10 years, the gestation period is 22 months, and interbirth intervals last up to 9 years (Buss and Smith, 1966). The close bond between mothers and their offspring can endure for 50 years. Males reach sexual maturity at 17 years (DiSilvestro, 1991), at which time they leave the family unit. At 30 years, a male is almost full size (3.7 meters at shoulder) and first experiences an annual condition of heightened sexual motivation, musth (Owens and Owens, 1992). There is only one musth male in an elephant population at one time because musth males are dominant and can suppress this breeding condition in other males (DiSilvestro, 1991).

Although reproduction is continuous throughout an elephant's lifetime (Laws et al., 1975), the peak of female elephant fecundity occurs at 30-40 years and steadily declines thereafter to 37 percent of the peak at 46-50 years, 25 percent at 51-55 years, and 0 percent after 55 years (Laws, 1966). Laws et al. (1975) estimated menopause in African elephants at 55 years, although Sukumar (1989) reported a pregnant 60-year-old cow.

The prime of life for an elephant is about 30-40 years (DiSilvestro, 1991). Old age begins around 50, and most elephants die by 60 (Fatti et al., 1980), although some have lived into their 70s (Freeman, 1980). Sikes (1967, 1971) believes that the upper limit of life span is 65 years and is determined by molar-teeth deterioration, so that old individuals cannot eat and survive. Elephants past 50 years usually have the temporal region of the skull depressed and sunken. This physical trait is a sign of old age but not an indication of failing health.

Major Roles of the Elderly

The first major role of the elderly in elephant populations is leadership. Elephant size determines dominance and is also age-dependent because elephants continue to grow throughout their lives. Therefore, older females tend to be the largest of their sex in the herd and, because elephants' social organization is matriarchal, the oldest females are usually the leaders (DiSilvestro, 1991; Redmond, 1991). Despite disease and deterioration, aging females still have an important role in elephant society, and the movements of the herd are adaptable to an aging animal (Freeman, 1980). If the matriarch is injured or killed, the family unit is lost and the animals are easily disbanded or fall prey to the same fate (e.g., poaching) in their confusion (Eltringham, 1982). When the family is approached by predators or other threatening situations, if the matriarch runs, the family runs; if she attacks, the family attacks (Hanks, 1973, 1979). The matriarch will also stand guard over any injured animal in her group, roaring loudly over the body while attempting to upright the animal.

Laws et al. (1975) noted that because of the overwhelmingly matriarchal structure of elephant populations, selective culling of old or barren cows is probably disadvantageous. It removes from the population the adult females with the lowest reproductive rate, which may be helpful for population control but, more seriously, removes the leaders. The elimination of their accumulated experience must add appreciably to the disturbance factor. Moreover, the removal of matriarchs may well lead to formation of larger groups with unfavorable effects on the habitats due to more intensified localized use.

The second major role of the elderly in elephant populations involves reproduction in males. Older males tend to be physically larger and possess larger, heavier tusks (Laws, 1966; Poole, 1987, 1994). Both traits have major influence on male mating success. Females prefer to mate with old bulls because consequently, offspring will inherit genes of long-lived, healthy adults, and old musth bulls will protect her from the harassment of young bulls (Lawley, 1994). After their matings, the older bull stays with the younger cow and guards or escorts her until the end of her estrous cycle, which provides her with some days of calm, free from male attentions, in which she hopefully will conceive (Owens and Owens, 1992; Lawley, 1994).

The importance of old bulls to the success of elephant reproduction eluded many early observers of elephant behavior when considering the impact of the harvest of the "big tuskers" in ivory trade (DiSilvestro, 1991). The old bulls no longer associated with the herd were interpreted as past their prime. However, they were in their prime, although solitary as almost all adult males are, and in search of estrous females from many different herds (Poole and Moss, 1981; DiSilvestro, 1991).

The third major role of elderly elephants involves essentially the collective knowledge of the matriarchs. In peaceful times, the matriarch decides where the family goes, when to move, and where and when to sleep. Seasonal movements are guided by the matriarch because she has retained knowledge of the optimal or long-forgotten food and water reserves from her long life (Shoshani, 1991). This she teaches to the younger animals (Eltringham, 1982). The solution to many problems of elephant daily life are learned rather than instinctual, making the matriarch, above all, the ultimate repository of essential survival skill that younger animals simply would not have had time to learn on their own (Lawley, 1994). As Laws et al. (1975) notes, "We feel that the dependence of a family unit upon its matriarch even in the most extreme of situations illustrates the great importance of the acquisition of experience and learning made possible by the evolution of longevity. We consider that this situation represents an evolutionary development that is now probably essential for the stability of elephant communities." The matriarch is a reservoir of "collective wisdom of the community" (Eltringham, 1982).

Primates

Ecological Background

Nonhuman primates are composed of 185 species comprising four main branches: prosimians (including lemurs, lorises, pottos, and bush babies), New World monkeys (including capuchins, marmosets, and night squirrel monkeys), Old World monkeys (including mandrills, guenons, baboons, and colobus monkeys), and great apes (including chimpanzees, orangutans, and gorillas) (Estes, 1991). With few exceptions (e.g., macaques and langurs in temperate Japan and China) primates are confined to the tropics, and 80 percent live in rain forests (Estes, 1991). Most nonhuman primates are arboreal or cliff-dwelling; only the gorilla sleeps on the ground (Estes, 1991).

Small primates, such as pottos and bush babies, feed primarily on small arthropods, but larger ones must rely on new leaves, buds, shoots, seed pods, and fruit. All monkeys and apes are sociable, and the majority live in female-bonded groups. Females never leave their home group, whereas males emigrate and have to join or take over another group before they can reproduce (Wrangham, 1980). Consequently, primate groups are typically female-biased (Clutton-Brock and Harvey, 1983; Clutton-Brock et al., 1977).

Mating systems differ among primate species (Figure 8-3). For example, langurs form large groups of unrelated individuals, consisting entirely of females and also one male that has dominant reproductive access. Other males remain on the periphery of the group awaiting a chance to challenge the dominant male. However, chimpanzees form groups that include more than one male that has access to breed. Within the large group, there is a coalition of several males that roams overlapping female ranges. Each female and her young offspring occupy a distinct range. This mating system allows males to have access to more females, yet no single male has ultimate control. Most primates breed relatively late in life, give birth to only one offspring at a time, have long gestation periods, and, in some species, breed at only one particular time of year.

Dunbar (1988) summarizes the six main types of social organizations in primates that include: solitary territorial animals, monogamous pairs, matrilines, one-male territorial troops, multi-male societies, and one-male harems. First, solitary territorial animals, such as the pottos, inherit their home ranges from their mothers. Female offspring often settle near their mother, who may donate part of her home range to successive female offspring. Males roam from female range to female range. Second, for monogamous primates (e.g., one lemur species and

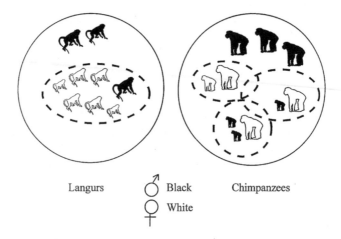

Langurs   ♂ Black   Chimpanzees
               ♀ White

FIGURE 8-3 Mating systems differ among primate species. Langur females live in small groups, and a single male may be able to prevent other males from joining the group. In chimpanzees, brothers defend a large joint territory, giving them access to more females, each of whom, with her juvenile offspring, lives in her own separate range within the larger territory.

possibly one guenon species), an obligatory pair bond is essential for offspring survival. Third, matrilines, or female kinship groups, consist of families of closely related females and one reproductively dominant male. Females forage separately at night but sleep together with the male during the day. This form of social organization is common in bush babies. Fourth, one-male territorial troops prevail among higher primates and are common in the blue monkey and black-white colobus. The resident male is the dominant member of the troop, and members may not necessarily be genetically related. Fifth, multi-male societies, typified by the savanna baboon, are found in species that forage in large troops in undefended home ranges. Social relations are complex and reflect kinship bonds, male coalitions, and male-female alliances. Finally, one-male harems are exemplified best in the hamadryas baboon and the gorilla. In this system a male may own two or more females for a period of time and remain in a separate bachelor group otherwise.

Reproduction, Life Span, and Aging

Most primates breed relatively late in life, give birth to only one offspring at a time, have long gestation periods, and, in some species, breed at only one particular time of year. A study by Caro et al. (1995) revealed that a significant postreproductive period in old females occurs in most nonhuman primate species, especially gorillas and chimpanzees.

The life spans of most nonhuman primates have been estimated conservatively, in that the recorded age represents the time in captivity. Thus the ages of animals captured in the wild are underestimated by their age at entry into captivity; the ages of those still living are underestimated by the time they will continue to live. Harvey et al. (1987) provide maximum longevity records of over 100 major primate species including the following: long-haired chimpanzee (*Pan troglodytes*; 44.5 yr), gorilla (*Gorilla gorilla*; 39.3 yr), (*Cercopithecus aethiops*; 31 yr), stumptail macaque (*Macaca arctoides*; 30 yr) hanuman langur (*Presbytis entellus*; 20 yr), and mouse lemur (*Microcebus murinus*; 15.5 yr). Cutler (1976) notes that the maximum life-span potential of primates is related to their postnatal developmental rate, length of general vigor, length of reproductive period, and time available for learning and teaching.

It is difficult to determine the age of primates in the wild, although the very old and senile individual can be identified by erosion and tartarization of teeth, deepening creases in facial skin, balding, changes in skin pigmentation and hair color, and weight loss (Hrdy, 1981).

Major Roles of the Elderly

The statement by Hrdy (1981) summarizes the beliefs of many scientists regarding elderly primates: "If one were to ask a primatologist how old animals behave in the wild the answer might well be 'They don't,' for it has long been thought that very few primates in natural habitats could evade predators and disease long enough to grow old. As a consequence little attention has been given to old animals in the vast literature on primate behavior."

The social rank of macaque females increases with age. For example, a daughter of a high-ranked female may adopt a home range overlapping her mother's range. When the mother dies, the young female gains access to resources from which she would otherwise be excluded (Clutton-Brock, 1991). Some studies show that feeding and reproductive skills also increase with age (Lack, 1968; De Steven, 1978), and the costs of rearing offspring may be greater for inexperienced adults than for older individuals (Clutton-Brock, 1991). Older females tend to be reproductively less active and may lead solitary lives, displaced from prime food sources and roosting sites. In contrast, older females of the gray-cheeked mangabey are fully integrated into the group but tend to be less active in grooming, embracing, and other individual social acknowledgments. Chalmers and Rowell (1971) observed that among old females, grooming decreased, while being groomed increased. Kinship ties in the macaque, *Macaca fascicularis*, preserve the rank of aging females, and only those that are senile drop in rank (Hrdy, 1981).

There is considerable evidence suggesting that leadership is a primary role of older individuals in primate groups. Old silverback gorillas make troop decisions including when and where to forage, rest, and sleep and arbitrate disputes within their harems (Stewart and Harcourt, 1987). However, the type of leadership is conditional upon the sex, ecological or social context (e.g., foraging, defense, etc.), and the mating system and overall life history of the species. In squirrel and toque monkeys, langurs, and gorillas, aging females are the most active in leading the troop movements.

A second important role of elderly females is care-giving. In geladas, aging females maintain their rank in association with their related female groups (matrilines) and act as "aunts" cuddling, carrying, and disciplining others' infants (Maxim, 1979). Researchers discovered that the presence of the grandmother of female vervets (small gray African monkey) in a captive socially living colony had a profound impact on the mortality rate of newborns. Specifically, (1) the presence of the infant's grandmother determined the level of risk; and (2) infant mortality for female vervets with grandmothers present was only 32 percent, whereas infant mortality for vervets without their grandmothers present was over double at 73 percent (Fairbanks and McGuire, 1986). In these circumstances, selection could be expected to favor females that terminate their reproductive life before the natural mortality rate rises steeply, particularly if reproduction would substantially increase the risk of mortality.

Even though the reproductive fitness is low in the elderly, their physical fitness may be relatively high, and thus their contributions to the group to which they belong may be in ways other than reproduction. For example, Hrdy (1981) suggested that in Japanese macaques the rank of the older females has a great potential effect on her genetic contribution to subsequent generations because her daughters inherit her rank. She referred to these as the "nepotists." Despite increasing feebleness with age, old females in high- and middle-ranking lines are still deferred to by their younger and more vigorous descendants (Figure 8-3). In contrast to the nepotistic system of macaques, hanuman langurs of India have a different breeding system, where females are more closely related to one another than females in a macaque troop. Hrdy (1981) showed that older, postreproductive langurs are low ranking but participate vigorously in defending the troop, advancing troop interests, and protecting and caring for infants and juveniles of close relatives. She referred to these as the "altruists." The concept of inclusive fitness offers an explanation for a ranking system that favors youthful females of high reproductive value combined with a defense system in which old females take great risks (Hamilton, 1964).

The rise and fall by age in the dominance hierarchy of three adult male chimpanzees from the long-term study by Goodall (1986) is shown in Figure 8-4. Several points merit comment. (1) It was not possible for either a young or a female chimpanzee to occupy the alpha position. (2) However, age alone does not assure a high position within the group. For example, Jomeo lived for 26 years but was always low ranking despite his superior weight and aggressiveness; one individual (Figan) occupied the alpha position for nearly a decade, and Evered occupied the

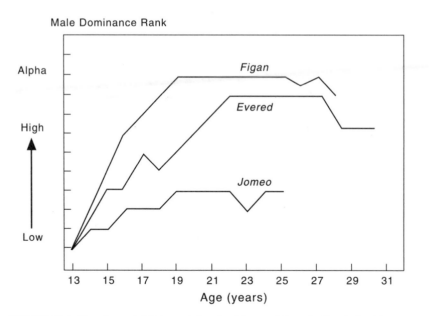

Male Dominance Rank

FIGURE 8-4 The rise and fall in social rank of three adult male Kasakela chimpanzees studied by Goodall (1986) in Gombe National Park, Kenya over a 25-year period.

beta position or a high rank also for nearly a decade. This provides stability to the entire group. (3) Also the beta position was held for a sustained period; the ranking males were almost certainly past their physical prime in their late 20s and early 30s and yet they maintained their rank out of "habit" and tradition.

One of the most important implications of the detailed longitudinal studies of individuals by Goodall and her coworkers is that they provide critical historical perspective on individuals at their older ages. For example, Goodall (1986) notes that, even when young, Figan showed signs of the qualities that would take him to the top of the male hierarchy. This included exploiting temporary ill health in older males and developing close supportive relationships with members of his family (e.g., high-ranking mother). Evered was motivated to attain high social rank but was at a disadvantage because he had no close ally. In contrast, Jomeo was apparently not motivated to attain high social status despite his apparent physical capabilities.

Cetaceans—Whales and Dolphins

Ecological Background

Cetacea consists of two extant suborders—Mysteceti, baleen whales, and Odontoceti, toothed whales (Carroll, 1988). Although both have evolved from a common archeocete ancestor (Carroll, 1988; Novacek, 1994; Gingerich et al., 1994), they drastically differ not only in feeding morphology but also in behavior (Figure 8-5; Table 8-1). Baleen whales are generally filter feeders, surviving on

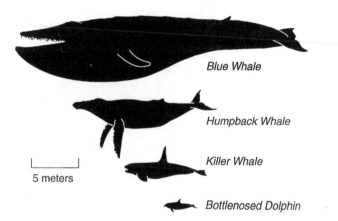

FIGURE 8-5 Body shape and scale for four species of cetaceans. Baleen whales, (e.g., the blue and humpback whales) tend to be larger than toothed whales (e.g., the killer whale and the bottlenosed dolphin). Not only do these groups differ by size, but also by life history.

TABLE 8-1 Comparative Life-History Traits of the Cetaceans

Life-History Trait	Baleen Whales	Toothed Whales
Social organization		
Structure	None	Communities with well-defined subgroups
Length of associations	Fleeting	Long-lasting
Migration	Seasonal	None
Feeding	Filter feeders	Active predators
Foraging	Individual grazing	Cooperative hunting
Communication	Only for mating	Highly developed, multi-purpose language
Mating/reproduction	Seasonal	Continuous
Care of offspring	Mother only	Mother and other adults
Juvenile development	Rapid	Normal

SOURCE: Based on Tyack (1986).

small planktonic crustacea and other small oceanic organisms, while toothed whales are active hunters of larger prey, including octopodes, sharks, and other whales. However, a fundamental difference between these groups lies in social organization. Baleen whales have virtually no social structure, and the only relations between individuals (usually mother-calf bonds or sexual encounters) are short-lived, never lasting more than 1 year and more often lasting only several hours (Tyack, 1986). In contrast, toothed whales generally live in complex social communities, consisting of adult females and young of both sexes, while coalitions of adult males travel between communities for access to females (Tyack, 1986; Wells, 1991). Other behavioral differences between the suborders, including migration, foraging, communication, mating, and offspring care, can be seen as artifacts of their social organizations. Therefore, analysis of the dichotomous life histories of baleen and toothed whales may give insight into why they live as long (or as briefly) as they do, and what the elderly members of their species contribute to the population.

Aging and Life Span

Age of cetaceans is usually determined by counting the annual layers of cementum or dentine in the teeth (Kasuya and Marsh, 1984), but this may be unreliable due to bone deterioration, especially in baleen whales (Tyack, 1986). However, the main obstacle to determining age of these animals is lack of specimens to study. Some detailed whaling records are kept, but for the most part, these are either inaccurate or not concerned with age. The only other source of information is from dead cetaceans beached on shore or recent captive specimens (Hayley, 1978). Thus, until recently when researchers have begun to track marine organisms for extended time periods, there have been only sketchy estima-

TABLE 8-2 Developmental Parameters of the Three Main Groups of
Cetaceans

Parameter	Baleen Whale	Toothed Whale	Dolphin/ Porpoise
Gestation period	11 mo	15-16 mo	10.5-12 mo
Intercalf interval	1-2 yr	3-5.8 yr	1-3 yr
Weaning			
Age	7-11 mo	Mean 1-5 yr	6-20 mo
		Max 13-15 yr	
Length	8.8-12.8 m	2.7-7 m	1-2 m
Sexual maturity			
Age	4-5 yr	13-17 yr	2.5-11.5 yr
Length	11.8-23.3 m	3.7-10.8 m	1.4-2.4 m
Adult			
Maximal age	82 yr	54.5 yr	27.5 yr
Maximal length	31 m	15 m	3.8 m

Note: For species in which male and female data were supplied, the average was used.
SOURCE: Adapted from Tyack (1986:Table 1); baleen whale maximum age is averaged from Table 8-3 in this paper.

tions of life span. However, these rough estimates are sufficient for examining general overall trends.

Specifically, investigators have attempted to define several life-history parameters for both baleen and toothed whales (Table 8-2). Baleen whales reach a length and age that is almost twice that of toothed whales. The ratio of longevity to length clearly increases from baleen whales to toothed whales and then increases dramatically in dolphins (Table 8-3). Specifically, the ratio of longevity to length ranges from 1.5 yr/m to 2.6 yr/m in baleens, from 1.8 yr/m to 2.9 yr/m in toothed whales, and reaches a maximum of 3.8 yr/m in the striped dolphin. The sperm whale (classified Odontoceti) shows a value much closer to those of Mysteceti, consistent with recent studies indicating sperm whales might be an intermediate of the two suborders (Milinkovitch et al., 1994).

Major Roles of the Elderly

It seems that toothed whales and, specifically, dolphins live much longer than would be predicted from their length. Thus, it can be construed that the occurrence of elderly organisms within odontocete communities is probably much greater than among the solitary baleen whales. From a fitness perspective, these old organisms would not seem to contribute to the reproductive fitness of a population; however, this may not be the case.

The sociality of toothed cetaceans has lead to the development of a specialized division of labor among the age classes. Therefore, it is apparent that the

TABLE 8-3 Relation of Longevity to Length in Cetaceans

Species	Common Name	Maximum Longevity (yr)	Length (m)	Ratio (yr/m)[a]
Baleen whales				
Balaenoptera acutorostrata	Minke whale	47	28	1.7
Balaenoptera borealis	Sei whale	74	47	1.6
Balaenoptera musculus	Blue whale	110	67	1.7
Balaenoptera physalus	Fin whale	114	45	2.6
Eschrichtius robustus	Gray whale	70	46	1.5
Megaptera novaeangliae	Humpback whale	77	46	1.7
Toothed whales				
Globicephala macrorhynchus	Pilot whale	49.5	17	2.9
Orcinus orca	Killer whale	50	24	2.1
Physeter catadon	Sperm whale	77	44	1.8
Dolphins				
Stenella coeruleoalba	Striped dolphin	34	9	3.8
Tursiops truncatus	Bottlenosed dolphin	35	9.8	3.6

[a]This ratio was calculated by dividing longevity by length.
Note: For species in which male and female data were supplied, the average was used.
SOURCE: Hayley (1978); pilot whale longevity from Leatherwood and Reeves (1978); data for striped dolphin length from Reilly (1978).

older animals in a group perform specific tasks not done by the younger animals. However, this is not apparent in the relatively less intelligent baleen species, in which parental care of young and social learning of offspring is not emphasized (Tyack, 1986). There are several roles that elderly odontocetes perform in their societies: guardian, aunt, and nurse.

First, both old male and old female dolphins are documented guarding or "baby-sitting" younger animals in their home groups. For example, in bottlenosed dolphins, an older male will not just pair with a juvenile, but will watch over that juvenile while the rest of the group forages (Wells, 1991). In a study by Johnson and Norris (1994), a very old Hawaiian spinner dolphin male was frequently seen with juveniles and in shore coves while the rest of the herd cruised the coast. This behavior suggests alloparenting because the old male and juveniles rest while most adults forage for food. This pairing can benefit the young dolphins in several ways: the young are protected from predators that wait to attack solitary members of the group, they are monitored so that they do not swim to unfamiliar waters and lose track of the herd, and possibly, they are taught adult behaviors from the old, experienced male. Norris and Pryor (1991) assert that a pilot whale's "principal biological contribution might be to learn, remember, and transmit what pilot whales need to know." By exercising these parent-like duties, the older male is allowing the younger parents to forage, an activity that the old male may not be able to do as efficiently. Therefore, there is a reciprocity in work allocation that requires the active involvement of all age classes (Tyack, 1986).

Old females in a group perform similar child care duties as old males. Specifically, elderly female dolphins act as "aunts" to other dolphin mothers before, while, and after a calf is born. During the birth, the aunt will be a midwife and even break the umbilical cord. After the calf is born, the aunt remains with the mother and calf, serving as a guardian to the young dolphin when the mother forages and rests (Tyack, 1986). In Atlantic bottlenosed dolphins, the grandmother will remain close to her daughter during pregnancy and assist in childbirth. Once the calf is born, the grandmother becomes a guardian to guide the infant through its early years (Caldwell and Caldwell, 1966). In killer whales, older females are thought to nurture the young of other females, creating a matriarchal bonding system (Brault and Caswell, 1993). Also, the oldest female in a Hawaiian spinner dolphin pod acts as a protector, herding the young away from dangerous obstructions (Johnson and Norris, 1994).

The high prevalence of postreproductive females within dolphin communities is significant. In a study on killer whales, a large proportion of females that had not bred for a long time were suggested to be postreproductive (Bigg, 1982, and cited in Kasuya and Marsh, 1984). Among all species, the only value possessed by the female sex is believed to be the ability to bear offspring. Once a mother has surpassed her reproductive prime, she becomes less and less important until she eventually dies. Therefore, it would seem that a menopausal female or one that has ceased to be fertile would certainly be ostracized from her group. However, within the odontocete cetaceans, postreproductive females play an active part in rearing young.

Not only do these females help watch, defend, and teach the younger animals, but, in fact, the postreproductive females nourish these young. Postreproductive female Hawaiian spinner dolphins can produce milk, enabling them to help the younger mothers feed their calves (Johnson and Norris, 1994). Also, in pilot whales, females have an exceptionally long postreproductive period, ceasing ovulation at about 40 years, although they often live until age 63. In Japanese fisheries, 25 percent of females captured are postreproductive and 25 percent of the postreproductive females are lactating. This information implies that females have switched their energies from bearing offspring to nurturing the ones already born, although whether these cetaceans suckle only their own offspring is unclear (Tyack, 1986). Continuous lactation of postreproductive pilot whales allows these whales to nurse other mothers' calves, which are unable to make the deep dive for food that is so characteristic of this species (Norris and Pryor, 1991). Thus, nonreproducing, yet lactating, females can be an important reservoir of nourishment for the young in the community, allowing younger mothers to put more energy into group activities in which older mothers may be less efficient.

In short, contrary to widely held beliefs, older animals that have passed their "prime" do exist in the wild and not just in extraordinary circumstances. This is evident in Cetacea, where the older males and females are essential to the optimal function of their community.

EXTENDED LONGEVITY AS A PREADAPTION FOR EUSOCIALITY

Success or failure in evolving particular mechanisms or structures often depends simply on the presence or absence of a previously existing structure, physiological process, or behavior pattern that is already functional in another context and available as a stepping-stone to the attainment of a new adaptation. This structure, process, or pattern is referred to as a preadaptation (Wilson, 1975; Holldöbler and Wilson, 1990). Preadaptations are often pervasive forces in the histories of all species, creating multiplier effects—such as fins evolving into limbs, limbs into forelegs, and forelegs into grasping appendages with digits. Preadaptations may reach all the way to brood care and advanced sociality by way of extended longevity—a requisite for the existence of both behaviors. Because of the importance of the concept of preadaptation in general and extended longevity in particular, the objective in this section is to examine the preadaptive role of extended longevity in the context of the evolution of eusociality in wasps.

Evolution of Eusociality in Wasps

Wasps are in the insect order Hymenoptera, which is thought to have evolved about 200 million years ago (Edwards, 1980). This order contains a wide variety of species including the sawflies, parasitic hymenopterans, and most extant social insect species, including social wasps, ants, and bees. Most social wasps, such as the yellow jackets and paper wasps, are in the superfamily Vespoidea, the majority of which construct a nest of papery material and progressively provision (i.e., feed as needed) their young. Vespoidea also contains a large number of solitary wasps, such as potter wasps and spider wasps, which first construct nests, find suitable prey, and sting and paralyze the prey. Then these insects bring the immobile prey back to the nest, lay an egg, seal the nest, and then repeat the process. This overall strategy is referred to as mass provisioning.

Extended Longevity in Wasps

One of the prerequisites for the evolution of eusociality in insects is generation overlap (i.e., the parents are alive when the offspring emerge as adults). Indeed, Evans and West-Eberhard (1970) conclude that an important factor explaining the lack of significant social evolution in sphecid wasps is the relatively short female life span, so that the adult lives of mothers and daughters rarely overlap. Significant preadaptations for this overlap include increased female longevity, multiple generations, and adult overwintering. The advantage of adults living throughout the winter is that female wasps can begin nesting earlier in the favorable season and be ready to mate as soon as the winter passes, rather than complete adult development, emerge, and mate as overwintering immatures would do (Matthew, 1991). The fact that virtually all social wasps and bees overwinter as adults suggests that this behavior might be a significant preadaptation for social development (Matthew, 1991).

Evolutionary Steps to Eusociality

Evans (1958) outlined 13 grades of social evolution in wasps, starting with the simplest and, presumably, most primitive and ending with worker-caste differentiation in large, complex colonies. These grades are said to follow the subsocial route, through which a single foundress gains enough longevity to coexist in the same nest as her female offspring (Hölldobler and Wilson, 1990). The parasocial route to eusociality arises when members of the same generation use a composite nest and cooperate in brood care. Recent evidence suggests eusociality appears to arise far more commonly from solitary or semisocial precursors favoring the familial route (Danforth et al., 1996). For brevity, we collapse Evans' 13 steps into the following five phases (Figures 8-6 and 8-7):

Phase I Solitary The ancestral type for the evolution of social wasps is thought to have been a parasitoid. A parasitoid is a hunter, searching for prey that it then

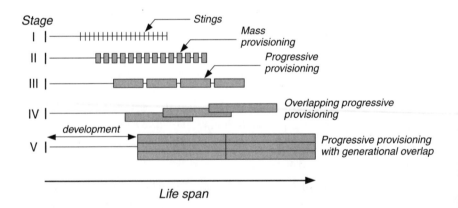

FIGURE 8-6 Schematic diagram of wasp evolution through five stages. Width of the horizontal bands indicates the duration of the association between parent and offspring. Vertical bands or blocks represent length of association between parent and individual offspring; for example, stage I shows short duration of association between a solitary parasitoid wasp and its offspring. The parasitoid lays eggs in a sequence of hosts but provides no parental care, thus "abandoning" each offspring directly after oviposition. Stage III indicates a longer association with progressive provisioning for each offspring; the parent wasp remains longer with each juvenile. Stage IV shows complete overlapping of generations. Note also that developmental time from egg to adult steadily increases from stage I to V (see also Figure 8-7).

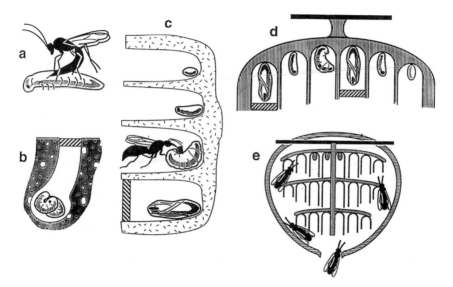

FIGURE 8-7 Likely stages for the evolution of eusociality in wasps (condensed from Evans, 1958). (*a*) Solitary parasitoid wasp laying egg in host. (*b*) Mass-provisioned chamber (paralyzed prey in sealed chamber with wasp egg). (*c*) Wasp feeding developing larva a piece of masticated caterpillar. (*d*) Foundress female lays egg in empty chamber and progressively provisions until daughters mature and can help. (*e*) Eusocial colony with distinct worker castes and age polyethism for nest construction, maintenance, nursing, and defense. SOURCE: *a-c* adapted from figure in Cowan (1991), *d* and *e* adapted from figure 14.43b and figure 14.43c, respectively, in Wenzel (1991).

temporarily paralyzes so that the prey can become a live incubator for its egg. The wasp egg hatches into a larva inside the prey, the larva consumes the prey, exits, and pupates.

Phase II Mass Provisioning An early subphase of mass provisioning occurs when the female paralyzes a prey, carries it to a previously constructed nest, lays her egg, and seals the nest. A later subphase occurs when the female brings multiple prey to the nest. She may have contact with some of her feeding offspring before sealing the nest and after delivering the last prey.

Phase III Progressive Provisioning The female brings more prey to the burrow, as needed, for the developing larva. She may remain in the nest with her offspring, adding some protection for the young. Later, females may begin to feed macerated food directly to the larvae. Here the degree of parental care strongly increases the bond between adult and offspring. The assumption is that progressive provisioning arose from delayed provisioning (Evans, 1966). Among sphecids, Evans (1966) suggests that progressively provisioning *Bembix* live two to four times as long as mass-provisioning *Gorytes*. As females spend longer periods sitting in the protected nest, different selective factors become important. Mortality due to accident and predation is likely to be reduced, there is selection to reduce rates of senescence, life span increases, and mothers are more likely to be alive when some of their offspring reach adulthood (Cowan, 1991).

Phase IV Generation Overlap/Primitive Eusociality The female's life is prolonged and overlaps that of the progeny that remain with her in the nest to form an extended family. Females at this phase lay eggs into an empty cell, a trait thought important in permitting evolution of the extended brood care of social wasps (Evans, 1958; Carpenter, 1991). The young females may construct more cells, lay eggs, and care for their own larvae. However, some females occasionally care for the brood of another female. These behaviors are important steps because the evolution of sociality is not possible without overlap of generations and, at least, rudimentary division of labor. Jayakar and Spurway (1966) believe that the ability to care for more than one cell and larva simultaneously is an important evolutionary step toward eusociality.

Phase V Caste Differentiation Extensive overlap of generations occurs because of extended life spans and because a clear division of labor and caste systems begins to emerge. Wasps have opportunities for fitness gain by associating with relatives of different generations (Cowan, 1991). Differential feeding of larvae occurs. Early progeny are workers, but some intermediate forms are present between these and true females. A single queen, usually the original foundress, is much more long lived than the workers and monopolizes oviposition, referred to as queen control. As long as the colony remains small and the life spans of reproductive individuals and helpers do not differ significantly, helpers may be expected to resist evolutionary specialization as workers because this would reduce or eliminate their chances to replace their mother as the sole reproductive female (Alexander et al., 1991).

As eusocial colonies become large and long-lasting, mothers become increasingly specialized as reproductives, and offspring specialize as workers and soldiers. As this happens, daughters have fewer opportunities to become replacement reproductives, both because the mother lives longer and because so many other individuals are available to replace the mother as well. Thus the identity of a queen's replacement becomes a sweepstakes, with each individual having a chance of, perhaps, one in 50,000 or one in a million (Alexander et al., 1991). One consequence of increased longevity as a preadaptation to sociality is that the stage is set for the evolution of large colonies that have certain advantages over smaller ones, including the ability to organize labor more efficiently, integrate colony activities, defend the nest more aggressively, and exert homeostatic control over physical conditions within the nest (Jeanne, 1991).

Evolution of Life Span in Eusocial Workers

Few uses of the disposable-soma theory of senescence (Kirkwood, 1985) are more apt than when this concept is applied to worker castes in social insects. The fact that honeybee workers are expendable is apparent from their sting and aggressive defensive behavior. Because honeybees' stings are barbed, their stings and adjacent tissues remain anchored in the skin of intruders, thereby creating a chemical alarm that guides other guards to the enemy (Seeley, 1985). Thus the gerontological question is not whether workers are "disposable," but rather how long they should live relative to the "needs" of the colony.

Insights into this question can be gained by considering the relationship of the number of births in a monogynous (single queen) colony (b_q), daily death rate of workers (d_w), and maximal colony size (N^*) as given in the equation (Carey, 1993):

$$N^* = \frac{b_q}{d_w} \qquad (1)$$

It is evident from this simple equation that colony size can increase by either increasing daily birth rate or decreasing daily death rate of workers. For example, if $b_q = 100$ eggs/day and $d_w = 0.10$, then $N^* = 1,000$. However, if either d_w decreased to 0.01 or b_q increased to 1,000, then the maximal colony size, N^*, would increase to 10,000 individuals. A more complete range of tradeoffs between birth and death rates for a fixed maximal colony size is given in Table 8-4. Primitive social-insect colonies probably maintain a modest colony size by evolving an increased life span of the as-yet-undifferentiated "worker" caste. This is because high egg production in queens requires a highly evolved system of food provisioning and propholaxis (liquid food exchange). At the early stages of the evolution of eusociality, it is probably easier to extend life span in all colony members. However, in more advanced groups, when queen longevity is several fold greater than workers, the worker life span is probably determined by needs of colony defense, predictability of food resources, and colony-maintenance requirements.

TABLE 8-4 Maximum Size of Social Insect Colonies Given Different Worker Life Expectancies and Queen Daily Egg Production

Life Expectation	Queen Daily Egg Production			
	100	1000	10,000	100,000
20 days	2,000	20,000	200,000	2,000,000
50 days	5,000	50,000	500,000	5,000,000
100 days	10,000	100,000	1,000,000	10,000,000
200 days	20,000	200,000	2,000,000	20,000,000

SOURCE: Carey (1993; tables 5-12).

DISCUSSION

General Themes

The overall theme of this paper is that, as a subgroup, the elderly play important roles in the cohesion and dynamics of groups, populations, and communities. They serve as care-givers, as guardians, as leaders, as stabilizing centers, as teachers, as sexual consorts, and as midwives. The elderly are at an evolutionary forefront when their brood-care behavior contributes to population fitness, which, in turn, may lead to evolution of sociality in insects and perhaps to other evolutionary pathways in other species. Virtually all behaviors exhibited by the elderly have an evolutionary basis, yet evolutionary aspects of behavior are seldom considered in the context of aging biology. Perhaps the time has come to expand the scope of gerontology and demography of aging to include behavioral to better incorporate the contributions of the elderly to the fitness of populations.

Another theme of this paper, particularly concerned with longevity as a preadaptation for the evolution of eusociality, is that it is important to distinguish between micro- and macroevolutionary aspects of aging and longevity change. Clearly, the evolutionary scale of change for fruit fly selection experiments (Rose, 1991) involving the cost of reproduction is different from changes involving the emergence of major taxonomic groups, new structures, physiological processes, or major adaptive shifts (i.e., eusocialty). It is important to recognize differences in evolutionary scales because the macroevolutionary scale provides context for broad differences in life spans, which may shed light on more subtle, microevolutionary differences. Cost of reproduction tradeoffs or metabolic-rate differences may help explain longevity constraints in microevolutionary settings but provide little insight into why, for example, bats and birds live longer than similarly sized mammals. Explanations for these life-span differences may have more to do with macroevolutionary causes, such as the evolution of sociality or changes in ecological factors, than with proximate factors, such as reproductive costs.

Biodemographic Perspectives on Life Span

In many species a substantial amount of energy is devoted to offspring care. Demographically, this results in reduction of birth rate. For example, Van Lawick-Goodall's (1976:86) description of the chimpanzee's early life is informative:

> The infant does not start to walk until he is six months old, and he seldom ventures more than a few yards from his mother until he is over nine months old. He may ingest a few scraps of solid food when he is six months, but solids do not become a significant part of his diet until he is about two years of age and he

TABLE 8-5 Partial List of Life-History Traits Associated with Extended
Longevity in Animals

Long gestation or developmental period
Small number of offspring per pregnancy, brood, or litter
Long interbirth intervals
Long period of offspring dependency
Intense parenting or brood care
Strong social bonds
Protracted learning period and increased learning potential
Home base, nest, or territory as locus
Monogamy/pair bonding
Enhanced sibling relationships

continues to nurse until he is between four-and-a-half and six years old. Moreover, while he may travel short distances...when he is about four years old, he
continues to make long journeys riding on his mother's back until he is five or six.

As Lovejoy (1981) notes, the extreme degree of parental investment has profound demographic consequences.

When the basic life-history patterns of humans are considered, noting that
chimpanzees often live 30-35 years in the wild and that species with intensive
parental care usually live substantially longer than species with little or no parental care, all the evidence suggests that the evolved life span of primitive humans
was severalfold greater than the life expectancy of 15-25 years (Hayflick, 1994).
For example, if the maturation period of early hominids was 15 years, the birth
interval was 5 years, and survival to adulthood was 30 percent to 50 percent (even
with intensive parental care), then a female must live 35 years just to replace
herself and her mate and 50 years to adequately care for her last-born child (i.e.,
the mother's death would substantially reduce the survival chances of several
dependent offspring, and even the survival chances of other members of the
group if she is involved in cooperative care of the young). If probability of
survival to adulthood was less than 30 percent and/or a percentage of the females
were sterile, then the last age of reproduction would increase to 40 years and life
span would increase to 55 years. This value is consistent with predictions of life
spans based on correlations between longevity, brain weight, and adult size
(Hayflick, 1994). Our approach combines biological and demographic logic with
perspectives on the life histories of other species. Table 8-5 contains a list of life-
history traits that appear to associate with increased longevity in many of these
species.

Gerontological and Demographic Implications

The perspectives provided by exploring the natural history and the roles of
the elderly in nonhuman populations have the potential to greatly expand the

scope of gerontology and the demography of aging by providing important ecological and biological context for these disciplines. Specifically, we have identified four different demographic and gerontological concepts that will benefit from further inquiry into the role of the elderly in nature. First, perspectives on the natural history of the elderly will provide a broader and deeper biological foundation for life-course analysis in demography, including the integration of concepts in demographic sociology (Riley and Riley, 1986), those in sociobiology (Wilson, 1975), and those in life-history theory (Roff, 1992).

Second, emphasis on research on the elderly in nonhuman species may encourage evolutionary biologists to reevaluate the evolutionary theories of aging and senescence. Theories may need to be reformulated to account for situations where the elderly contribute a disproportionate share of genes to the next generation. Emphasis on the importance of the elderly at the population level will also provide important context for studies concerning adaptive demography or the optimal age/stage/size composition of various social groups (Oster and Wilson, 1978), as well as for the rate of genetic change in age-structured populations (Rose, 1991; Charlesworth, 1994).

Third, the concept "roles" of the elderly provide an organizational theme for interdisciplinary aspects of aging. For example, retirement has been referred to by social demographers as a "roleless role," lacking content and sure rewards (Riley and Riley, 1986). But social scientists have no biological foundation upon which to construct theories of social roles, just as many biologists have long thought that very few animals in natural habitats could evade predators and disease long enough to grow old.

Fourth, in humans, the role of the elderly at the oldest ages is becoming almost synonymous with the role of elderly women. The aging society is increasingly becoming a society of older women, often widows. Our future studies will examine whether this feminization of the elderly is general, whether there are gender-specific roles of the elderly, and, if so, how and why these exist. Indeed, infant and juvenile care given by older "aunts" appears to be fairly common across many species. Thus, the literature on inclusive fitness theory (Hamilton, 1964) can be brought to bear on the development of aging theory and the behavioral traits of the elderly. These concepts have not yet been introduced to the gerontological literature; they are clearly fundamental to a deeper understanding of how older caregivers help perpetuate their own genes.

ACKNOWLEDGMENTS

We thank Lynn Kimsey and Robert Jeanne for their insights and help with wasp evolution, and Claudia Graham and Shin-min Tsai for graphics. We are particularly indebted to the undergraduates who enrolled in our University of California at Davis research course on the role of the elderly in nature: Karen Abalos, Harold Amogan, Sophie Betts, Alicia Cook, Kimberly Day, Hoa Giang,

Sandra Lara, Sarah Mertz, Sakura Nakahara, Phuoc Nguyen, Janel Rodas, Nancy Toy, Jennifer Schmidt, Duc Vo, and Elmer Yee. We also thank Stephen Helfand for his suggestions. The research was supported by the National Institute on Aging (Grant AG08761-01) and a Duke University Pilot Project Program grant from the Center for Demographic Studies.

REFERENCES

Alcock, J.
  1993   *Animal Behavior: An Evolutionary Approach*, 5th ed. Sunderland, MA: Sinauer Associates, Inc.
Alexander, R.D., K.M. Noonan, and B.J. Crespi
  1991   The evolution of eusociality. In P.W. Sherman, J.U.M. Jarvis, and R.D. Alexander, eds., *The Biology of the Naked Mole-Rat*. Princeton, NJ: Princeton University Press.
Allee, W.C.
  1931   *Animal Aggregations: a Study in General Sociology*. Chicago: University of Chicago Press.
Bigg, M.
  1982   An assessment of the killer whale (*Orcinus orca*) stocks off Vancouver Island, British Columbia. *Report of the International Whaling Commission* 32:655-670.
Blest, A.D.
  1963   Longevity, palatability and natural selection in five species of New World saturniid moth. *Nature* 197:1183-1186.
Bonner, J.T.
  1980   *The Evolution of Culture in Animals*. Princeton, NJ: Princeton University Press.
Brault, S., and H.C. Caswell
  1993   Pod-specific demography of killer whales (*Orcinus orca*). *Ecology* 75(5):1444-1544.
Buss, I.O.
  1961   Some observations on food habits and behavior of the African elephant. *Journal of Wildlife Management* 25(2):131-148.
  1990   *Elephant Life: Fifteen Years of High Population Density*. Ames, IA: Iowa State University Press.
Buss, I.O., and N.R. Smith
  1966   Observations on reproduction and breeding behavior of the African elephant. *Journal of Wildlife Management* 30(2):375-385.
Caldwell, M.C., and D.K. Caldwell
  1966   Epimeletic (care-giving) behavior in Cetacea. In K. Norris, ed., *Whales, Dolphins, and Porpoises*. Berkeley, CA: University of California Press.
Carey, J.R.
  1993   *Applied Demography for Biologists, with Special Emphasis on Insects*. New York: Oxford University Press.
Caro, T.M., D.W. Sellen, A. Parish, R. Frank, D.M. Brown, E. Voland, and M. Borgerhoff Mulder
  1995   Termination of reproduction in nonhuman and human female primates. *International Journal of Primatology* 16(2):205-220.
Carpenter, J.M.
  1991   Phylogenetic relationships and the origin of social behavior in the Vespidae. In K.G. Ross and R.W. Matthew, eds., *The Social Biology of Wasps*. Ithaca, NY: Comstock Publishing Associates.
Carroll, R.L.
  1988   *Vertebrate Paleontology and Evolution*. New York: W.H. Freeman and Company.

Caswell, H.
    1989   *Matrix Population Models.* Sunderland, MA: Sinauer Associates, Inc.
Cavalli-Sforza, L.L., and M.W. Feldman
    1981   *Cultural Transmission and Evolution: A Quantitative Approach.* Princeton, NJ: Princeton University Press.
Chalmers, N.R., and T.E. Rowell
    1971   Behavior and female reproductive cycles in a captive group of mangabeys. *Folia Primatologica* 14:1-14.
Charlesworth, B.
    1994   *Evolution in Age-Structured Populations,* 2nd ed. London: Cambridge University Press.
Clutton-Brock, T.H.
    1991   *The Evolution of Parental Care.* Princeton, NJ: Princeton University Press.
Clutton-Brock, T.H., and P.H. Harvey
    1983   The functional significance of variation in body size among mammals. *Special Publication, American Society of Mammalogists* 7:632-663.
Clutton-Brock, T.H., P.H. Harvey, and B. Rudder
    1977   Sexual dimorphism, socionomic sex ratio and body weight in primates. *Nature* 269:797-800.
Coulson, J.C.
    1966   The influence of the pair-bond and age on the breeding biology of the kittiwake gull, *Rissa tridactla. Journal of Animal Ecology* 35:269-279.
Cowan, D.P.
    1991   The solitary and presocial Vespidae. In K.G. Ross and R.W. Matthew, eds., *The Social Biology of Wasps.* Ithaca, NY: Comstock Publishing Associates.
Cutler, R.G.
    1976   Evolution of longevity in primates. *Journal of Human Evolution* 5:169-202.
Danforth, N.J., L. Neff, and P. Baretto-Ko
    1996   Nestmate relatedness in a communal bee, *Perdita texana* (Hymenoptera:Andrenidae), based on DNA fingerprinting. *Evolution* 50:276-284.
Deevey, E. S., Jr.
    1947   Life tables for natural populations of animals. *Quarterly Review of Biology* 22:283-314.
De Steven, D.
    1978   Clutch size, breeding success and parental survival in the tree sparrow (*Iridoprocne bicolor*). *Evolution* 34:278-291.
Diamond, J.
    1996   Why women change. *Discover* 17:131-137.
DiSilvestro, R.L.
    1991   *The African Elephant: Twilight in Eden.* New York: John Wiley and Sons, Inc.
Douglas-Hamilton, I.
    1987   African elephants: population trends and their causes. *Oryx* 21:11-24.
Dugatkin, L.A.
    1995   Formalizing Allee's ideas on dominance hierarchies: an intrademic selection model. *The American Naturalist* 146(6):954-960.
Dunbar, R.I.M.
    1988   *Primate Social Systems.* London: Christopher Helm.
Edwards, R.
    1980   *Social Wasps. Their Biology and Control.* East Grinstead, England: Rentokil Limited.
Eltringham, S.K.
    1982   *Elephants.* Poole: Blandford Press.
Estes, R.D.
    1991   *The Behavior Guide to African Mammals, Including Hoofed Mammals, Carnivores, and Primates.* Berkeley, CA: University of California Press.

Evans, H.E.
 1958   The evolution of social life in wasps. *Proceedings of the 10th International Congress on Entomology, (Montreal, 1956)* 2:449-457.
 1966   *The Comparative Ethology and Evolution of the Wasps.* Cambridge, MA: Harvard University Press.
Evans, H.E., and M.J. West-Eberhard
 1970   *The Wasps.* Ann Arbor, MI: University of Michigan Press.
Fairbanks, L.A., and M.T. McGuire
 1986   Age, reproductive value, and dominance-related behaviour in vervet monkey females: cross-generational influences on social relationships and reproduction. *Animal Behavior* 34:1710-1721.
Fatti, L.P., G.L. Smuts, A.M. Starfield, and A.A. Spurdle
 1980   Age determination in African elephants. *Journal of Mammology* 61(3): 547-551.
Finch, C.E., and R.E. Ricklefs
 1991   Age structure of populations. *Science* 254:779.
Freeman, D.
 1980   *Elephants: the Vanishing Giants.* Hong Kong: Bison Books Limited.
Gingerich, P.D., S.M. Raza, M. Arif, M. Anwar, and X. Zhou
 1994   New whale from the Eocene of Pakistan and the origin of cetacean swimming. *Nature* 368:844-847.
Goodall, J.
 1986   *The Chimpanzees of Gombe.* Cambridge, MA: Belknap Press.
Gosling, L.M.
 1982   A reassessment of the function of scent marking in territories. *Zeitschrift fur Tierpsychologie* 60:89-118.
Greenberg, B.
 1947   Some relations between territory, social hierarchy, and leadership in the green sunfish (*Lepomis cyanellus*). *Physiological Zoology* 20:267-299.
Guhl, A.M.
 1968   Social inertia and social stability in chickens. *Animal Behaviour* 16(2,3):219-232.
Guhl, A.M., and W.C. Allee
 1945   Some measurable effects of social organization in flocks of hens. *Physiological Zoology* 17:320-347.
Hamilton, W.D.
 1964   The genetical evolution of social behavior. *Journal of Theoretical Biology* 7:1.
 1966   The moulding of senescence by the natural selection. *Journal of Theoretical Biology* 21(1):12-45.
Hanks, J.
 1973   Population dynamics of the African elephant (*Loxodonta africana*). *Journal of Zoology (London)* 169:29-38.
 1979   *The Struggle for Survival: The Elephant Problem.* New York: Mayflower Books.
Harvey, P.H., R.D. Martin, and T.H. Clutton-Brock
 1987   Life histories in comparative perspective. In B.B. Smuts, D.L. Cheney, R.M. Seyfarth, R.W. Wrangham, and T.T. Struhsaker, eds., *Primate Societies.* Chicago: University of Chicago Press.
Hayflick, L.
 1994   *How and Why We Age.* New York: Ballantine Books.
Hayley, D.H.
 1978   Cetaceans. In D. Hayley, ed., *Marine Mammals of Eastern North Pacific and Arctic Waters.* Seattle, WA: Pacific Search Press.

Hölldobler, B., and E. O. Wilson
  1990   *The Ants.* Cambridge, MA: Belknap Press of Harvard University Press.
Hrdy, S.H.
  1977   *The Langurs of Abu.* Cambridge, MA: Harvard University Press.
  1981   "Nepotists" and "altruists": the behavior of old females among macaques and langur monkeys. In P.T. Amoss and S. Harrell, eds., *Other Ways of Growing Old: Anthropological Perspectives.* Stanford, CA: Stanford University Press.
Izquierdo, J.I.
  1991   How does *Drosophila melanogaster* overwinter? *Entomolgia Experimentalis et Applicata* 59:51-58.
Jayakar, S.D., and H. Spurway
  1966   Re-use of cells and brother-sister mating in the Indian species *Stenodynerus miniatus* (Sauss.) (Vespidae: Eumenidae). *Journal of the Bombay Natural History Society* 63:378-398.
Jeanne, R.L.
  1991   The swarm-founding Polistinae. In K.G. Ross and R.W. Matthews, eds., *The Social Biology of Wasps,* Ithaca, NY: Comstock Publishing Associates.
Johnson, C.M., and K.S. Norris
  1994   Social behavior. In K.S. Norris, B. Wursig, R.S. Wells, and M. Wursig, eds., *The Hawaiian Spinner Dolphin.* Berkeley, CA: University of California Press.
Kasuya, T., and H. Marsh
  1984   Life history and reproductive biology of the short-finned pilot whale, *Globicephala macrorhynchus,* off the Pacific Coast of Japan. *Report of the International Whaling Commission* (Special Issue) 6: 259-310.
Kirkwood, T.B.L.
  1985   Comparative and evolutionary aspects of longevity. In C.E. Finch and E.L. Schneider, eds., *Handbook of the Biology of Aging,* 2nd ed. New York: Van Nostrand Reinhold Co.
Kluijver, H.N., and L. Tinbergen
  1953   Territory and the regulation of density in titmice. *Archives Néerlandaises de Zoologie, Leydig* 10(3):265-289.
Lack, D.
  1968   *Ecological Adaptations for Breeding in Birds.* London: Methuen and Company.
Lawley, L.
  1994   *The World of Elephants.* New York: Freidman/Fairfax Publishers.
Laws, R.M.
  1966   Age criteria for the African elephant, *Loxodonta a. africana. East African Wildlife Journal* 4:1-37.
  1970   Elephants as agents of habitat and landscape change in East Africa. *Oikos* 21:1-15.
Laws, R.M., I.S.C. Parker, and R.C.B. Johnstone
  1975   *Elephants and their Habitats: The Ecology of Elephants in North Bunyoro, Uganda.* Oxford: Clarendon Press.
Leatherwood, S., and R.R. Reeves
  1978   Porpoises and Dolphins. In D. Haley, ed., *Marine Mammals of Eastern North Pacific and Arctic Waters.* Seattle, WA: Pacific Search Press.
Lotka, A.J.
  1907   Relation between birth rates and death rates. *Science* 26:12-22.
Lovejoy, C.O.
  1981   The origin of man. *Science* 211:341-350.
Matthew, R.W.
  1991   Evolution of social behavior in Sphecid wasps. In K.G. Ross and R.W. Matthew, eds., *The Social Biology of Wasps.* Ithaca, NY: Comstock Publishing Associates.

Maxim, P.E.
  1979   Social behavior. In D.M. Bowden, ed., *Aging in Nonhuman Primates*. New York: Van
          Nostrand Reinhold Company.
Medawar, P.B.
  1957   *The Uniqueness of the Individual, 2nd ed*. New York: Dover Publications, Inc.
Milinkovitch, M.C., A. Meyer, and J.R. Powell
  1994   Phylogeny of all major groups of cetaceans based on DNA sequences from three mito-
          chondrial genes. *Molecular Biology and Evolution* 11(6): 939-944.
Norris, K.S., and K. Pryor
  1991   Some thoughts on grandmothers. In K. Pryor and K.S. Norris, eds., *Dolphin Societies:
          Discoveries and Puzzles*. Berkeley, CA: University of California Press.
Novacek, M.J.
  1994   Whales leave the beach. *Nature* 368:807.
Oster, G., and E.O. Wilson
  1978   *Caste and Ecology in the Social Insects*. Princeton, NJ: Princeton University Press.
Owens, D., and M. Owens
  1992   *The Eye of the Elephant*. Boston, MA: Houghton Mifflin Company.
Poole, J.H.
  1987   Elephants in musth, lust. *Natural History* November:46-55.
  1994   Sex differences in the behavior of African elephants. In R.V. Short and E. Balaban, eds.,
          The Differences Between the Sexes. Cambridge: Cambridge University Press.
Poole, J.H., and C.J. Moss
  1981   Musth in the African elephant, *Loxodonta africana*. *Nature* 292:830-831.
  1989   Elephant mate searching: group dynamics and vocal and olfactory communication. *Sym-
          posia of the Zoological Society of London* 61:111-125.
Redmond, I.
  1991   With elephants underground. In R. Orenstein, ed., *Elephants: Saving the Gentle Giants*.
          Toronto, Canada: Key Porter Books Ltd.
Reilly, S.B.
  1978   Pilot whale. In D. Hayley, ed., *Marine Mammals of Eastern North Pacific and Arctic
          Waters*. Seattle, WA: Pacific Search Press.
Riley, M.W.
  1979   Introduction. Life-course perspectives. In M.W. Riley, ed., *Aging From Birth to Death:
          Interdisciplinary Perspectives* Vol. I. AAAS Symposium 30. Boulder, CO: Westview
          Press.
Riley, M., and J. Riley, Jr.
  1986   Longevity and social structure: the added years. *Daedalus* 115:51.
Roff, D.
  1992   *The Evolution of Life Histories*. New York: Chapman and Hall.
Rose, M.
  1991   *Evolutionary Biology of Aging*. New York: Oxford University Press.
Rosenberg, A.
  1992   Altruism: theoretical contexts. In E.F. Keller and E.A. Lloyd, eds., *Keywords in Evolu-
          tionary Biology*. Cambridge, MA: Harvard University Press.
Seeley, T.
  1985   *Honeybee Ecology*. Princeton, NJ: Princeton University Press.
Shoshani, J.
  1991   Last of a noble line. In R. Orenstein, ed., *Elephants: Saving the Gentle Giants*. Toronto,
          Canada: Key Porter Books Ltd.

Sikes, S.K.
  1967   The African elephant, *Loxodonta africana*: a field method for the estimation of age. *Journal of Zoology (London)* 154:235-248.
  1971   *The Natural History of the African Elephant*. New York: American Elsevier Publishing Company, Inc.
Silverstone, B.
  1996   Older people of tomorrow: a psychosocial profile. *The Gerontologist* 36:27-32.
Stewart, K.J., and A.H. Harcourt
  1987   Gorillas: variation in female relationships. In B.B. Smuts, D.L. Cheney, R.M. Seyfarth, R.W. Wrangham, and T.T. Struhsaker, eds., *Primate Societies*. Chicago: University of Chicago Press.
Strickberger, M.W.
  1996   *Evolution*, 2nd ed. Boston, MA: Jones and Bartlett Publishers.
Sukumar, R.
  1989   *The Asian Elephant: Ecology and Management*. Cambridge: Cambridge University Press.
Timiras, P.S.
  1994   *Physiological Basis of Aging and Geriatrics*, 2nd ed. Boca Raton, FL: CRC Press.
Tyack, P.
  1986   Population biology, social behavior, and communication in whales and dolphins. *Trends in Ecology and Evolution* 1(6):144-150.
Van Lawick-Goodall, J.
  1976   Continuities between chimpanzee and human behavior. In G.L. Isaac and E.R. McCown, eds., *Human Origins: Louis Leakey and the East African Evidence*. Menlo Park, CA: Benjamin.
Wells, R.S.
  1991   The role of long-term study in understanding the social structure of a bottlenose dolphin community. In K. Pryor and K.S. Norris, eds., *Dolphin Societies: Discoveries and Puzzles*. Berkeley, CA: University of California Press.
Wenzel, J.W.
  1991   Evolution of nest architecture. In K.G. Ross and R.W. Matthews, eds., *The Social Biology of Wasps*. Ithaca, NY: Comstock Publishing Associates.
Williams, G.C.
  1957   Pleiotropy, natural selection and the evolution of senescence. *Evolution* 11:11-21.
Wilson, E.O.
  1975   *Sociobiology: the New Synthesis*. Cambridge, MA: Harvard University Press.
Wrangham, R.W.
  1980   An ecological model of female-bonded primate groups. *Behaviour* 75:262-300.

9

Postreproductive Survival

Steven N. Austad

POSTREPRODUCTIVE SURVIVAL IN NATURE

Women in modern societies can expect to live nearly one-third of their adult lives in a postreproductive state. Whether this phenomenon is relatively new in human experience or whether it represents something that has been a part of human life for millennia may be relevant to understanding medical and social issues surrounding postmenopausal life. One approach to an understanding of the human significance of menopause is to examine it comparatively. How commonly is postreproductive life found in nature, and under what circumstances is it found? Is there a reason to assume that humans are somehow special in this regard?

Some of the special pleading for a novel evolutionary explanation for complete reproductive cessation and a long postreproductive life in human females derives from the misimpression that the more rapid senescent decline in reproductive capacity in women relative to men is a life-history feature unique to humans (Hill and Hurtado, 1991; Lancaster and King, 1992). On the contrary, such a pattern is common among well-maintained captive species such as laboratory rats (Austad, 1994) (see Figure 9-1).

This pattern is not surprising given the dynamics of oocyte formation and depletion in mammals. With possibly a few exceptions, female mammals do not exhibit continuous oocyte formation. Oocyte formation is terminated either before birth or shortly after, so there is a finite oocyte pool that is gradually depleted during life (see Finch, 1990, for details). Given this constraint on oocyte numbers, it would make evolutionary sense to assume that natural selection would ensure that sufficient oocytes were produced initially and that the rate of deple-

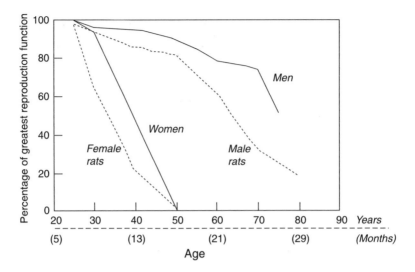

FIGURE 9-1 Comparison between humans and captive rats in sex-specific reproductive senescence.

tion is such that oocytes would be available at least as long as animals could expect to live *under natural conditions* (that is, under the conditions that this physiology evolved) unless there were some adaptive advantage to ceasing reproduction before death.

Consistent with this logic, physiologically postreproductive individuals are very rarely found in nature except in a few species (described below). This is not to say that long intensive field studies will not occasionally identify postreproductive individuals (e.g., Waser, 1978), only that they should always be rare. A typical example is the study of great tits (*Parus major*) in Wytham Woods near Oxford, U.K., where analysis of demographic data collected over 18 years suggests that 7-year-old females and 8-year-old males may be physiologically postreproductive. But for every thousand females or males fledged, only four females and two males will survive to postreproductive ages, respectively (McCleery and Perrins, 1988).

By contrast, male gamete production is continuous throughout life. Therefore under captive conditions in which the major sources of natural mortality are removed as life span is much extended, it is not surprising that males continue to be reproductively competent somewhat longer than females.

While it is true that menopause in nonhuman primates occurs only near the end of life under captivity (van Wagenan, 1972; Nozaki et al., 1995), this may reflect more about the current state of primate husbandry than about differences among primates in reproductive cessation.

A type of postreproductive condition that is much more common in nature than physiological reproductive cessation, especially among strongly polygynous species, is age-related, behaviorally imposed reproductive cessation. For instance, when aging males can no longer successfully defend a harem against younger male competitors, reproduction ceases, not from senile sterility but from lack of opportunity. This is apparently true for red deer (*Cervus elaphus*) stags at age 11 or greater on the Scots island of Rhum (Clutton-Brock et al., 1988). In this type of case, postreproductive individuals are not necessarily expected to be rare. Thus, fully 20 percent of all red deer stags born on Rhum are still alive at an age when at least some individuals are behaviorally postreproductive (Clutton-Brock et al., 1988). The loss of blatantly physical competitive ability with age is explicable from standard analyses of the evolution of senescence. It requires no special interpretation and will not be discussed further.

In striking contrast to the rarity of physiologically postreproductive individuals in nature, such animals are often common in captivity (vom Saal and Finch, 1988). This fact is not surprising. Animals in captivity are protected from food and water shortages, environmental extremes, predators, and many pathogens. Consequently, they live much longer than in nature and, in fact, can frequently outlive the period over which natural selection has molded their reproductive physiology to remain intact. A well-documented example of this situation is the house mouse (*Mus musculus*), which in nature lives about 4 months, on average, and has 90 percent mortality by 9-10 months of age (Phelan and Austad, 1989). In the laboratory, of course, house mice average 2+ years of life (Myers, 1978), and females begin becoming postreproductive near the end of their first year of life, about the time they would almost certainly be dead in nature. Some information suggests that wild-type house mouse females can remain reproductively active until almost 2 years (Sacher and Hart, 1978).

Among our closest relatives, the other primates, a similar condition prevails—physiologically postreproductive individuals are rare to nonexistent in nature but occur in significant numbers in captivity. Japanese (*Macaca fuscata*) and rhesus macaques (*Macaca mulatta*), for instance, begin to experience female reproductive decline at about age 20 and undergo menopause at about 27 and 30 years, respectively (Nozaki et al., 1995; van Wagenan, 1972). But even in human-protected and food-provisioned semi-natural populations, median survival is less than 5 and 10 years, respectively, with maximum survival less than 25 years (Dunbar, 1986). Therefore, as in other mammals, the commonness of captive postreproductive survival is a consequence of increased captive longevity with no evolutionary significance. These animals were simply not physiologically designed for such a long survival.

Significantly though, there do seem to be at least a few species in nature in which postreproductive survival is relatively common. The best-documented example is female short-finned pilot whales, *Globicephala macrorhynchus*, in which 24 percent of all females born have been reported to live past the physiological end of reproduction (Marsh and Kasuya, 1984; see Table 9-1). The life

TABLE 9-1 Paleo-humans Compared with Cetaceans Known to Have a
Natural Postreproductive Life

Trait	Human	Killer Whale	Pilot Whale
Proportion living to postreproductive ages (%)	5-25[a]	29	24
Life expectancy at end of reproduction (years)	3-22	26	14
Age at maturity (years)	15-19	15	9-18
Period of obligatory offspring care (years)	10-12	?	?

[a]Lower estimates for humans come from paleodemographers, who estimate age at death from osteological cues, whereas higher estimates come from the study of modern hunter-gatherers. Conclusions of these two groups of researchers dramatically differ. SOURCES: Marsh and Kasuya (1984), Kasuya and Marsh (1984), and Olesiuk et al. (1990).

expectancy of females at the end of their reproductive lives is 14 years (Kasuya and Marsh, 1984). Although not confirmed by ovarian histology, as in the pilot whales, detailed long-term observations and demographic analyses of resident killer whales along the northwestern coast of North America suggest that in a stable population about 30 percent of females born will live to become postreproductive and that their life expectancy at the end of reproduction will be more than 25 years (Olesiuk et al., 1990). A significant female postreproductive life is also suspected in several other species of toothed whales (Marsh and Kasuya, 1986). Life expectancy and maximum reported age is dramatically shorter in males relative to females in both pilot and killer whales.

In neither of these cetacean species is there any evidence that mortality rates have plunged recently, so this long period of postreproductive life does seem to be a product of natural selection rather than an artifact of a recent rapid increase in longevity.

Several hypotheses have been advanced to explain common postreproductive female survival; all assume that at some age it becomes more evolutionarily advantageous to redirect energy from continued personal reproduction to facilitating the survival and/or reproduction of existing offspring. Note that these hypotheses agree in predicting that postreproductive individuals will be actively involved in helping younger individuals.

The logic of hypotheses for adaptive postreproductive survival is that as the risk of reproductive failure and/or death increases with age in species with an extended obligatory period of postnatal parental care, there will eventually come an age when the expected fitness gain of attempted personal reproduction will be lower than that available from redirecting energy toward rearing the last-born offspring to independence and/or assisting already-independent progeny with *their* reproduction. Specific quantitative models of adaptive menopause reveal that the conditions under which it is favored are stringent, however, requiring enormously effective assistance of young individuals by postreproductive females (Hill and Hurtado, 1991; Rogers, 1993).

Although relatively little is known about the social system of pilot whales or killer whales, existing knowledge *is* consistent with such adaptive hypotheses. Pilot whales live in breeding schools of a few to a few dozen individuals, with females thought to remain in their natal school throughout their lives. Therefore breeding schools are matrilineal kin groups. Females mature at 9 years of age (range: 7-12) and produce an average of four to five calves before ceasing reproduction at 30-40 years of age (Kasuya and Marsh, 1984). Males are probably functionally mature by age 16 but may not mate for several years after this. Calves of young females are nursed for 2+ years, but as females approach the end of reproduction, the duration of nursing increases substantially, so that postreproductive mothers wean their daughters at ages up to 8 years and wean their sons at up to 15 years. In either case, weaning occurs as the reproductive age of the calf is approached—long past the end of their mother's reproductive potential.

Killer whales similarly live in multigenerational groups. Pods averaged 10-26 individuals in the northern and southern coastal study populations (Olesiuk et al., 1990), and *neither* males nor females are thought to emigrate from their natal pod (Bigg et al., 1990). Both sexes reach sexual maturity at about 15 years of age. Females produce a calf at about 6-year intervals and become postreproductive at about age 40. Information about lactational duration of older females specifically or other types of parental care in killer whales is lacking, although that lactation is known to last for only about 2 years in younger mothers, and calves travel and rest close to their mothers for at least 6 years. When a female has a second calf before the previous one is sexually mature, an "auntie" (who may be postreproductive) will assume a pseudomaternal role and spend a great deal of time with the older calf (Haenel, 1986).

The potential growth and survival advantages of reliable maternal resources to their own offspring is self-evident, and postreproductive females are likely to have three or more generations of kin in the same social group. Simultaneous assistance to several generations of descendant and nondescendent kin is therefore possible. It is notable in this regard that one of the other whale species with suggestions of postreproductive female life (the sperm whale, *Physeter macrocephalus*) also lives in stable cohesive multigenerational female kinship groups (Marsh and Kasuya, 1986).

Modern human females, of course, also have a widespread and extensive postreproductive life. However whether this postreproductive life is an adaptive consequence of natural selection, as in short-finned pilot whales, or is a non-adaptive artifact of the rapid increase in longevity over the past few centuries analogous to the postreproductive life of captive animals has been controversial (for an alternative interpretation from that found here, see Nesse and Williams, 1994). The potential significance of this issue is not merely abstract or trivial. If menopause represents an artifact of modern life, then it also probably represents an uncontrolled degenerative loss of homeostasis associated with senescence. In this case, one cannot assume that the normal menopausal hyposteroidal state will facilitate optimum health. Hormonal intervention may be expected to improve overall postreproductive health. Indeed, the ability of postmenopausal hormone-replacement therapy to mitigate some life-threatening conditions, such as accelerated bone thinning and an accelerating risk of cardiovascular disease (Marshburn and Carr, 1994), and reduce overall mortality rate (Gura, 1995; Ettinger et al., 1996) might be considered evidence for this interpretation. In this case, there is also no reason to suppose that an uncontrolled degenerative loss of homeostasis will proceed similarly from species to species, and there is no reason to suppose that rodent or even primate models of the postreproductive state will provide revealing mechanistic details of the postreproductive state in humans.

On the other hand, if menopause *is* an adaptive physiological state molded by evolution to maximize fitness in the face of generalized senescence, then natural selection would presumably have tailored postreproductive physiology to the hyposteroidal state, suggesting that medical interventions to alleviate menopausal conditions should be approached with considerably more caution.

To what extent did humans in our evolutionary past have life histories similar to those of modern cetaceans with a known postreproductive existence (Table 9-1)?

Any hypothesis of adaptive human menopause requires at least two types of supporting evidence. First, it must be established that humans before recent medical and public health advances lived long enough for menopausal years to be a common part of life. Otherwise, selection would have no opportunity to favor the putative adaptations of postmenopausal existence. Second, it must be established that postreproductive females can provide sufficient help to their younger kin to offset the reproduction they forfeited when menopause occurred. That there is considerable consistency in the age of menopause (about 45-50 years, on average) across cultures and environments does not seem relevant to this issue, given the rather deterministic dynamics of mammalian oocyte depletion.

The evidence relevant to preagricultural survival is dichotomous. Researchers studying living peoples without apparent access to the obvious benefits of modern medicine and hygiene such as the !Kung San of the Kalahari Desert or the Aché of the Paraguayan forests find that as many as 30-40 percent of women survive into their postreproductive years (Hill and Hurtado, 1991) (Figure 9-2) and that life expectancy at the age of menopause is about 20 years. On the other hand, paleodemographers, who estimate the demography of past human periods such as among Paleolithic hunter-gatherers (Weiss, 1973) or primitive agricultur-

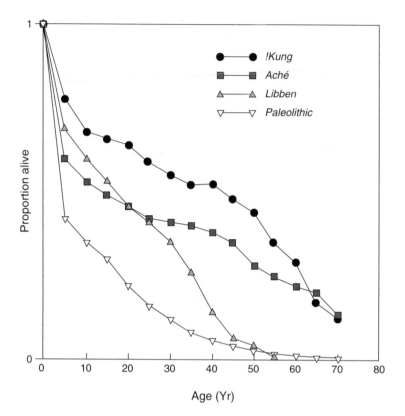

Age (Yr)

FIGURE 9-2 Survivorship estimates of some living (!Kung and Aché) and nonliving (Libben and Paleolithic) nontechnological populations. Estimates for living populations were made from personal interviews; estimates for nonliving populations were made from osteological examination of cemetary remains. SOURCES: Lovejoy et al. (1977), Howell (1979), Weiss (1973), and Hill and Hurtado (1991).

alists (Lovejoy et al., 1977) reach just as unanimous a conclusion that humans until recently did not live into their postreproductive years except very rarely. This disagreement may be unresolvable. Living nontechnological peoples may be more influenced by modernity than researchers imagine, or conversely there may be systematic errors in the age estimation of very old skeletal remains. With such a fundamental contradiction in evidence, this aspect of the adaptive menopause hypothesis must await further evidence.

The second aspect of the hypothesis—whether postreproductive females, if alive, could provide sufficient help to kin to offset their own potential reproduction—has been approached primarily from a theoretical perspective. For instance, a model by Hill and Hurtado (1991), combined with the demography they collected from the forest-dwelling Aché suggested that even given the higher estimates of human survival that anthropologists studying modern hunter-gatherers find, postreproductive women did not provide enough assistance to offset the potential personal reproduction lost due to menopause. The model assumed that hypothetical women who did not undergo menopause would still experience a reproductive decline, such that fertility by age 65 would be 43 percent of maximum fertility and that increased maternal death risk at later ages had a trivial demographic impact. Nevertheless, the authors were hesitant to conclude that menopause was nonadaptive and theorized that *if* in the past older women could have improved the survival of their children and grandchildren more than they were doing at present, *if* they also improved the survival of relatives in addition to their own children and grandchildren, and *if* older women were more likely than observed to die in childbirth, then evolution might indeed have favored an adaptive menopause. A ringing endorsement of adaptive menopause this clearly isn't!

A somewhat different approach was used by Rogers (1993), who used the particularly detailed demographic information from Chinese farmers in turn-of-the-century Taiwan as a surrogate demographic model of Paleolithic human life to ask mathematically exactly how much help postreproductive mothers would have had to provide to their children for adaptive menopause to have evolved. His analytical model addressed effects on both survival and fertility for several generations of descendents. He assumed that the costs of continued fertility past menopause were due to either an increased probability of death during childbirth, a reduced ability of a mother to care for her older existing offspring, or a combination of both of these effects. His analysis revealed that the presence of a postmenopausal "mother" would have had to double the number of children all of *her* children had and completely eliminate infant deaths for evolution to have produced menopause by natural selection. As in Hill and Hurtado's model, the conditions favoring adaptive menopause seemed unlikely to hold. Unfortunately, whales have not been similarly analyzed to date.

Although this issue must remain unresolved at present, there is certainly no compelling reason to believe that human menopause is the adaptive result of selection for reproductive cessation. We seem to resemble laboratory mice more than killer whales.

THE ROLE OF THE ELDERLY IN NATURE

This thesis is not to say that elderly humans and other mammals do not have specialized roles in nature. But we need an instructive definition of what "elderly" means. If, as was formerly often assumed, animals did not exhibit senescence in nature (as measured by a mortality rate unrelated to age), then the concept of elderly is meaningless, because no matter what age an animal achieves, its expectation of further life remains undiminished. However, measurable senescence among mammals and birds now appears widespread in nature (Promislow, 1991; Holmes and Austad, 1995), so that even though a postreproductive existence or the type of extreme senile debilitation found in captive animals and some elderly humans still appears rare, older animals often clearly have reduced expectation of life compared with younger animals. Thus in many natural populations, demographic studies allow the definition of ages beyond which animals will probably not survive, at which the likelihood of death is substantially increased, and those ages might sensibly be considered elderly, regardless of whether those animals are obviously debilitated at that time in life.

Given this definition of elderly, animals that acquire or accumulate important resources such as food caches, complex and costly burrow systems or nests, or foraging and breeding territories during their lifetime will inevitably influence their own reproductive success and the ultimate genetic structure of populations by the manner in which those resources are disposed of as they approach the end of life—specifically, whether those resources will be available to offspring.

The material value of some of these resources are considerable. For instance, all bannertail kangaroo rats (*Dipodomys specabilis*) require mounds in which to live. These mounds consist of an intricate burrow system and massive quantities of hoarded seeds. Mounds persist for much longer than the life of any individual, probably for decades. Construction of new mounds requires as long as 2 years (Best, 1972) and thus is rarely initiated (Holdenreid, 1957). Therefore sharing such a mound or somehow bequeathing it to one's offspring obviates their need to obtain a mound of their own.

Possible scenarios of the transfer of important material resources include (1) preventing adult offspring from making use of the resource at all, which I will call *evicting them*; (2) *sharing* the resource with adult offspring, which has the effect of *bequeathing* it upon their death; or (3) *relinquishing* resources to their offspring, while they are still alive and thereby sacrificing their own prospects to those of their offspring. Scenario 1 is most costly to offspring in terms of energy and risk associated with achieving independence. This risk can be substantial, particularly for small mammals. Female water voles (*Arvicola terrestris*), for instance, suffer 86 times the risk of predation when dispersing as when remaining in their natal home range (Leuze, 1980). Scenario 2 will be minimally costly to a parent and maximally beneficial to offspring if the expectation of continued parental life is low. Thus this pattern might be expected when overall mortality rates are high. In a high-mortality environment, the effect of resource transfer converges in scenario 2 and scenario 3. However, if a parent is likely to continue living, scenario 3 can be more or less costly than 2, depending upon the quality of the resources relinquished relative to those held. I will discuss representative examples of each of these scenarios in turn.

Eviction of Young from Resources Controlled by the Elderly

Any parentally forced dispersal from the parental home range would fall into this classification. Eviction not only has the effect of preventing one generation from acquiring resources accumulated by the previous generation but also it places them at substantial risk while searching for new resources. In fact, when large amounts of resources are accumulated during one generation, parents will probably allow their offspring access to these resources well into adult life, unless their own life expectancy is still substantial. On the other hand, when life expectancy *is* still substantial, one might expect parental eviction of offspring to avoid direct competition for those resources. Indeed there is an encyclopedic literature (summarized in Baker, 1978) on the timing and extent of forced dispersal, but elderly individuals are by definition those with low life expectancy. Therefore, I expect that eviction of offspring will be rare among elderly animals. Systematic information on this sort of question has not been collected, mainly because field biologists have assumed that senescence is irrelevant to animals in the wild.

Bequeathing Resources to Young

Some mammals, at least occasionally, share access to valuable material resources with their offspring. For instance, bannertail kangaroo rat females frequently allow offspring, potentially of either sex, to share their home mounds (Jones, 1987). Thus a 3- or 4-year-old female who has a low life expectancy and shares a mound with her offspring is ultimately making a decision to bequeath them that mound. In a population in southeastern Arizona, 37 percent of males remained in their natal mound into adulthood, and 70 percent of these remained throughout their lives. Twenty-three percent of females remained in their natal mounds into adulthood, and 72 percent of these remained for their entire lives. Because mound improvement and renewing of cached seeds occur throughout life, resources acquired during the lifetime of females are passed along to their offspring. No information exists on whether males bequeath mounds to their offspring (Jones, 1987); however, it is improbable that males of this polygynous species can even recognize their own offspring.

In many species, this sort of resource bequeathing is sex-biased. As a gross generality, males are more apt to be bequeathed valuable resources such as nests, dens, or territories in birds, whereas females are more apt to inherit such resources in mammals (Greenwood, 1980). Thus in many communally breeding birds that defend valuable territories, territory ownership is passed down male lineages. For instance, among stripe-backed wrens (*Campylorhynchus nuchalis*), 60 percent of breeding males gained breeding status on their natal territory compared with 3 percent of breeding females (Rabenold, 1990). Conversely, among black-tailed prairie dogs (*Cynomys ludovicianus*) in Kansas, 98 percent of females bred in their natal coterie compared with 0 percent of males. The advantages of male-biased versus female-biased dispersal are still unresolved, but such dispersal is assumed to be related to aspects of mating system (Greenwood, 1980; Waser and Jones, 1983). It is generally assumed that dispersal of one sex is necessary to avoid close inbreeding between parents and offspring or among siblings (Shields, 1982).

Relinquishing Resources to Offspring

Even if life expectancy is low, there is some finite chance of survival through one or more additional breeding episodes. In spite of this, adults of some species relinquish some or all of their existing resources to their offspring. For instance, adult female black bears (*Ursus americanus*) frequently shift their territories away from areas that overlap with their daughters, effectively reducing their own foraging area (Rogers, 1987). Daughters that are the recipients of territory in this manner grow at a faster rate than females that must acquire their own territory. Female wood rats sometimes completely abandon their middens to their young (Fitch and Rainey, 1956), apparently an even larger personal sacrifice than in black bears, but the consequences for either mother or daughter have not been investigated.

Because field biologists have generally not been interested in problems of aging, little evidence as to the adaptive nature of intergenerational resource transfer has accumulated. The possibilities are intriguing, however. For instance, if in a species such as the banner-tailed kangaroo rat, in which parents sometimes allow offspring to share their mound and sometimes do not, it is possible that such a decision is based on the life expectancy or senescent stage of that parent. Thus, parents that have begun to senesce and are consequently not likely to live much longer, would be more likely to allow mound sharing as a form of bequeathing the mound to their offspring. This sort of senescence-related question has yet to be specifically addressed by field biologists. To the extent that it is addressed in the coming years, a generalized theory of the ecology of resource transfer across generations may emerge.

REFERENCES

Austad, S.N.
    1994   Menopause: an evolutionary perspective. *Experimental Gerontology* 29:255-263.
Baker, R.R.
    1978   *The Evolutionary Ecology of Animal Migration.* London: Hodder and Stroughton.
Best, T.L.
    1972   Mound development by a pioneer population of the banner-tailed kangaroo rat *Dipodomus spectabilis bailey* Goldman, in eastern New Mexico. *America Midland Naturalist* 87:201-206.
Bigg, M.A., P.F. Olesiuk, G.M. Ellis, J.K.B. Ford, and K.C. Balcomb III
    1990   Social organization and geneology of resident killer whales (*Orcinus-orca*) in the coastal waters of British Columbia Canada and Washington State USA. *Report of the International Whaling Commission* (Special Issue 12). Cambridge, England: International Whaling Commission.

Clutton-Brock, T.H., S.D. Albon, and F.E. Guinness
1988   Reproductive success in male and female red deer. In T.H. Clutton-Brock, ed., *Reproductive Success*. Chicago: University of Chicago Press.

Dunbar, R.I.M.
1986   Demography and reproduction. In B.B. Smuts, D.L. Cheney, R.M. Seyfarth, R.W. Wrangham, and T.T. Struhsaker, eds., *Primate Societies*. Chicago: University of Chicago Press.

Ettinger, B., G.D. Friedman, T. Bush, and C.P. Quesenberry, Jr.
1996   Reduced mortality associated with long-term postmenopausal estrogen therapy. *Obstetrics and Gynecology* 87:6-12.

Finch, C. E.
1990   *Longevity, Senescence, and the Genome*. Chicago: University of Chicago Press.

Fitch, H.S., and D.C. Rainey
1956   Ecological observations on the wood rat, *Neotoma floridana*. *University of Kansas Publications, Museum of Natural History* 8:499-533.

Greenwood, P.J.
1980   Mating systems, philopatry and dispersal in birds and mammals. *Animal Behaviour* 28:1140-1162.

Gura, T.
1995   Estrogen: key player in heart disease among women. *Science* 269:771-773.

Haenel, N.J.
1986   General notes on the behavioral ontogeny of Puget Sound killer whales and the occurrence of allomaternal behavior. In B.C. Kirkevold and J.S. Lockard, eds., *Behavioral Biology of Killer Whales*. New York: Alan R. Liss.

Hamilton, W.D.
1966   The moulding of senescence by natural selection. *Journal of Theoretical Biology* 12:12-45.

Hill, K., and A.M. Hurtado
1991   The evolution of premature reproductive senescence and menopause in human females: an evaluation of the "grandmother hypothesis." *Human Nature* 2:313-350.

Holdenreid, R.
1957   Natural history of the banner-tailed kangaroo rat in New Mexico. *Journal of Mammalogy* 38:330-350.

Holmes, D.J., and S.N. Austad
1995   Birds as animal models for the comparative biology of aging: A prospectus. *Journal of Gerontology and Biological Science* 50A:B59-B66.

Howell, N.
1979   *Demography of the Dobe !Kung*. New York: Academic Press.

Jones, W.T.
1987   Dispersal patterns in kangaroo rats. In B.D. Chepko-Sade and Z.T. Halpin, eds., *Mammalian Dispersal Patterns*. Chicago: University of Chicago Press.

Kasuya, T., and H. Marsh
1984   Life history and reproductive biology of the short-finned pilot whale, *Globicephala macrorhynchus*, off the Pacific Coast of Japan. *Report of the International Whaling Commission* (Special Issue 6).

Lancaster, J.B., and B.J. King
1992   An evolutionary perspective on menopause. In V. Kerns and J.K. Brown, eds., *In Her Prime*. Urbana and Chicago: University of Illinois Press.

Leuze, C.C.K.
1980   The application of radio tracking and its effect on the behavioral ecology of the water vole, *Arvicola terrestris*. In C.J. Amlamer and D.W. MacDonald, eds., *A Handbook on Biotelemetry and Radio Tracking*. New York: Springer.

Lovejoy, C.O., R.S. Meindl, T.R. Pryzbeck, T.S. Barton, K.G. Heiple, and D. Kotting
1977   Paleodemography of the Libben Site, Ottawa County, Ohio. *Science* 198:291-293.
McCleery, R.H., and C.M. Perrins
1988   Lifetime reproductive success of the great tit, *Parus major*. In T.H. Clutton-Brock, ed., *Reproductive Success*. Chicago: University of Chicago Press.
Marsh, H., and T. Kasuya
1984   Changes in the ovaries of the short-finned pilot whale, *Globicephala macrorhynchus*, with age and reproductive activity. *Report of the International Whaling Commission* (Special Issue 6).
1986   Evidence for reproductive senescence in female cetaceans. *Report of the International Whaling Commission* (Special Issue 8).
Marshburn, P.B., and B.R. Carr
1994   The menopause and hormone replacement therapy. In W.R. Hazzard, E.L. Bierman, J.P. Blass, W.H. Ettinger, and J.B. Halter, eds., *Principles of Geriatric Medicine and Gerontology*, 3rd ed. New York: McGraw-Hill.
Myers, D.D.
1978   Review of disease patterns and life span in aging mice: genetic and environmental interactions. *Birth Defects: Original Article Series* 14:41-53.
Nesse, R.M., and G.C. Williams
1994   *Why We Get Sick: The New Science of Darwinian Medicine*. New York: Times Books.
Nozaki, M., F. Mitsunaga, and K. Shimizu
1995   Reproductive senescence in female Japanese monkeys (*Macaca fuscata*): Age- and season-related changes in hypothalamic-pituitary-ovarian functions and fecundity rates. *Biology of Reproduction* 52:1250-1257.
Olesiuk, P.F., M.A. Bigg, and G.M. Ellis
1990   Life history and population dynamics of resident killer whales *(Orcinus orca)* in the coast waters of British Columbia and Washington State. *Report of the International Whaling Commission* (Special Issue 12). Cambridge, England: International Whaling Commission.
Phelan, J.P., and S.N. Austad
1989   Natural selection, dietary restriction, and extended longevity. *Growth, Development and Aging* 53:4-6.
Promislow, D.E.L.
1991   Senescence in natural populations of mammals: A comparative study. *Evolution* 45:1869-1887.
Rabenold, K.N.
1990   *Campylorhynchus* wrens: The ecology of delayed dispersal and cooperation in the Venezuelan savanna. In P.B. Stacey and W.D. Koenig, eds., *Cooperative Breeding in Birds*. Cambridge, U.K.: Cambridge University Press.
Rogers, A.R.
1993   Why menopause? *Evolutionary Ecology* 7:406-420.
Rogers, L.L.
1987   Factors influencing dispersal in the black bear. In B.D. Chepko-Sade and Z.T. Halpin, eds., *Mammalian Dispersal Patterns*. Chicago: University of Chicago Press.
Sacher, G.A., and R.W. Hart
1978   Longevity, aging and comparative cellular and molecular biology of the house mouse, *Mus musculus*, and the white-footed mouse, *Peromyscus leucopus*. *Birth Defects: Original Article Series* 14:71-96.
Shields, W.
1982   *Philopatry, Inbreeding, and the Evolution of Sex*. Albany, NY: State University of New York Press.

van Wagenan, G.
 1972   Vital statistics from a breeding colony: Reproduction and pregnancy outcome in *Macaca mulatta. Journal of Medical Primatology* 1:3-28.
vom Saal, F.S., and C.E. Finch
 1988   Reproductive senescence: Phenomena and mechanisms in mammals and selected vertebrates. In E. Knobil and J. Neill et al., eds., *The Physiology of Reproduction*. New York: Raven Press, Ltd.
Waser, P.M.
 1978   Postreproductive survival and behavior in a free-ranging female mangabey. *Folia Primatologica* 29:142-160.
Waser, P.M., and W.T. Jones
 1983   Natal philopatry among solitary mammals. *Quarterly Review of Biology* 58:355-390.
Weiss, K.M.
 1973   Demographic models for anthropology. *Society for American Archaeology Memoirs* 27:1-186.

10

The Evolution of the Human Life Course

Hillard Kaplan

INTRODUCTION

This paper presents a theory of evolution of the human life course. Compared to other primates and mammals, there are at least three distinctive characteristics of human life histories: (1) an exceptionally long life span, (2) an extended period of juvenile dependence, and (3) support of reproduction by older postreproductive individuals. Because most hominid evolution occurred in the context of a hunting and gathering life style and because all well-studied hunting and gathering groups exhibit those three characteristics, the theory considers the aspects of the traditional human way of life that might account for their evolution. It proposes that those three features of the human life course are interrelated outcomes of a feeding strategy emphasizing nutrient-dense, difficult-to-acquire foods. The logic underlying this proposal is that effective adult foraging requires an extended developmental period during which production at young ages is sacrificed for increased productivity later in life. The returns to investment in development depend positively on adult survival rates, favoring increased investment in mortality reduction. An extended postreproductive, yet productive, period supports both earlier onset of reproduction by next-generation individuals and the ability to provision multiple dependent young at different stages of development. A postreproductive period depends upon menopause. Menopause may have evolved to facilitate postreproductive investment in offspring. Alternatively, it may be the result of other selective forces, such as the costs of maintaining viable oocytes for many decades. Even if menopause is the result of other selective forces, the theory may still account for the extension of life span beyond the reproductive period.

The paper begins with a basic description of available data on longevity in traditional hunting and gathering societies and the age profile of food production and consumption. These data are compared to information available on nonhuman primates with particular emphasis on chimpanzees, our closest living relatives.[1] This discussion is followed by consideration of the comparative feeding and reproductive ecologies of humans and nonhuman primates. A model is then presented to outline the major tradeoffs involved in life-history evolution. The model shows that investments in foraging efficiency and mortality reduction coevolve and affect the age pattern of investments in reproduction. Several different approaches to the evolution of menopause are then considered. The paper concludes with a discussion of the implications of the theory for historical, current, and future trends in human development and longevity.

HUMAN AND NONHUMAN PRIMATE LIFE HISTORIES: FUNDAMENTAL CHARACTERISTICS

Mortality and Longevity

Survival curves for four traditional groups and chimpanzees are presented in Figure 10-1. The Aché are a hunting and gathering group, living in the subtropical forests of eastern Paraguay, who made first peaceful contact with outsiders in the 1970s and now practice a mixed economy of hunting, gathering, horticulture, and wage labor (see Hill and Hurtado, 1996, for a detailed description of their way of life and demography as hunter-gatherers; for further information on diet and activities, see Hawkes et al., 1982; Hawkes et al., 1987; Hill and Kaplan, 1988a, b; Hill and Hawkes, 1983; Hill et al., 1985; Kaplan and Hill, 1985; Hurtado et al., 1985). The Hiwi live in the Venezuelan savanna and rely primarily on hunting and gathering roots for their subsistence (for ethnographic information on the Hiwi, see Hurtado and Hill, 1987, 1990, 1992; Hurtado et al., 1992). The !Kung were hunter-gatherers with various degrees of contact and economic relationships with other groups until the 1970s and now practice a mixed economy of hunting, gathering, farming, and wage labor (for ethnographic information on the !Kung, see Blurton Jones, 1986, 1987; Blurton Jones and Konner, 1976; Blurton Jones et al., 1994a, b; Blurton Jones et al., 1989; Draper, 1975, 1976; Draper and Cashdan, 1988; Harpending and Wandsnider, 1982; Howell, 1979; Konner and Shostak, 1987; Konner and Worthman, 1980; Lee, 1979, 1984, 1985; Lee and DeVore, 1976; Schrire, 1980; Wiessner, 1982a, b; Wilmsen, 1978, 1989; Yellen, 1976). The Yanomamo practice a mixed economy of hunting, gathering and horticulture; many Yanomamo groups have yet to make peaceful contact with outsiders (Chagnon, 1974, 1983, 1988; Hames, 1983, 1992;

---

[1]Although gorillas and bonobos (pygmy chimpanzees) may be as closely related to humans as common chimpanzees, the demographic and behavioral data on the latter are much more complete.

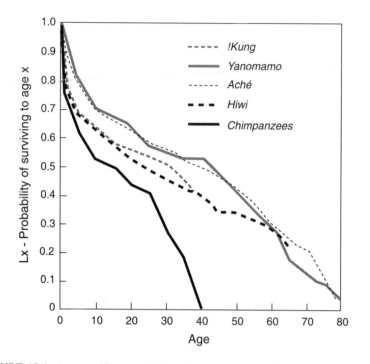

FIGURE 10-1 Age-specific probabilities of survival among human foragers and chimpanzees. SOURCE: !Kung (Howell, 1979); Yanomamo (Melancon, 1982); Aché (Hill and Hurtado, 1996); Hiwi (Hill and Hurtado, unpublished data from Kim Hill); chimpanzees (Goodall, 1986, and Courtenay and Santow, 1989).

Melancon, 1982). The chimpanzees are those living in the Gombe nature reserve (for dietary and life-historical information on chimpanzees at Gombe, see Courtenay and Santow, 1989; Goodall, 1986; Silk, 1978, 1979; Teleki, 1973; Wrangham, 1974, 1977; Wrangham and Smuts, 1980). Although sample size and methods of data collection vary among the four human groups, the survival curves show remarkable convergence. Although infant mortality rates vary, with Hiwi being the highest and Yanomamo the lowest, adult mortality rates between the ages of 20 and 45 are almost identical, about 1.5 percent per year. For that reason the survival curves are parallel to one another during the adult period. Chimpanzee survival curves, however, diverge dramatically from the human curves, due to a quite distinct adult mortality profile. For example, while both Hiwi and chimpanzees have about equal probability of reaching age 15, the conditional probability of reaching age 45, having reached age 15, is near zero for chimpanzees in the wild and about 75 percent among the Hiwi (see also Lancaster and King, 1992, for supporting data from other groups). Adult mortality rates among chimpanzees over age 25, living at the Gombe reserve, are about 7.9

percent per year (Goodall, 1986; Courtenay and Santow, 1989), about five times as high as among the four traditional human societies. Even gorillas, with much larger body sizes, do not live much longer than chimpanzees and have an adult mortality rate of about 5 percent per year (Harcourt and Fossey, 1981).

The most reliable estimates of adult mortality rates available for a pre-contact hunting and gathering group are derived from Aché research (Hill and Hurtado, 1996), because of the research focus on producing accurate measures of age and accounting for all adults that lived during the twentieth century. Figure 10-2 shows the age-specific mortality rate of Aché males and females. Adult mortality rates remain low and do not rise significantly until the seventh decade of life, where the rate climbs to 5 percent per year and reaches 15 percent per year by age 75. It should be mentioned that the data displayed in Figure 10-2 deviate somewhat from the age-specific mortality profile predicted by the Gompertz model (see Finch et al., 1990; Finch and Pike, 1996). According to that model, which is quite robust in predicting the mortality profiles of many animal populations (see references cited in Finch et al., 1990), human adult mortality rates are expected to double about every 8 years (ibid:903). The slow rate of increase in mortality during early and middle adulthood estimated for the Aché may be due to small sample size. Alternatively, it may be that age-related increases in mor-

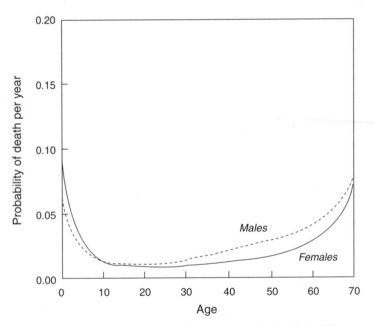

FIGURE 10-2 Aché age-specific probability of death, smoothed with logistic regression. SOURCE: Hill and Hurtado (1996:Fig. 6.2). Copyright 1996 by Water de Gruyter, Inc., New York.

tality due to physical deterioration are swamped by causes of death due to accidents, snake bite, warfare, and predation by jaguars that impact on all adult age classes equally and may even occur more frequently in young adults (see Hill and Hurtado, 1996:table 5.1).

In any case, once a child reaches adult age, the prospect of surviving to a reasonably old age is high. For example, a woman who reaches the average age of first reproduction (age 19) has about a 50 percent chance of reaching age 65.[2] This suggests that living well past the age of last reproduction is a common experience for human females. This survival probability distinguishes our species from almost all other mammals, with the notable exception of some whales (discussed by Austad, in this volume) and contrasts markedly with chimpanzees.

Feeding Ecology and the Life Cycle of Productivity

Although there is a great deal of variability in the diets of both hunting and gathering groups and nonhuman primate species, there appears to be a fundamental difference in the age schedules of production and consumption between humans and their primate relatives. Human children remain dependent on their parents until well into their teen years and sometimes until they are over 20 years old. Data collected with !Kung san also indicate that children under age 15 acquire very little food (Draper, 1976:209-213; Draper and Cashdan, 1988; Lee, 1979:236), spending less than 3 minutes per hour engaged in productive labor. Hill and Hurtado's data on Hiwi children (Kaplan, Hill, Hurtado, and Lancaster, unpublished work) show that boys do not produce as much food as they consume until about age 18 and girls do not do so until they are postreproductive.

Detailed information on the foraging behavior of children is also available for the Hadza, hunter-gatherers living in a mixed savanna woodland habitat in the Eastern Rift Valley of Tanzania (see Woodburn, 1968, 1972, 1979, for general ethnographic information; for data on food production by age, see Blurton Jones, 1993; Blurton Jones et al., in press; Blurton Jones et al., 1994a, b; Hawkes et al., 1989, 1991, 1995, 1996). In the above series of papers by Blurton Jones, Hawkes, and O'Connell, the authors report that Hadza children can be very productive, especially when compared to !Kung children. Nevertheless, Hadza girls do not produce as much as they consume until about 15 years of age, and boys produce about half as much as they consume through 18 years of age (Blurton Jones et al., in press:figure 5).

In contrast with the low productivity of children in hunter-gathering groups, postreproductive and middle-aged people, especially women, appear to work very hard and produce much food. Among the Hadza, postreproductive women

---

[2]While estimates derived from some prehistoric mortuary samples show much lower adult survival rates, there is good reason to believe that inaccuracies due to aging of materials and the sampling properties of the distribution of found remains make them unreliable.

spend 22-52 percent more time in food acquisition than reproductive-age women (depending on the season), and 90-275 percent more time than unmarried girls (Hawkes et al., 1989:figure 2 and table 1). Among the !Kung, while work effort appears to decline with age during the adult years, people over 60 work almost as many hours as younger adults (Lee, 1979:table 9.5).

Quantitative data on food production and food consumption through the life course (measured in units of calories per day) are available for three different traditional groups: Piro, Machiguenga and Aché (see Figures 10-3a - 10-3c; and Kaplan, 1994, for details). The Piro and Machiguenga practice a mixed economy of swidden horticulture, hunting, fishing, and gathering. There is considerable similarity in the age profiles of the three groups. First, children produce much less than they consume, and production does not exceed consumption until 18-20 years of age. Childhood and even adolescence are characterized by very low rates of food production. Second, production exceeds consumption well past the reproductive period into old age. This is particularly evident among the Piro and Machiguenga. Unfortunately, sample sizes for older Aché men and women are extremely low, due to high rates of death associated with disease at first contact. However, data on Aché men show that they produce about twice as much as they consume in their fifties, but in their sixties they produce about a third of what they consume.

This pattern contrasts markedly with age profiles of production among non-

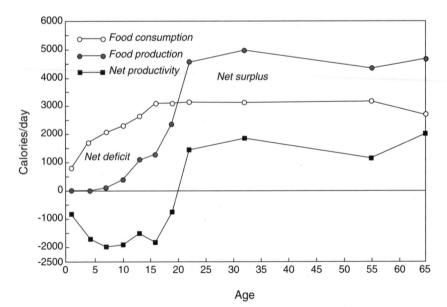

FIGURE 10-3a Machiguenga food production and consumption by age: both sexes combined.

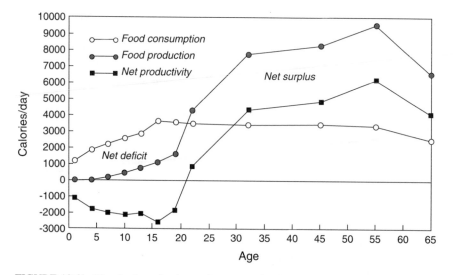

FIGURE 10-3b Piro food production and consumption by age: both sexes combined.

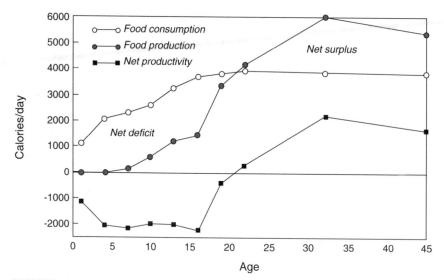

FIGURE 10-3c Aché food production and consumption by age: both sexes combined.
SOURCE: Kaplan (1994).

human primates. Virtually all nonhuman primates follow the standard mammalian pattern. The period of infancy is one of complete nutritional dependence on the mother. The second, juvenile period, from weaning to the onset of reproduction, is characterized by almost exclusive self-feeding. There is no significant period of nonlactational parental provisioning among nonhuman primates. The third, adult period begins with reproduction but includes no significant period of postreproductive productivity before ending in death. These differences between humans and nonhuman primates are summarized in Table 10-1.

My proposal is that these differences are linked to dietary differences. A close examination of the feeding ecology of human hunter-gatherers, when compared to that of nonhuman primates, yields some revealing patterns. The major difference between human and nonhuman primate diets is in the importance of nutrient-dense, difficult-to-acquire (i.e., skill- and/or strength-intensive) food resources (see Figure 10-4). While the diets of nonhuman primates vary considerably by species and by local ecology, most feed, to various degrees, on leaves, fruits, and insects, supplemented in some cases by small amounts of hunted meat and tree gums (Oates, 1987; Terborgh, 1983). Humans, in contrast, rarely feed on leaves. When people do consume leaves, it is as a low-calorie supplement to calorie-dense foods (David Tracer, personal communication) as a source of micronutrients. Humans also avoid most fruits consumed by primates living in the same area. When people eat fruits, these fruits tend to be large and ripe, whereas nonhuman primates feed on a much larger array of small and unripe fruits as well. The bulk of the food acquired by human foragers is derived from difficult-to-extract, nutrient-dense plant foods and hunted game.

Calorically, the most important plant foods for humans are roots, seeds, palm fiber, and nuts. Among the Hadza, roots are the most important plant food. The \\ekwa roots (*Vigna frutescens*), which provide the bulk of the carbohydrate calories in the diet, are found deep in rocky soil, from which "extraction is a lengthy subterranean jigsaw puzzle, sometimes involving the removal of heavy boulders and encounters with scorpions" (Blurton Jones, 1993). Although Hadza researchers do not report actual amounts of roots acquired as a function of age, they do report return rates per hour of work for \\ekwa root digging. Until about age 10, children acquire less than 200 kcal/hr, and then returns increase steadily by about 125 kcal/hr/yr until the age of 18 when they acquire about 1100 kcal/hr

TABLE 10-1 Life History Stages

Mammals/Primates	Traditional Humans
Infancy	Infancy
Independent prereproductive, juvenile	Dependent, prereproductive juvenile
Adult, reproductive	Adult, reproductive
	Postreproductive, productive
	Frail elderly (very short until recently)
Death	Death

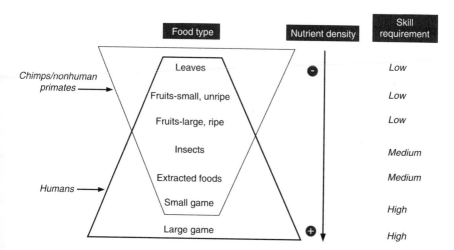

FIGURE 10-4 The feeding ecology of humans and other primates.

of work (Blurton Jones et al., in press:figure 2). Reproductive-aged and postreproductive women acquire 1500 and 1670 Kcal/hr, respectively. A similar pattern is found among Hiwi hunter-gatherers, for whom roots are also the most important plant food.

Among some !Kung groups, mongongo nuts are reported to be the plant food staple (Lee, 1979). While the nuts are easy to collect, several factors appear to limit the productivity of children (see Blurton Jones et al., 1989, 1994a,b for an in-depth analysis). First, mongongo nut groves are often found quite distant from water sources (about 10 km) where camps are located (Blurton Jones et al., 1994a,b). This requires a great deal of endurance and the ability to walk far without much water (ibid.). In addition, extraction of nut meat requires skill. According to experimental data on nut-cracking rates (Blurton Jones et al., 1994a), most children under the age of 9 are unable to crack the nuts safely. Children aged 9-13 cracked 120 nuts per hour, teens aged 14-17 cracked 241 nuts per hour, and adults cracked 314 nuts per hour. Bock, who worked with villagers in the Okavango delta who practiced a mixed economy of hunting, fishing, gathering, horticulture, and animal husbandry, found that mongongo cracking rates peak at age 35 for women (Bock, 1995).

The most important plant food among the Aché is palm starch. Extraction of palm starch requires felling the tree, cutting a vertical window down the length of the trunk to expose the pulp, and then pounding the pulp into mush. This is a difficult task involving both strength and skill, and women do not reach peak productivity at palm-fiber extraction until age 35 (A.M. Hurtado, unpublished data). Again, Aché girls less than 15 years of age rarely pound palm fiber.

Seeds, an important plant food staple in Australia and the North American

Great Basin (e.g., O'Connell and Hawkes, 1981; O'Connell et al., 1983; Steward, 1938), also require much processing to extract the nutrients (Simms, 1984). Meat is also an important part of human diets. Whereas meat accounts for no more than 5 percent of total caloric consumption (and usually much less) in any nonhuman primate, hunted and fished foods account for between 15 and 100 percent of total calories consumed among human foragers (Kelly, 1995:table 10-3.1). Although there is no comparative, quantitative database on the factors affecting hunting ability in humans, my own observations hunting with four South American groups suggest that hunting, as practiced by those peoples, is a very skill-intensive activity. Because people are slow runners, they rely on knowledge of prey behavior to find and kill prey. Conversations with men among the Aché, Piro, Machiguenga, and Yora foragers suggest to me that they have detailed knowledge of the reproductive, parenting, grouping, predator avoidance, and communication patterns of each prey species, and this takes decades to learn. For example, in a test with wildlife biologists, an Aché man could identify the vocalizations of every bird species known to inhabit his region and claimed to know many more, which the biologists have yet to identify (Kim Hill, personal communication). After most hunts, details of the hunt and the prey's behavior are discussed and often recounted again in camp. Even the stomach and intestinal contents of the animal are examined to determine its recent diet for future reference. In addition, knowledge of predator behavior may also be very important. Villagers in Botswana reported to me that one reason why teens hunt little is because they are at risk of predation themselves. According to some informants, the ability to detect potential predators such as lions, hyenas, and leopards and then escape them requires years to learn. It should be mentioned, however, that available empirical data do not allow us to assess the relative impacts of skill, knowledge, strength, endurance, and ambition on hunting returns. Those impacts may vary across ecologies and individuals.

Nevertheless, the age patterning of hunting success is striking. Figure 10-5 shows the age distribution of hunted calories acquired per day among the Aché. Fifteen- to seventeen-year-old boys acquired 440 calories of meat per day, 18- to 20-year-olds acquired 1,530 calories, and 21- to 24-year-olds acquired 3,450 calories, whereas 25- to 50 year olds acquired about 7,000 calories of meat per day. The fourfold increase between 18 and 25 years of age exists in spite of the fact that by age 18, young men are hunting about as much as fully adult men. This pattern is not unique to the Aché. From independent samples acquired in different !Kung camps, both Lee (1979) and Draper (1976) report that men under age 25 acquired very little meat and were considered incompetent hunters. Among the Hadza, although boys spend much time pursuing game, their returns are quite low. Blurton Jones et al. (1989) report that during 31 observation days the total meat production for Hadza boys was about 2 kg, mostly composed of small-to-medium-sized birds. This is less than the daily production of a single adult Hadza man, who acquires a mean of 4.6 kg per day (Hawkes et al., 1991).

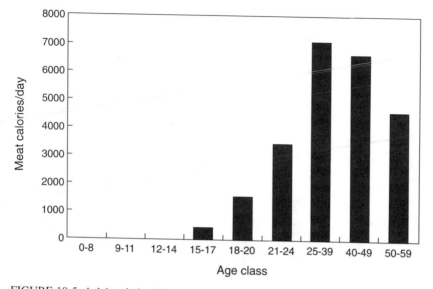

FIGURE 10-5 Aché male hunting acquisition.

Fruit collection, in contrast, is the least skill-intensive activity in human foraging. Fruits are also the most important food acquired by children. In fact, most variability in children's food acquisition, both within and among hunting and gathering societies, appears to be due to access to fruits. In an insightful series of papers comparing !Kung and Hadza foraging (Blurton Jones, 1993; Blurton Jones et al., 1989, 1994a, b, and in press), the authors show that foraging return rates and especially access to fruits close to camp sites are the critical determinant of the higher food acquisition by Hadza children. Not only are there more fruits close to Hadza camps than close to !Kung camps but also the environment near !Kung camps is more dangerous for children due to poor long-range visibility (ibid.). In addition, Hadza children acquire more food and spend more time foraging during seasons when fruits are abundant (Blurton Jones, 1993; Blurton Jones et al., in press; Hawkes et al., 1996). In fact, Hadza children can provide as much as 50 percent of their total calories when fruits are in season (Blurton Jones et al., 1989). Similarly, one area (Bate) where !Kung children were reported to forage more often did have fruit and nut trees nearby (Blurton Jones et al., 1994b:205). Fruits also explain dramatic variation in Aché children's foraging. When fruits are in season, food production increases more than five-fold for children under age 14 (Figure 10-6). For older teens who are stronger and more skilled, the effect is less dramatic.

The effects of ease of acquisition also apply to meat. When meat resources are collectable, children can also be very productive. For example, among the Machiguenga and Piro, streams are frequently dammed and poisoned with roots.

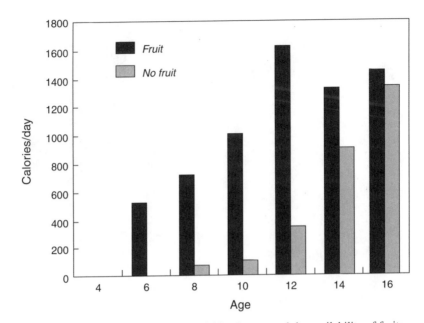

FIGURE 10-6 Aché children's food acquisition by age and the availability of fruits.

Fish float to the surface and can be collected easily by children. Even though these fish poisoning events occur less than twice a month, they account for almost half of all meat calories that girls under age 16 acquire and about 20 percent of meat acquired by boys.

A similar pattern of effects can be found among chimpanzees. The few, difficult-to-acquire foods consumed by chimpanzees are not acquired by young, weaned individuals and are shared by mothers with their offspring (Silk, 1978). These are termites and ants (which are "fished" with a stick) (ibid.), nuts that are cracked with stones, and game (Teleki, 1973). Thus, those foods that are easy to procure are acquired by human and chimpanzee young alike, and those foods difficult to extract or procure are not acquired by the young of either species and are provisioned by parents. The principal difference then is that human diets are composed primarily of large, nutrient-dense, low-fiber, difficult-to-acquire foods, whereas nonhuman primate diets are composed primarily of foods that are easily collected. As a result, human children are provisioned.

The Relationships Between Feeding Ecology,
Reproductive Ecology and Life Span

Table 10-2 summarizes some major differences in the life-history character-istics of humans and chimpanzees interrelated by the theory. We begin with the

TABLE 10-2 Ape and Human Reproductive Ecology

Characteristic	Apes	Humans
Feeding ecology	Less skill-intensive, lower quality	More skill-intensive higher quality
Age of independence	Weaning	18
Number of dependent young	Single	Multiple
Energy for lactation	Supported by increased food consumption during lactation	Fat storage supporting uninterrupted brain growth
Work effort following birth	Increased	Decreased with support of others
Adult life span	Long for mammals of similiar body size; No postreproductive period	Exceptionally long; Potential postreproductive period about as long as reproductive period

differences in feeding ecology and the juvenile period discussed above. Those features have important effects on reproductive ecology.

First, most primates have only one dependent young at a time. Humans have multiple dependent young due to the fact that the length of the dependency period is much greater than the interbirth interval. At some stage in the life course it is likely that a family will contain children of about 15, 11, 7, and 3 years of age.

A second important difference between humans and other primates, including the great apes, is the energetic support for lactation. Most primates support lactation through increased food acquisition during the entire lactation period, using a "pay-as-you-go" financing strategy. Humans, in contrast, store large quantities of energy during pregnancy to support lactation. Fat stored in the hips and buttocks during pregnancy is specifically designed to support lactation (Rebuffe-Scrive et al., 1985). That fat is accessed in response to prolactin, which, in turn, is produced in response to nipple stimulation and serves to "order the next meal" (Short, 1984). The storage of fat during pregnancy may be related to birth seasonality as well. Humans exhibit significant seasonality in births when there is regular fluctuation in the food supply (Ellison, 1990, 1995; Ellison et al., 1989; Huffman et al., 1978; Hurtado and Hill, 1990; Leslie and Fry, 1989; Lunn et al., 1984; Prentice and Whitehead, 1987). When net energy flow to women (energy consumed less energy expended) is low, women are much less likely to conceive. Perhaps food availability to support fat storage during pregnancy is more critical to human birth seasonality than is food availability after weaning (the latter appears the more critical among baboons (Altmann, 1980).

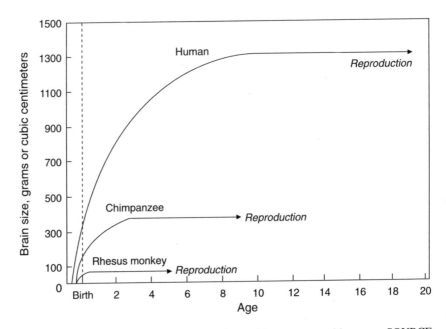

FIGURE 10-7 Brain growth in rhesus monkeys, chimpanzees, and humans. SOURCE: Lancaster (1986). Reprinted by permission

The storage of fat during pregnancy as a preparation for lactation may be a direct result of our feeding ecology. Human brains grow more than twice as fast and twice as long as chimpanzee brains (see Figure 10-7). In fact, during the first year of life, as much as 65 percent of all resting energetic expenditure is used to support the maintenance and growth of the brain (Holliday, 1978). It is highly likely that our large, flexible brain is a necessary component of the feeding strategy focusing on high-quality, difficult-to-acquire foods. It is also possible that the fat storage system for lactation evolved to produce a nonfluctuating, uninterrupted flow of energy to sensitive, fast-growing brains (this set of hypotheses is due to Jane Lancaster, personal communication; see also Lancaster, 1986).

The third important difference between apes and humans is that among humans, individuals other than the child's mother also provide the energy used to nurse and provision children. In fact, nursing women in the hunting and gathering groups for which the information is available work fewer hours than women who are not nursing an infant; this is true of the Aché (Hurtado, 1985), the Hiwi (Hurtado et al., 1992), the Efe (Peacock, 1985), and for women with young infants among the Hadza (Hawkes et al., 1996).

Support of reproduction in humans is derived from many sources. Most obvious is the provisioning of women and children by men, particularly the child's father or the woman's husband. However, another important source of support is provided by postreproductive individuals, particularly the child's grandparents (see Hawkes et al., 1989, 1996; Kaplan, 1994). The data on age-specific food production and consumption presented in Figure 10-3 reveal some important trends. First reproduction occurs at an age when women and their husbands are just able to support themselves; the extra food and energy needed to support the offspring must come from elsewhere. During the peak period of child dependence, when there could be four or five dependent children, adults do not acquire enough food to support the net needs of their children (i.e., including the child's own food production). Postreproductive and nonreproductive individuals support the reproduction of young people and families with high-dependency ratios.

In addition to providing direct food assistance, older women often help their daughters and daughters-in-law in caring for young babies and even older children. Grandmothers can be particularly helpful with vulnerable first-born children whose mothers are inexperienced.[3] After infancy, children often sleep with their grandparents and sometimes live with them in separate residences from their parents. For example, among the Machiguenga 16 percent of all children were residing in their grandmother's hut.

Older men, as their physical strength begins to wane, still give advice in hunts and shift their work effort toward plant foods and tool making. They also provide political assistance in marriage, dispute resolution, and friendship formation.

In this sense the extended juvenile period, early reproduction relative to productivity, and high-dependency ratios depend on the existence of older, postreproductive and yet productive individuals. The exceptionally low adult mortality rates before age 60 appear an integral component of the skills-based food niche.

A GENERAL MODEL FOR THE EVOLUTION OF LIFE HISTORIES

The above discussion presented a specific theory for the evolution of human life-history characteristics. In this section, I embed that theory in a more general analysis of the determinants of life histories. Figure 10-8 illustrates the basic model underlying the analysis. This model builds upon and integrates two distinct literatures: life-history theory in biology (particularly Blurton Jones, 1987, 1993; Charlesworth, 1994; Charnov, 1993; Gadgil and Bossert, 1970; Hamilton, 1966; Kirkwood, 1981; Kozlowski and Weigert, 1986; Pennington and Harpending, 1988; Rogers, 1990, 1994; Rogers and Blurton Jones, 1992; Smith and Fretwell, 1974; and Stearns, 1992) and human capital and fertility theory in economics (particularly Becker, 1975, 1991; Becker and Barro, 1988; Ben-Porath, 1967; Mincer, 1974; Willis, 1973, 1987).

---

[3]In fact, coresident grandmothers improve outcomes for low-birth-weight babies even in our own society (Pope et al., 1993).

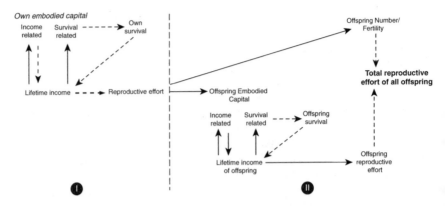

FIGURE 10-8 Decision model for the life history of investments. The first part of the figure depicts the tradeoff between current and future reproductive effort. The second part represents the tradeoff between quantity and reproductive value (quality) of offspring. The solid arrows depict investment options, and the dashed arrows depict the impacts of investments.

The figure depicts two fundamental life-history tradeoffs. The first is the tradeoff between current and future reproduction; the second is the tradeoff between quantity and quality of offspring. Natural selection is expected to act on those tradeoffs so as to maximize the long-term representation of the genes underlying life-history traits. The traits associated with highest fitness are expected to vary with ecological factors affecting the shape of those tradeoffs.

The concept of embodied capital (Kaplan et al., 1995), borrowed from the concept of human capital developed in economics, can be useful in the analysis of the tradeoffs. Development can be seen as a process in which individuals and their parents invest in a stock of embodied capital. In a physical sense, embodied capital is organized somatic tissue. In a functional sense, embodied capital includes strength, immune function, coordination, skill, knowledge, all of which affect the profitability of allocating time and other resources to alternative activities such as resource acquisition, defense from predators and parasites, mating competition, parenting, and social dominance. Because such stocks tend to depreciate with time due to physical entropic forces and to direct assaults by parasites, predators, and conspecifics, allocations to maintenance such as feeding, cell repair, and vigilance, can also be seen as investments in embodied capital.

Figure 10-8 begins with lifetime income. By income, I mean the total value of time allocated to alternative activities, such as resource acquisition, child care, rest, etc. At each age, an individual's income will be a function of his or her embodied capital. Income can be invested directly in reproductive effort or in embodied capital. Embodied capital, in turn, can be divided into stocks affecting the ability to acquire the resources for reproduction and stocks affecting the probability of survival.[4]

The solid arrows depict investment options. The dotted arrows depict the impacts of investments. Investments in income-related capital, such as in growth, physical coordination, skills and knowledge, affect lifetime income through the value or productivity of time in the future. Investments in survival-related capital, such as immune function, predator defense, and tissue repair, affect lifetime income through increasing the expected life span of earnings. However, an organism that does not reproduce leaves no descendants. Thus, the optimization problem acted upon by natural selection is to allocate lifetime income among investments in future income, survival, and reproductive effort at each age so as to maximize total allocations to reproduction.

The optimum strategy will be the one that maximizes resources for reproduction over the life course (see Charnov, 1993; Kirkwood, 1981; Kozlowski and Weigert, 1986; and Stearns, 1992, for theoretical treatments). The "decision rule" under selection involves allocating resources to be used for current reproductive effort and those that will be used to increase future reproductive effort. The tradeoff results from the fact that allocations to current reproductive effort utilize resources which could be allocated to increasing survival or to increasing productivity in the future. Within each broad area of allocations, there are subproblems that must be solved. For example, energy invested in the production of antibodies to infection cannot be invested in cell repair, growth, or even other antibodies. Similarly, time invested in learning one skill competes with time allocated to learning other skills.

The subproblem involving the allocation of reproductive effort is the quantity-quality tradeoff. Individuals can invest not only in capital embodied in their own soma but also in the capital embodied in offspring. However, such allocations decrease resources available for the production of other offspring and hence decrease the total quantity of offspring produced with a given amount of income. The second part of Figure 10-8 shows the relationships between investments and outcomes for two generations. Here, both the parent and the offspring can invest in the offspring's survival- and income-related capital. The optimization problem for the parent is then to allocate investments in fertility and in embodied capital of offspring so as to maximize the total lifetime allocations by offspring to their own reproductive effort (summed over all offspring). If individuals in each generation allocate investments in their own and offspring-embodied capital optimally, then the "dynastic" fitness of the lineage is maxi-

---

[4]Some forms of capital, such as body size and strength, may affect both income and mortality rates. In this case, the total effect of increases in such stocks would include effects on both income and survival.

mized (see Kaplan, 1996, for a theoretical treatment). The multigenerational decision path is illustrated in Figure 10-9.

In this model the diversity of life histories is due to the fact that the shape of the relationships between investments and outcomes varies ecologically. For each major class of mortality (predation, disease, intraspecific violence, accidents, starvation), there will be variable relationships between the probability of dying from it and investments by the organism. For example, the density and characteristics of predators, in interaction with the characteristics of the organism, determine the relationship between allocations and the probability of being eaten. Some organisms, such as bivalve mollusks, tortoises, and porcupines, apparently benefit significantly from allocations to predator defense and live long lives. Feeding niche appears to interact with the benefits to investments in mortality reduction. Birds, bats, and primates appear to lower predation rates by spending less time in terrestrial habitats and by being able to escape to aerial strata (Austad and Fischer, 1991).

There is also ecological variability in the benefits to investment in income-related capital. The relationships between body size and productivity depend on feeding niche. The value of knowledge, skill, and information-processing ability depends on the type of foods exploited. Grazing animals probably benefit much less from investments in learning than do species who eat more variable or difficult-to-capture foods.

In addition to factors affecting the shape of each relationship between investments and outcomes, the quantitative analysis of this model shows that optimal investment in each component depends, in part, on investments in other components and in the effects of those investments (Kaplan, 1996; see also Blurton

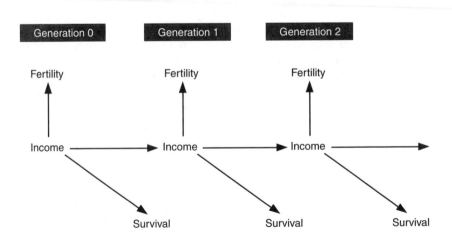

FIGURE 10-9 Multigenerational recursion for fitness effects of parental investment.

Jones, 1993, and Rogers and Blurton Jones, 1992). One result is that the value of investments in income-related capital depends on the probability of surviving to future ages (Kaplan et al., unpublished work; see also Ben-Porath, 1967).[5] If the expected future life span is short, it pays little to invest in future earnings, favoring allocation of resources to current reproduction instead. The corollary is also true. The value of investments in survival depends on expected future income. If income is increasing through time, higher investments in survival are favored (for a related result, see Hamilton, 1966, and Charlesworth, 1994:chapter 5). Another result is that the value of allocations to each form of mortality reduction depends on the probability of dying from other causes. For example, if one is likely to die from predation, it pays less to invest in cell repair and immune function, which would affect future condition and the likelihood of dying from disease. Low probabilities of predation are probably an important determinant of why birds, bats, and primates allocate more resources to maintaining physical condition and senesce at late ages for their body size (Austad and Fischer, 1991, 1992; Kirkwood, 1981; Kirkwood and Rose, 1991), as do some animals living on islands with few predators (Austad, 1993). Lastly, the model also suggests that optimal investments in offspring survival and offspring income are complementary and positively associated (Kaplan, 1996).

These general results can be applied to the specific model of human life-history presented above. The nature of our feeding niche increases the value of both one's own and parental investment in income-related capital. Because many investments in income-related capital do not mature fully until after the age of 25, the value of investments in survival increases in order to realize the dividends from investments in income. The low productivity of hunter-gatherer children probably reflects both investment in skills and investments in survival. For example, boys in many hunting and gathering societies spend a great deal of time hunting very small animals. They achieve very low returns from those activities and could probably acquire more food by collecting. This is evidently an investment in future income. However, it also appears to be the case that adults restrict children to safe places (Draper, 1976; Blurton Jones et al., 1994b). When hunter-gatherers make camps in which they will reside for more than a few days, a great deal of effort is spent clearing the area of all underbrush. This is the safe zone, especially for very young children. Moreover, informants among both the !Kung (ibid.) and the Aché (Kim Hill, personal communication) report that they prefer to leave children in camp rather than to take them foraging. The food the children could collect on those foraging trips is apparently less valuable than the risks and costs associated with taking them along.[6] Such effects appear to be ecologically variable, however. The comparative analysis of children's behavior and parental

---

[5]Becker (1975) and Ben-Porath (1967) obtain similar results in the analysis of investments in human capital.

[6]In fact, young offspring interfere with maternal food collection in both humans (Hurtado, 1985; Hurtado et al., 1992) and nonhuman primates (Altmann, 1980).

protectiveness among the !Kung and Hadza (Blurton Jones et al., 1994a, b) shows that the danger in the environment predicts both children's behavior and parental concerns. Blurton Jones (1993) suggests that high fertility, high parental demands for children's labor, and lowered parental protectiveness among the Hadza are all correlated responses to an environment that poses less risks to children.

It is also possible that our feeding niche directly and indirectly contributes to high rates of return on investments in survival. First, modern hunter-gatherers present a formidable challenge to predators. People have been reported to take kills away from predators among the !Kung and Hadza (Blurton Jones and Konner, 1976; O'Connell et al., 1988). Second, the high-quality foods people consume (especially those rich in protein and fat) may facilitate more effective immune responses to disease and lower mortality. Third, the food-sharing pattern characteristic of the hunting and gathering way of life may allow sick and injured individuals to recover without suffering the downward spiral of decreased energy intake and increased illness experienced by many other animals [see Kaplan and Hill, 1985, theory and data about the relationship between hunter-gatherer diets and food sharing; Lawrence Sugiyama (visiting lecture, Department of Anthropology, University of New Mexico) has explicitly developed the theory regarding the role of food sharing in buffering the risks associated with physical injury]. The interaction of increased returns to income-related capital and greater resistance to predation and disease may be directly responsible for our long life span and delayed senescence.[7]

In the light of this model, we should not expect to see people living longer than they are productive under traditional conditions. Although data on old-age mortality among hunter-gatherers are few and based on small samples, it appears that many people reach age 60, but much fewer reach age 70. Although the evidence is anecdotal, my experience with traditional peoples suggests that death and decline of productivity occur about the same time in older people. The frail elderly period, as a life stage that endures for many years and is experienced by significant numbers of people, is probably a very recent occurrence and may even be rare in modern societies (Finch, 1996:498).

MENOPAUSE, LONGEVITY, AND THE POSTREPRODUCTIVE PERIOD

The existence of a long postreproductive period in humans has attracted the attention of numerous biologists and anthropologists (e.g., Alexander, 1974;

---

[7]It should be mentioned, however, that humans engage in a great deal of warfare, which itself may be a product of our feeding niche, both because of cooperative activities and because hunting requires large territories (see Divale and Harris, 1976; Harris, 1977, for the proposition that warfare in Amazonia is due to protein and game scarcity; see Chagnon and Hames, 1979, for a critique of this position). In any case, we lack the empirical data to assess the effects of our feeding niche on mortality rates through warfare.

Austad, in this volume; Gaulin, 1980; Hamilton, 1966; Hawkes et al., 1989; Hill and Hurtado, 1991; Lancaster and King, 1992; Rogers, 1993; Trivers, 1972; Williams, 1957). According to one view, this interest is misplaced. Some argue that the existence of a postreproductive period in humans is a novel effect due to very recent (within the past few hundred years), environmentally induced increases in the life span (Austad, in this volume; Washburn, 1981; Weiss, 1981). Under the traditional conditions in which humans evolved, people rarely lived longer than the reproductive period. However, that view is based upon the analysis of skeletal data and not on direct measurements of age-specific death rates with living humans. Although empirical data on adult mortality rates in traditional foraging groups are scarce, available data suggest that a significant proportion of females who reach adulthood will live to undergo menopause (see Figure 10-1 and Lancaster and King, 1992). Apparently a significant postreproductive period has existed under traditional conditions and requires explanation.

Those who assume the existence of a postreproductive period have addressed the problem from the perspective of the evolution of menopause. Taking the length of the human life span as a given, they have asked what kinds of selective forces could result in the evolution of menopause. Selection for cessation of reproduction has been seen as a solution to a tradeoff between investment in the reproductive value of existing kin and the production of additional descendants.

Both parts of the tradeoff have received some consideration. First, it may be the case that the offspring of older women will be of low reproductive value. This may be due to increased chances of producing an impaired offspring or to the high probability of parental death during the long juvenile period. If older mothers produce less viable offspring, either due to genetic abnormalities or to decreased survival after parental death, the costs of menopause could be low. Second, older people have many descendent kin, whose survival and reproduction may be improved from investment. By ceasing to reproduce, old people can use their time and resources to invest in the reproduction of kin. This second possibility has been labeled the grandmother hypothesis, because it has focused on assisting children in the production and raising of grandchildren. If costs are low and benefits are high, menopause could maximize biological fitness.

Attempts to test the grandmother hypothesis with empirical data (Hill and Hurtado, 1991; Rogers, 1993) have yielded largely negative results. However, problems with estimating the shape of the tradeoff between investment in descendants and the production of additional offspring render the rejection of the hypothesis premature (see Hill and Hurtado, 1996; Austad, in this volume; Hawkes et al., 1996, for useful discussions).

The grandmother hypothesis is consistent with the difficult-to-acquire-foods hypothesis for the evolution of the extended juvenile period and the long life span. It may be the feeding ecology of humans that favors reproductive cessation and investment in descendant kin. However, each hypothesis could be true while the other is not. This can be seen by reframing the problem of the postreproductive life span. One could ask, "Given that humans cease to reproduce in their early to late forties, why do they live so long?" This focuses the question on the evolution of the long life span and shows that both menopause and longevity require explanation (Hawkes et al., 1996, have independently come to a similar conclusion).

Several possible ancestral conditions may be considered. One possibility is that the ancestral condition is a somewhat longer reproductive period and a shorter life span. Selection, due to an increased value of grandparenting, could direct additional resources toward longevity and investment in descendant kin, at the expense of shortening the reproductive period. If this were true, the grandmother hypothesis could account for both menopause and the long life span.

Another possible ancestral condition is the same life span as is found currently but no cessation of reproduction. In that case, the tradeoff is solely between production of offspring and investment in existing kin. Selection due to increased benefits from grandparenting could produce menopause. The long life span of humans for their body size would then require another explanation.

A third possible ancestral condition is a short life span, ending at about the same time as, or before, menopause occurs today but with no menopause. In this case, selection could favor the increase in life span without a concomitant increase in the length of the reproductive period. One possible scenario for such a selection regime is that different tradeoffs are involved in the evolution of the reproductive period than in the life span.

With respect to the reproductive period, it appears that the physiological cause of menopause is the depletion of oocytes due to the process of follicle decay, known as atresia (vom Saal et al., 1994).[8] Mammalian females begin life with their full complement of germ cells, and this process of follicle decay seems to be a very general feature of mammalian reproductive physiology (ibid., Finch, 1994). Follicle decay appears to exhibit a constant exponential decline through life, with an acceleration just before menopause—with menopausal women having essentially no viable oocytes left (Richardson et al., 1987:figure 3). The main difference between humans and other mammals, except for some whales, is that total loss of oocytes occurs in human females well before most have died and before other organs senesce (Austad, in this volume, and Hill, 1993).

It is possible that the main constraints on the reproductive life span are the number of germ cells at the outset and the rate of follicle decay. There is

---

[8]There is some confusion in discussions of menopause, due to definitional issues. Many mammals, including primates, show evidence of decreasing fecundity and ovarian function late in life (Caro et al., 1995; Gould et al., 1981). If such evidence is considered to be indicative of menopause, then it is fairly common. On the other hand, other authors have been interested in the evolution of menopause as a postreproductive period of significant duration. If this latter definition is used, then it is quite rare (see Austad, in this volume, for a related discussion).

evidence that rates of oocyte loss are under genotypic influence in different laboratory strains of mice (Finch and Nelson, 1994:figure 6). Perhaps the costs of increasing the length of the reproductive period are allocations to increasing follicle number or follicle viability. Those costs may decrease energy available for reproduction early in life. Thus the tradeoff may be between early reproduction and late reproduction rather than between late reproduction and investment in descendant kin.

If the optimal solution to that tradeoff is to only produce enough eggs and to maintain them at the observed rate so that reproduction is only possible to about age 45, we are then left with the problem of explaining the evolution of the life span after age 45. Perhaps, the tradeoff here is not between producing more offspring in old age and investing in descendants but between living longer to invest in descendant kin and early reproduction. In this case, selection might favor allocating more resources to survival and maintenance during the reproductive period at the expense of a lower reproduction rate. The benefit of the longer life would be gained through increased reproduction of descendant kin. This idea is displayed in Figure 10-10; the bold line depicts (in stylized form) the classic age-specific fertility pattern seen in noncontracepting populations without delayed marriage (for review, see Wood, 1994). The dashed line below the bold line represents the fertility rates that would be achieved without the help of older individuals, primarily parents. The difference in the heights of those two lines is the increased reproduction due to assistance. The solid line below the bold line represents the alternative fertility rate that would be achieved without the allocations necessary to survive past menopause and without assistance from kin.

Of course, the two effects are simultaneous: the effect of kin assistance requires the loss of peak reproduction in order to live longer. The costs and benefits are distributed across two generations. The younger generation receives the benefits of assistance from parents, and the older generation pays the costs of lower peak reproduction in order to live longer. The older generation received the benefits from their parents, in turn. If the benefits of kin assistance outweigh the reproductive costs of higher adult survival rates and greater expenditures on maintenance, such a system of intergenerational transfers could evolve. This system is consistent with the feeding ecology model discussed above. Thus, it is possible that a long life span evolved, even though an increase in the reproductive period did not, due to different costs and benefits.

Available data do not allow us to distinguish among these and possibly other evolutionary scenarios. Each of these possibilities requires investigation and test. For example, tests of the third scenario require that we understand the costs of maintaining a viable egg supply for more than 45-50 years and the costs of maintaining our bodies in better condition than our closest primate relatives. In any case, we must recognize that two explanations are required: one for long life span and another for menopause.

It is also important to ask why human males both live long and sometimes

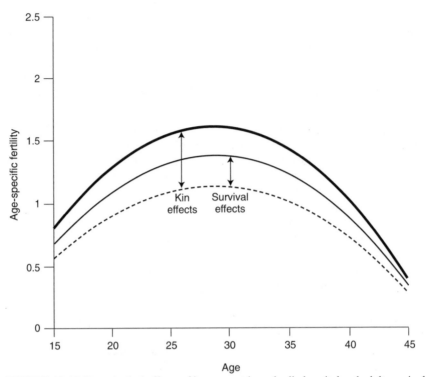

FIGURE 10-10 Hypothetical effects of investment in embodied capital and adult survival on fertility (with intergenerational assistance).

continue to reproduce in middle and old age. Aché data show that men evidence major declines in fertility after age 50 (Hill and Hurtado, 1996). However, we do not know the generality of this pattern across foraging groups, whether Aché men do not actively seek new reproductive opportunities in favor of grandparental investment, or whether they are simply not chosen as partners by women. It is possible that there is a great deal of variation in men's strategies both within and among societies. Greater focus on the mating and kin investment behavior of middle-aged and older men and on their impacts for survival and reproductive success of offspring and other kin in traditional societies is clearly necessary. An understanding of men's behavior may help solve the riddle of long life and menopause.

HISTORICAL, CURRENT, AND FUTURE TRENDS IN MORBIDITY AND MORTALITY

The general life-history model presented above predicts that increased returns to investments in embodied capital affecting either income or survival will be associated with greater longevity. This prediction has a number of implications for understanding recent changes in health-related investments, current variability in morbidity and mortality within populations, and future trends in expected life spans. However, before the discussion of those implications, it is important to consider the evolution of short- and long-term responses to ecological variation.

The traditional view of evolutionary processes underlying adaptation is that in a given environmental context, natural selection favors certain genetic variants over others, with each genetic variant corresponding to a phenotypic trait. Populations adapt and remain adapted to the environment through directional and stabilizing selection, respectively. Recently, the concepts of phenotypic plasticity and evolved norms of reaction have become increasingly important in biologists' understanding of adaptation. Under many conditions genotypes are thought to code for mechanisms that translate environmental inputs into phenotypic outputs rather than for an invariant response. For example, the reproductive rate of most plants and animals varies positively with energy availability (due to environmental conditions associated with temperature, rainfall, prey density, population density, etc.—for mammalian examples, see Wade and Schneider, 1992).

Norms of reaction to environmental and individual conditions evolve because the optimal phenotype varies with conditions and because genetic variants coding for the ability to modify phenotype adaptively sometimes can compete more effectively against variants that produce the same phenotype in all environments. However, such phenotypic plasticity is costly. Humans, whose behavioral phenotypes are at the extreme of plasticity, have a long developmental period of low productivity, precisely because it takes so long to "program" the brain with environmental information. Thus, each organism represents a compromise between the benefits and costs of phenotypic plasticity.

The nature of this compromise determines how organisms will respond to environmental variation. In general, it can be expected that organisms will respond flexibly and adaptively to environmental variation commonly experienced in the evolutionary history of the organism and respond less adaptively or even nonadaptively to environmental variation outside the range of common experience. The concepts of long- and short-run profit maximization/cost minimization in the economics of the firm are a convenient analogy. Some inputs in the production process, such as materials and labor, can be adjusted easily in the short run. Other inputs, such as plant size and other forms of physical capital, require longer periods for adjustment. Over the short run, a firm can adjust inputs to a given range of variation in the demand for products and still maximize profits. However, large increases or decreases in demand will probably reduce profits in the short run, until the fixed inputs can be adjusted in the long run.

Norms of reaction can be analyzed in a similar way. A norm of reaction can be optimal for a given range of environmental variation. Thus, many organisms can respond adaptively to seasonal and year-to-year variation in environmental conditions. However, substantial changes in the environment may select for a new norm of reaction, and this will occur over the longer run because it requires change in the distribution of genotypes in the population.

The most basic features of the psychological and physiological mechanisms underlying our set of responses to environmental variation evolved in the context of a hunting and gathering ecology. Given that environmental dangers, disease threats, food supply, and the importance of skill in food acquisition are likely to have varied across hunter-gatherer ecologies, we can expect that optimal life-history allocations would have varied as well. For example, food-intake rates undoubtedly varied through time, across habitats, and as a function of population density. The ability to alter allocations to survival, maintenance, reproductive effort, fertility, and parental investment in response to changing net energy-intake rates must have been under selection.

Part of the response system is under physiological control. The probability of having a fecund menstrual cycle varies positively with seasonal variation in net food-intake rates in food-limited populations (Ellison, 1990, 1995; Ellison et al., 1989; Huffman et al., 1978; Hurtado and Hill, 1990; Leslie and Fry, 1989; Lunn et al., 1984). In children, disease rates decrease and growth rates increase with increased food and protein intake, indicating a distribution of the extra food to several functions (for review, see Hill and Hurtado, 1996:chapter 10 and table 10-1). Part of the response system is under behavioral control. Both parents and children exert control over the introduction of weaning foods. Age-specific exposure to environmental risks of accident, intraspecific aggression, and predation depends, in part, on activity regimes. Because the behavioral and physiological responses interact in determining the final outcome (e.g., rates of breast feeding and food intake interact in determining probability of an ovulatory menstrual cycle), it is likely that selection would have produced a coordinated physiological/psychological response system that yields adaptive life-history adjustment in relation to changing conditions characteristic of hunter-gatherer ecologies.

Most people today live under very different conditions. What kinds of responses do we expect in relation to modern environments and to variability within modern environments? Very little is known about the answer to this question. It is perhaps the most fundamental question facing the social, behavioral, and medical sciences today. One working assumption is that environmental variation in modern societies qualitatively similar to variation in hunter-gatherer societies should produce similar responses to what would be expected under traditional conditions. The response to the changing importance of skill and education in the last century may be one such example.

The *central prediction* of the life-history model presented above is that payoffs to investment in income-related capital interact positively with payoffs to investment in survival in determining allocations to reproductive effort and embodied capital. One theory of the demographic transition (the dramatic reduction in fertility that occurred in Europe and America about 100 years ago) is that it is the result of the emergence of skills-based labor markets as the dominant economic institution (Kaplan, 1996; Kaplan et al., 1995). This theory proposes that payoffs to investment in education increased radically with the emergence of labor markets and technological growth spurred by the industrial revolution. As a result, parents lowered fertility to invest in more skilled children.

The theory can be extended to consider the relationship between investments in income-related educational capital and investments in mortality reduction. In modern labor markets, increased education is not only associated with increased income but also with higher rates of income growth through the life course (Mincer, 1974; see Figure 10-11). According to the life-history model, the increased value of investments in education and growth in income through the life course should favor increased investment in longevity. The increased investments in public and private health that we have witnessed in the past century may be explainable as direct outgrowths of increased payoffs to investment in skill. As a corollary, the improvements in health and survival also increased the value of investments in income growth, due to the increased duration of returns from those investments.

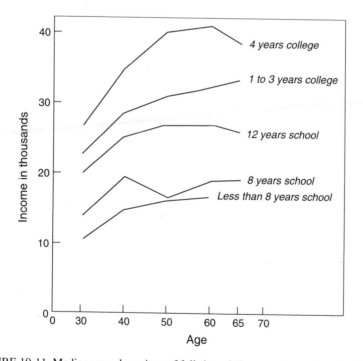

FIGURE 10-11 Median annual earnings of full-time, full-year male workers in 1985 as a function of education and age. SOURCE: U.S. Bureau of the Census (1985).

This view differs considerably from standard demographic transition theory, which explains fertility reduction as a result of reductions in infant and juvenile mortality. The standard theory sees fertility reduction as an equilibrating response to maintain population stability in the face of changing mortality regimes. The capital-investment theory explains lower fertility, increased survival rates, and increased investment in skills as coordinated responses to a changing economic system.

The same logic predicts the observed correlation between old-age survival and education found today. Health-promoting and health-reducing behaviors (exercise, diet, cigarette smoking, drug and alcohol use) are closely associated with education. Perhaps the reason for this association is not the increased information available to educated people but the increased value of longevity associated with an increase in income growth through the life course (of course, many other possible causal processes may be responsible for this association). Because morbidity associated with behavior represents a significant portion of resources spent in health care, an understanding of the factors determining the relative values of present consumption and future longevity is of great practical importance.

Finally, it is also the case that access to food resources is virtually unlimited for many people today. This food availability is outside the range of anything experienced by traditional peoples in the past. This availability may mean that our evolved allocation mechanisms are not designed to respond to unlimited food access. Perhaps the increases in longevity and the increased health of very old people that have occurred in the last several decades are at the bounds of our adaptive flexibility. Even though we have enough food energy to allocate additional resources to maintenance, we appear to store that energy as fat rather than to use it to prevent aging from occurring. Our evolutionary history probably did not design our allocation system to respond adaptively to the virtually unlimited food supply and ability to combat illness through medicine, characteristic of modern developed nations. It may be that large, future increases in the healthy human life span will require major manipulation of our evolved allocation system, either through genetic engineering or chemical interventions.

SUMMARY AND CONCLUSIONS

This paper has addressed the evolution of the human life course from the perspective of competing allocations to reproduction, growth, skill development, health, and maintenance. Compared to other primates and mammals, there are three distinctive characteristics of human life histories: (1) an exceptionally long life span, (2) an extended period of juvenile dependence, and (3) support of reproduction by older postreproductive individuals. The theory presented here proposes that those three features of the human life course are interrelated outcomes of a feeding strategy emphasizing nutrient-dense, difficult-to-acquire foods. The logic underlying this proposal is that for humans, effective adult foraging requires an extended developmental period during which production at young ages is sacrificed for increased productivity later in life. The returns to investment in development depend positively on adult survival rates, favoring increased investment in mortality reduction. An extended postreproductive, yet productive, period supports both earlier onset of reproduction by next-generation individuals and the ability to provision multiple dependent young at different stages of development.

Two distinct possibilities regarding the evolution of the postreproductive period were considered. One is that menopause evolved to facilitate postre-productive investment in offspring. The other is that reproductive senescence evolved due to the costs of maintaining viable oocytes and that increased longev-ity evolved, in spite of menopause, to support the reproduction of descendants.

This theory was developed as part of a more general theory of the evolution of life histories. Two major tradeoffs were considered. First, resources can be invested in either current or future reproductive effort. Investments in future reproductive effort include both those that enhance survival and increase future income (in a general sense). Age-specific allocations that maximize the lifetime allocation to reproductive effort will be favored by natural selection. Second, there is a tradeoff between quantity and quality of offspring. The specific model of human life-history evolution proposes that compared to other primates, tradi-tional human ecology favored higher levels of investment in both future repro-duction and quality of offspring.

It is useful to think of short- and long-term responses to various environ-ments and, hence, various optimal allocation regimes. Natural selection can favor the evolution of physiological and psychological mechanisms that facilitate short-term adjustments to environmental variation. The degree of phenotypic plasticity that evolves will represent a compromise between the costs and benefits of flexible responses and also reflect the range of environmental variation expe-rienced by the organism. Humans clearly demonstrate a high degree of adaptive flexibility, mediated through both physiology and behavior. Although the mecha-nisms underlying our response system evolved in the context of a hunting and gathering way of life, this evolved flexibility is apparent in our recent history as well. Changes in investments in income-related capital, mortality reduction, and maintenance associated with the demographic transition may reflect increased returns to those investments, stimulated by the increasing importance of skills-based competitive labor markets. Similarly, within developed countries, those that have more to gain from investments in education also invest more in longev-ity and health.

Long-term adjustments occur when one short-term response system is com-petitively more effective than another response system. In general, this would occur when environments change sufficiently so that the ancestral response sys-tem produces unfavorable outcomes. We cannot expect natural selection to have altered our response system in relation to the contingencies of modern environments, given their very recent appearance. With respect to contemporary issues, such as aging, fertility, and development, the fundamental theoretical issue faced by the social, behavioral, and medical sciences is how to build models of an ancient, but flexible, response system in a very novel environment.

REFERENCES

Alexander, R.D.
    1974   The evolution of social behavior. *Annual Review of Ecology and Systematics* 5:325-383.
Altmann, J.
    1980   *Baboon Mothers and Infants.* Cambridge, MA: Harvard University Press.
Austad, S.N., and K.E. Fischer
    1991   Mammalian aging, metabolism, and ecology: Evidence from the bats and marsupials. *Journal of Gerontology* B47-B53.
    1992   Primate longevity: Its place in the mammalian scheme. *American Journal of Primatology* 28:251-61.
    1993   Retarded senescence in an insular population of Virginia opossums (*Didelphis virginiana*). *Journal of Zoology (London)* 229:695-708.
Becker, G.S.
    1975   *Human Capital*, 2nd ed. New York: Columbia University Press.
    1991   *A Treatise on the Family* Enl. ed. Cambridge, MA: Harvard University Press.
Becker, G.S., and R.J. Barro
    1988   A reformulation of the economic theory of fertility. *Quarterly Journal of Economics* 103(1):1-25.
Ben-Porath, Y.
    1967   The production of human capital and the life cycle of earnings. *Journal of Political Economy* 75:352-365.
Blurton Jones, N.
    1986   Bushman birth spacing: a test for optimal interbirth intervals. *Ethology and Sociobiology* 4:145-147.
    1987   Bushman birth spacing: Direct tests of some simple predictions. *Ethology and Sociobiology* 8:183-203.
    1993   The lives of hunter-gatherer children: Effects of parental behavior and parental reproductive strategy. Pp. 309-326 in M.E. Pereira and L.A. Fairbanks, eds., *Juvenile Primates.* Oxford: Oxford University Press.
Blurton Jones, N., K. Hawkes, and J. O'Connell
    1989   Modeling and measuring the costs of children in two foraging societies. Pp. 367-390 in V. Standen and R.A. Foley, eds., *Comparative Socioecology: The Behavioral Ecology of Humans and Other Mammals.* London: Basil Blackwell.
In press   Why do Hadza children forage? In N.L. Segal, G.E. Weisfeld, and C.C. Weisfeld, eds., *Genetic, Ethological and Evolutionary Perspectives on Human Development. Essays in honor of Dr. Daniel G. Freedman.* American Psychological Society.
Blurton Jones, N., K. Hawkes, and P. Draper
    1994a   Foraging returns of !Kung adults and children: Why didn't !Kung children forage? *Journal of Anthropological Research* 50(3):217-248.
    1994b   Differences between Hadza and !Kung children's work: Original affluence or practical reason? Pp. 189-215 in E.S. Burch, Jr. and L.J. Ellanna, eds., *Key Issues in Hunter-Gatherer Research.* Oxford: Berg.

Blurton Jones, N., and M. Konner
1976   !Kung knowledge of animal behavior. Pp. 325-348 in R.B. Lee and I. DeVore, eds., *Kalahari Hunter-Gatherers*. Cambridge, MA: Harvard University Press.

Bock, J.
1995   The Determinants of Variation in Children's Activities in a Southern African Community. Ph.D. dissertation. University of New Mexico.

Caro, T.M., D. Sellen, A. Parish, R. Frank, D. Brown, E. Voland, and M. Borgerhoff Mulder
1995   Termination of reproduction in nonhuman and human female primates. *International Journal of Primatology* 16:205-220.

Chagnon, N.
1974   *Studying the Yanomamo*. New York: Holt, Rinehart and Winston.
1983   *Yanomamo: The Fierce People*, 3rd ed. New York: Holt, Rinehart and Winston.
1988   Life histories, blood revenge, and warfare in a tribal population. *Science* 239:985-992.

Chagnon, N., and R. Hames
1979   Protein deficiency and tribal warfare in Amazonia: New data. *Science* 20(3):910-913.

Charlesworth, B.
1994   *Evolution in Age-Structured Populations*, 2nd ed. Cambridge: Cambridge University Press.

Charnov, E.L.
1993   *Life History Invariants*. Oxford: Oxford University Press.

Courtenay, J., and G. Santow
1989   Mortality of wild and captive chimpanzees. *Folia Primatologica* 52:167-177.

Divale, W., and M. Harris
1976   Population, warfare and the male supremacist complex. *American Anthropologist* 78:521-538.

Draper, P.
1975   !Kung women: Contrasts in sexual egalitarianism in foraging and sedentary contexts. Pp. 77-109 in R. Reiter, ed., *Toward an Anthropology of Women*. New York: Monthly Review Press.
1976   Social and economic constraints on child life among the !Kung. Pp. 199-217 in R.B. Lee and I. DeVore, eds., *Kalahari Hunters and Gatherers*. Cambridge, MA: Harvard University Press.

Draper, P., and E. Cashdan
1988   Technological change and child behavior among the !Kung. *Ethnology* 27:339-365.

Ellison, P.
1990   Human ovarian function and reproductive ecology: New hypotheses. *American Anthropologist* 92:933-954.
1995   Understanding natural variation in human ovarian function. In R.I.M. Dunbar, ed., *Human Reproductive Decisions: Biological and Social Perspectives*. London: MacMillan.

Ellison, P.T., N.R. Peacock, and C. Lager
1989   Ecology and ovarian function among Lese women of the Ituri forest. *American Journal of Physical Anthropology* 78:519-526.

Finch, C.E.
1994   The evolution of ovarian oocyte decline with aging and possible relationships to Down syndrome and Alzheimer disease. *Experimental Gerontology* 29:299-304.
1996   Biological bases for plasticity during aging of individual life histories. D. Magnusson. Pp. 488-512 in *The Lifespan Development of Individuals: Biological and Psychosocial Perspectives, a Synthesis*. Cambridge: Cambridge University Press.

Finch, C.E., and J.F. Nelson
1994   Genotypic influences on reproduction and reproductive aging in mice: Influences from alleles in the *H-2* complex and other loci. Pp. 93-108 in D.K. Sarkar and C.D. Barnes,

eds., *The Reproductive Neuroendocrinology of Aging and Drug Abuse.* Boca Raton, FL: CRC Press.

Finch, C.E., and M.C. Pike
1996　Maximum life span predictions from the Gompertz mortality model. *Journal of Gerontology* 51A(3):B183-B194.

Finch, C.E., M.C. Pike, and M. Witten
1990　Slow mortality rate accelerations during aging in animals approximate that of humans. *Science* 249:902-905.

Gadgil, M., and W.H. Bossert
1970　Life historical consequences of natural selection. *American Naturalist* 104:1-24.

Gaulin, S.
1980　Sexual dimorphism in the human post-reproductive lifespan: Possible causes. *Human Evolution* 9:227-232.

Goodall, J.
1986　*Chimpanzees of Gombe: Patterns of Behavior.* Cambridge, MA: Harvard University Press.

Gould, K.G., M. Flint, and C.E. Graham
1981　Chimpanzee reproductive senescence: A possible model for the evolution of menopause. *Maturitus* 3:157-166.

Hames, R.
1983　The settlement pattern of a Yanomamo population bloc: A behavioral ecological interpretation. Pp. 393-427 in R.B. Hames and W.T. Vickers, eds., *Adaptive Responses of Native Amazonians.* New York: Academic Press.
1992　Variation in paternal investment among the Yanomamo. Pp. 85-110 in B. Hewlett, ed., *Father-Child Relations: Cultural and Biosocial Contexts.* Chicago: Aldine de Gruyter.

Hamilton, W.D.
1966　The moulding of senescence by natural selection. *Journal of Theoretical Biology* 12:12-45.

Harcourt, A.H., and D. Fossey
1981　Demography of Gorilla gorilla. *Journal of Zoology, (London)* 195:215-233.

Harpending, H., and L. Wandsnider
1982　Population structure of Ghanzi and Ngamiland !Kung. *Current Developments in Anthropological Genetics* 2:29-50.

Harris, M.
1977　*Cannibals and Kings.* New York: Random House.

Hawkes, K., H. Kaplan, K. Hill, and A.M. Hurtado
1987　Aché at the settlement: Contrast between farming and foraging. *Human Ecology* 15(2):133-161.

Hawkes, K., K. Hill, and J. O'Connell
1982　Why hunters gather: Optimal foraging and the Aché of eastern Paraguay. *American Ethnologist* 9:379-398.

Hawkes, K., J. O'Connell, and N. Blurton Jones
1989　Hardworking Hadza grandmothers. Pp. 341-366 in V. Standen and R.A. Foley, eds., *Comparative Socioecology: The Behavioral Ecology of Humans and Other Mammals.* London: Basil Blackwell.
1991　Hunting income patterns among the Hadza: Big game, common goods, foraging goals and the evolution of the human diet. Pp. 243-251 in A. Whiten and E. Widdowson, eds., *Foraging Strategies and Natural Diet of Monkeys, Apes and Humans.* Proceedings of the Royal Society of London 334. Oxford: Clarendon Press.
1995　Hadza children's foraging: Juvenile dependency, social arrangements and mobility among hunter-gatherers. *Current Anthropology* 36:688-700.

1996   Hadza Women's Time Allocation, Offspring Provisioning, and the Evolution of Long
        Post-Menopausal Lifespans. Unpublished manuscript. Department of Anthropology,
        University of Utah, Salt Lake City, UT 84112.
Hill, K.
1993   Life history theory and evolutionary anthropology. *Evolutionary Anthropology* 2(3):78-
        88.
Hill, K., and K. Hawkes
1983   Neotropical hunting among the Aché of eastern Paraguay. Pp. 139-188 in R. Hames and
        W. Vickers, eds., *Adaptive Responses of Native Amazonians.* New York: Academic
        Press.
Hill, K., and A.M. Hurtado
1991   The evolution of reproductive senescence and menopause in human females. *Human
        Nature* 2(4):315-350.
1996   *Aché Life History: The Ecology and Demography of a Foraging People.* New York:
        Aldine de Gruyter.
Hill, K., and H. Kaplan
1988a   Tradeoffs in male and female reproductive strategies among the Aché, part 1. Pp. 277-
        290 in L. Betzig, P. Turke, and M. Borgerhoff Mulder, eds., *Human Reproductive Behav-
        ior.* Cambridge: Cambridge University Press.
Hill, K., and H. Kaplan
1988b   Tradeoffs in male and female reproductive strategies among the Aché, part 2. Pp. 291-
        306, in. L. Betzig, P. Turke, and M. Borgerhoff Mulder, eds., *Human Reproductive
        Behavior.* Cambridge: Cambridge University Press.
Hill, K., H. Kaplan, K. Hawkes, and A.M. Hurtado
1985   Men's time allocation to subsistence work among the Aché of eastern Paraguay. *Human
        Ecology* 13:29-47.
Holliday, M.A.
1978.   Body composition and energy needs during growth. Pp. 117-139 in F. Falker and J. M.
        Tanner, eds., *Human Growth.* Vol. 2. New York: Plenum.
Howell, N.
1979   *Demography of the Dobe !Kung.* New York: Academic Press.
Huffman, S. L., A.M.K. Chowdhury, J. Chakborty, and W.H. Mosley
1978   Nutrition and postpartum amenorrhea in rural Bangladesh. *Population Studies* 32:251-260.
Hurtado, A. M.
1985   Women's Subsistence Strategies among Aché Hunter-Gatherers of Eastern Paraguay.
        Ph.D. dissertation, University of Utah.
Hurtado, A., K. Hawkes, K. Hill, and H. Kaplan
1985   Female subsistence strategies among Aché hunter-gatherers of eastern Paraguay. *Human
        Ecology* 13:1-28
Hurtado, A., and K. Hill
1987   Early dry season subsistence ecology of the Cuiva foragers of Venezuela. *Human Ecol-
        ogy* 15:163-187.
1990   Seasonality in a foraging society: Variation in diet, work effort, fertility and the sexual
        division of labor among the Hiwi of Venezuela. *Journal of Anthropological Research*
        46:293-345.
1992   Paternal effect on offspring survivorship among Aché and Hiwi hunter-gatherers: Impli-
        cations for modeling pair-bong stability. Pp. 31-55 in B. Hewlett, ed., *Father-Child
        Relations: Cultural and Biosocial Contexts.* New York: Aldine de Gruyter.
Hurtado, A., K. Hill, H. Kaplan, and I. Hurtado
1992   Trade-offs between female food acquisition and child care among Hiwi and Aché forag-
        ers. *Human Nature* 3(3):185-216.

Kaplan, H.
1994   Evolutionary and wealth flows theories of fertility: Empirical tests and new models. *Population and Development Review* 20(4):753-791.
1996   A theory of fertility and parental investment in traditional and modern human societies. *Yearbook of Physical Anthropology* 39:91-135.

Kaplan, H., and K. Hill
1985   Food sharing among Aché foragers: Tests of explanatory hypotheses. *Current Anthropology* 26(2):223-245.

Kaplan, H., J.B. Lancaster, J.A. Bock, and S.E. Johnson
1995   Does observed fertility maximize fitness among New Mexican men? A test of an optimality model and a new theory of parental investment in the embodied capital of offspring. *Human Nature* 6:325-360.

Kelly, R.L.
1995   *The Foraging Spectrum.* Washington, DC: Smithsonian Institution Press.

Kirkwood, T.B.L.
1981   Repair and its evolution: Survival versus reproduction. Pp. 165-189 in C.R. Townsend and P. Calow, eds., *Physiological Ecology: An Evolutionary Approach to Resource Use.* Oxford: Blackwell.

Kirkwood, T.B.L., and M.R. Rose
1991   Evolution of senescence: Late survival sacrificed for reproduction. Pp. 15-24 in P.H. Harvey, L. Partridge, and T.R.E. Southwood, eds., *The Evolution of Reproductive Strategies.* Cambridge: Cambridge University Press.

Konner, M., and M. Shostak
1987   Timing and management of birth among the !Kung: Biocultural interaction in reproductive adaptation. *Current Anthropology* 2:11-28.

Konner, M., and C. Worthman
1980   Nursing frequency, gonadal function, and birth spacing among !Kung hunter-gatherers. *Science* 207:788-791.

Kozlowski, J., and R.G. Weigert
1986   Optimal allocation of energy to growth and reproduction. *Theoretical Population Biology* 29:16-37.

Lancaster, J.B.
1986   Human adolescence and reproduction: An evolutionary perspective. Pp. 17-38 in J.B. Lancaster and B.A. Hamburg, eds., *School-Age Pregnancy and Parenthood.* New York: Aldine de Gruyter.

Lancaster, J.B., and B. King
1992   An evolutionary perspective on menopause. Pp. 7-15 in V. Kerns and J. Brown, eds., *In Her Prime: New Views of Middle-Aged Women.* Chicago: University of Illinois Press.

Lee, R.B.
1979   *The !Kung San: Men, Women and Work in a Foraging Society.* Cambridge: Cambridge University Press.
1984   *The Dobe !Kung.* New York: Rinehart and Winston.
1985   Work, sexuality, and aging among !Kung women. Pp. 23-35 in J. Brown and V. Kerns, eds., *In Her Prime: A New View of Middle-Aged Women.* South Hadley, MA: Bergin and Garvey.

Lee, R.B., and I. DeVore, eds.
1976   *Kalahari Hunter-Gatherers: Regional Studies of the !Kung San and Their Neighbors.* Cambridge, MA: Harvard University Press.

Leslie, P.W., and P.H. Fry
1989   Extreme seasonality of births among nomadic Turkana pastoralists. *American Journal of Physical Anthropology* 79:103-115.

Lunn, P., S. Austin, A.M. Prentice, and R. Whitehead
1984   The effect of improved nutrition on plasma prolactin concentrations and postpartum infertility in lactating Gambian women. *American Journal of Clinical Nutrition* 39:227-235.

Melancon, T.
1982   Marriage and Reproduction among the Yanomamo Indians of Venezuela. Ph.D. dissertation, Pennsylvania State University.

Mincer, J.
1974   *Schooling, Experience and Earnings.* Chicago: National Bureau of Economic Research.

Oates, J.F.
1987   Food distribution and foraging behavior. Pp. 197-209 in B.B. Smuts, D.L. Cheney, R.M. Seyfarth, R.W. Wrangham, and T.T. Struhsaker, eds., *Primate Societies.* Chicago: University of Chicago Press.

O'Connell, J.F., and K. Hawkes
1981   Alyawara plant use and optimal foraging theory. Pp. 99-125 in E. Smith and B. Winterhalder, eds., *Hunter-Gatherer Foraging Strategies.* Chicago: Chicago University Press.

O'Connell, J.F., K. Hawkes, and N. Blurton Jones
1988   Hadza scavenging: Implications for Plio-Pleistocene hominid subsistence. *Current Anthropology* 29:356-363.

O'Connell, J., P. Latz, and P. Barnett
1983   Traditional and modern plant use among the Alyawara of central Australia. *Economic Botany* 37:80-109.

Peacock, N.R.
1985   Time Allocation, Work and Fertility Among Efe Pygmy Women in the Ituri Forest of Northeast Zaire. Ph.D. dissertation, Harvard University.

Pennington, R., and H. Harpending
1988   Fitness and fertility among Kalahari !Kung. *American Journal of Physical Anthropology* 77:303-319.

Pope, S.K., L. Whiteside, J. Brooks-Gunn, K. Kelleher, V. Rickert, R. Bradley, and P. Casey
1993   Low-birth-weight infants born to adolescent mothers. *Journal of the American Medical Association* 269:1396-1400.

Prentice, A., and R. Whitehead
1987   The energetics of human reproduction. *Symposia Zoological Society of London* 57:275-304.

Rebuffe-Scrive, M., L. Enk, N. Crona, P. Lonnroth, L. Abrahamsson, U. Smith, and P. Bjorntorp
1985   Fat cell metabolism in different regions in women—effect of menstrual cycle, pregnancy and lactation. *Journal of Clinical Investigation* 75:1973-1976.

Richardson, S.J., V. Senikas, and J.F. Nelson
1987   Follicular depletion during the menopausal transition: Evidence for accelerated loss and ultimate exhaustion. *Journal of Clinical Endocrinology and Metabolism* 65(6):1231-1237.

Rogers, A.
1990   The evolutionary economics of human reproduction. *Ethology and Sociobiology* 11:479-495.
1993   Why menopause? *Evolutionary Ecology* 7:406-420.
1994   Evolution of time preference by natural selection. *American Economic Review* 84(3):460-481.

Rogers, A., and N. Blurton Jones
1992   Allocation of Parental Care. Unpublished manuscript. Department of Anthropology, University of Utah, Salt Lake City, UT 84112.

Schrire, C.
  1980   An inquiry into the evolutionary status and apparent identity of San hunter-gatherers. *Human Ecology* 8:9-32.
Short, R.V.
  1984   Breast feeding. *Scientific American* 250:35-41.
Silk, J.B.
  1978   Patterns of food-sharing among mother and infant chimpanzees at Gombe National Park, Tanzania. *Folia Primatologica* 29:129-141.
  1979   Feeding, foraging, and food sharing behavior in immature chimpanzees. *Folia Primatologica* 31:12-42.
Simms, S.
  1984   Aboriginal Great Basin Foraging Strategies: An Evolutionary Approach. Ph.D. dissertation. University of Utah.
Smith, C.C., and S.D. Fretwell
  1974   The optimal balance between size and number of offspring. *American Naturalist* 108:499-506.
Stearns, S.
  1992   *The Evolution of Life Histories*. Oxford: Oxford University Press.
Steward, J.H.
  1938   *Basin Plateau Aboriginal Sociopolitical Groups*. Bureau of American Ethnology Bulletin 120. Washington, DC.
Teleki, G.
  1973   *The Predatory Behavior of Wild Chimpanzees*. Lewisburg, PA: Bucknell University Press.
Terborgh, J.W.
  1983   *Five New World Primates: A Study in Comparative Ecology*. Princeton, NJ: Princeton University Press.
Trivers, R. L.
  1972   Parental investment and sexual selection. Pp. 136-179 in B. Campbell, ed., *Sexual Selection and the Descent of Man*. Chicago: Aldine.
U.S. Bureau of the Census
  1985   Money income of households, families and persons in the United States, 1985. Current Population Reports. Series P-60, No. 156, Table 35. Washington, DC: U.S. Department of Commerce.
vom Saal, F.S., C.E. Finch, and J.F. Nelson
  1994   Natural history and mechanisms of reproductive aging in humans, laboratory rodents, and other selected vertebrates. Pp. 1213-1314 in E. Knobil and J.D. Neill, eds., *The Physiology of Reproduction*, 2nd ed. New York: Raven Press.
Wade, G., and J. Schneider
  1992   Metabolic fuels and reproduction in female mammals. *Neuroscience and Biobehavioral Reviews* 16:235-272.
Washburn, S. L.
  1981   Longevity in primates. Pp. 11-29 in J. March and J. McGaugh, eds., *Aging, Biology and Behavior*. New York: Academic Press.
Weiss, K. M.
  1981   Evolutionary perspectives on human aging. Pp. 25-58 in P. Amoss and S. Harrell, eds., *Other Ways of Growing Old*. Stanford, CA: Stanford University Press.
Wiessner, P.
  1982a   Measuring the impact of social ties on nutritional status among the !Kung San. *Social Science Information* 20:641-678.

Wiessner, P.
  1982b Risk, reciprocity, and social influences on !Kung San economics. Pp. 61-84 in E. Leacock
         and R.B. Lee, eds., *Politics and History in Band Societies*. Cambridge: Cambridge Uni-
         versity Press.
Williams, G. C.
  1957   Pleiotropy, natural selection and the evolution of senescence. *Evolution* 11:398-411.
Willis, R.J.
  1973   A new approach to the economic theory of fertility behavior. *Journal of Political
         Economy* 81:S14-S64.
  1987   Wage determinants: A survey and reinterpretation of human capital earnings functions.
         Pp. 525-602 in O. Ashenfelter and R. Layard, eds., *Handbook of Labor Economics*.
         Amsterdam: North Holland.
Wilmsen, E.N.
  1978   Seasonal effects of dietary intake on Kalahari San. *Federation of American Societies for
         Experimental Biology, Proceedings* 37:65-72.
  1989   *Land Filled with Flies*. Chicago: University of Chicago Press.
Wood, J.
  1994   *Dynamics of Human Reproduction: Biology, Biometry, and Demography*. New York:
         Aldine de Gruyter.
Woodburn, J.C.
  1968   An introduction to Hadza ecology. Pp. 49-55 in R.B. Lee and I. DeVore, eds., *Man the
         Hunter*. Chicago: Aldine de Gruyter.
  1972   Ecology, nomadic movement and the composition of the local group among hunters and
         gatherers: An east African example and its implications. Pp. 193-206 in P.J. Ucko, R.
         Tringham, and G.W. Dimbleby, eds., *Man, Settlement and Urbanism*. London:
         Duckworth.
  1979   Minimal politics: The political organization of the Hadza of north Tanzania. Pp. 244-266
         in W. Snack and P. Cohen, eds., *Politics and Leadership: A Comparative Perspective*.
         Oxford: Clarendon Press
Wrangham, R.W.
  1974   Artificial feeding of chimpanzees and baboons in their natural habitat. *Animal Behaviour*
         22:83-94.
  1977   Feeding behaviour of chimpanzees in Gombe National Park, Tanzania. Pp. 504-537 in H.
         Clutton-Brock, ed., *Primate Ecology*. New York: Academic Press.
Wrangham, R.W., and B.B. Smuts
  1980   Sex differences in the behavioural ecology of chimpanzees in the Gombe National Park,
         Tanzania. *Journal of Reproductive Fertility Supplement* 28:13-31.
Yellen, J.
  1976   Settlement pattern of the !Kung: An archaeological perspective. Pp. 48-72 in R.B. Lee
         and I. DeVore, eds., *Kalahari Hunter-Gatherers*. Cambridge, MA: Harvard University
         Press.

11

Intergenerational Relations and the Elderly

Ronald D. Lee

INTRODUCTION

Recent essays on the role of the elderly in nature (Carey and Gruenfelder, Austad, in this volume) describe a variety of animal behaviors across the life cycle. This note is prompted by the thought that these animal behaviors have interesting links and counterparts in human behaviors. In it I will consider some of these links, particularly those that have an intergenerational aspect. Specifically, I will discuss (1) various estimates of the prevalence of post-reproductive and elderly women in human stationary populations, (2) the role of elders as repositories of knowledge that may benefit their kin or larger group, (3) transfer flows of resources from members of one age group to members of another, and (4) transfers of assets to children at the death of their parent or inter vivos.

PREVALENCE OF THE ELDERLY IN HUMAN POPULATIONS—
ACTUAL, HISTORICAL, AND PROJECTED

According to Austad (in this volume), physiologically postreproductive indi-viduals are generally very rare in nature, although for some particular species such as toothed whales they are quite prevalent. Austad indicates that 24 percent of female short-finned pilot whales survive past the physiological reproductive age, at which point their remaining life expectancy is 14 years. In some killer whale populations, about 30 percent of females are postreproductive, and postre-productive life expectancy is over 25 years.

It is interesting to compare these figures to human populations. Austad (in this volume) takes the view that the evidence on human survival in preagricultural populations is dichotomous, with paleodemographic data indicating that "humans until recently did not live into their postreproductive years except very rarely," while other data indicate much higher proportions of postreproductive females in the populations. He suggests that the disagreement in these estimates may be unresolvable.

A brief survey of the evidence may be useful. To begin with, we must operationalize "post reproductive." In developed countries, the mean age at menopause ranges from 47 to 50 years, but menopause comes some years after the effective cessation of the ability to bear children. In noncontracepting agricultural populations, the mean age at last birth is usually in the range of 39 to 41 years (Bongaarts, 1983:124-127). The mean age at last birth for the forest dwelling Aché hunters and gatherers is slightly higher (42.1 years; Hill and Hurtado, 1996:254) and for the !Kung is substantially lower (35.4 years; Howell, 1979:130). Nonetheless, many females in noncontracepting populations continue to bear children after age 40, so it is preferable to use age 45 for present purposes. By this age, about 70 percent of couples are sterile (Bongaarts, 1983:126), although often the sterility of the couple is due to sterility of the male rather than the female.

Evidence for survival in high-mortality populations comes from a variety of sources that include skeletal data, contemporary preagricultural populations who retain traditional life styles, high-mortality agricultural populations, and extrapolation from agricultural populations using statistical methods to generate model life-table systems.

There are many estimates of mortality based on skeletal (paleodemographic) data. These estimates have well-known weaknesses that arise from differences by age in the probability that a dead person will be represented by bones in the collection, difficulty in ascribing an age at death to the bones, distortions due to nonstationarity of the age distribution of the population giving rise to the specimens, etc. There is a very wide range in estimated life expectancies from skeletal data (Hassan, 1981), with some analysts reporting very low life expectancies, far lower than those estimated for contemporary preagricultural groups, whereas others estimate mortality at levels consistent with those for contemporary groups. Table 11-1 gives one estimate based on a combination of the model life-table methods developed by Weiss (1973) for preagricultural populations (here assuming that 60 percent of births survive to age 15), with an estimate of life expectancy at age 15 of 21.2 years presented as an average for a large body of paleodemographic data reviewed by Hassan (1981:118). The implied life expectancy at birth is 23 years.

The next column is based on a model life table with a life expectancy at birth of only 20 years and with an age pattern of mortality based on extrapolation from high-mortality agricultural populations analyzed by Coale and Demeny

TABLE 11-1 Postreproductive Females in Stationary Populations

	Paleo Average[a]	High Mortality[b]	High Mortality[c]	Aché[d]	!Kung[e]	Modern Industrial[f]	U.S. in in 2065[g]
Life expectancy at birth (years)	23	20	20	37	30	79	90
Prop surviving to age 45 (%)	0.17	0.21	0.18	0.46	0.35	0.96	0.997
Life expectancy at age 45 (years)	14	17	16	22	20	36	45
Pop 45+ as Prop of total female pop (%)	0.10	0.18	0.15	0.28	0.23	0.44	0.50
Prop surviving to age 65 (%)	0.05	0.08	0.06	0.28	0.17	0.85	0.965
Life expectancy at age 65 (years)	7	8	8	10	9	19	27
Pop 65+ as Prop of total female pop (%)	0.01	0.03	0.02	0.08	0.05	0.20	0.28

[a]This is interpolated from Weiss (1973) model life tables with survival to age 15 assumed to be 0.6, and with life expectancy at 15 set equal to the average given by Hassan (1981) for the Paleolithic studies he reviews, which was 21.2 years.

[b]Based on Coale and Demeny (1983), model west female life tables and stable populations with growth rate 0.

[c]Based on Preston et al. (1993) model life table for females.

[d]Calculated from data in Hill and Hurtado (1996:196-198). These data are explicitly for the forest dwelling period, not the later reservation period when mortality was lower.

[e]Based on Howell (1979), which I interpret to mean that it is appropriate to use Coale-Demeny model west life table with life expectancy at birth of 30 years to characterize !Kung mortality in the past; recent !Kung mortality has been much lower.

[f]Based on the U.S. female life table for 1990, according to data of the Social Security Administration (1992:34-35).

[g]Based on Carter and Lee (1992), who forecast mortality using statistical time-series analysis and some modeling assumptions; they forecast somewhat larger gains in life expectancy than do either the Social Security Administration or the U.S. Census Bureau.

Note: Pop = population; Prop = proportion.

SOURCES: Weiss (1973), Hassan (1981), Coale and Demeny (1983), Hill and Hurtado (1996), Howell (1979), U.S. Social Security Administration (1992), Carter and Lee (1992).

(1983).[1] Even in this case, 18 percent of the stationary female population would be postreproductive. In both these life tables, which describe extremely high mortality, there are still substantial numbers of postreproductive women, and the life expectancy of women surviving to age 45 is still an additional 14 to 17 years. There are very few elderly women, however.

The Hassan-Weiss life table has a radically different shape than those in the Coale-Demeny model life-table system: child mortality is lower, and adult mortality is higher. In the Coale-Demeny system, the lowest life expectancy at age 15 for females is about 31 years, and that corresponds to about 41 percent of births surviving to age 15, for an overall life expectancy at birth of 20 years. However, the Coale-Demeny model life tables for life expectancies of 20 to 30 years are mainly extrapolations from life tables with life expectancies of 33 years or higher, and the method of extrapolation has been criticized as exaggerating the mortality of children and understating the mortality of adults (Bhat, 1987; Preston et al., 1993). Preston et al. (1993) have developed a new set of model life tables for high-mortality populations, which are better based empirically and which avoid the methodological problems of the Coale-Demeny tables at low life expectancies. These model life tables have a shape between that of the Hassan-Weiss and Coale-Demeny life tables, as shown in the third column of Table 11-1. At a life expectancy at birth of 20 years, 44 percent survive to age 15, with a remaining life expectancy of 27 years.

It is true that there are some analysts of some skeletal collections who conclude that mortality was higher than these three life tables suggest and that the proportion of female births surviving to age 45 was lower (e.g., Lovejoy et al., 1977; Weiss, 1973). Others, analyzing similar collections, conclude that life expectancy was substantially higher than these life tables suggest (see the many life tables described in Hassan, 1981). Hassan (1981:121) sums up his survey with the view that "It is premature, pending further evaluation of the age distribution of prehistoric skeletal populations, to affirm that prehistoric mortality was greater than that for ethnographic hunter-gatherers." Which leaves open the possibility that it may have been greater.

The leading demographic studies of contemporary hunter-gatherer populations are for the Aché and the !Kung. Howell (1979:116) concluded that the !Kung had a life expectancy at birth of about 30 years in the past, although in recent years it appears to have been much higher. She also found that the !Kung

---

[1] It may be questioned whether these model life tables, based as they are on extrapolation from the experience of modern high-mortality agricultural populations, are appropriate for preagricultural populations. Hill and Hurtado (1996:192), for example, argue that they are not. However, they appear to overstate their case in this regard. They base their conclusion on the selection of a Coale-Demeny table to match infant mortality, rather than on the best overall fit. It is readily seen that within the west female family, matching on either e_0 or e_{10}, both of which indicate a level-8 model table with $e_0 = 37.5$, gives a vastly superior fit to the level 13 ($e_0 = 50$), which Hill and Hurtado (1996:217) use to draw their conclusions.

data were fit reasonably well by Coale-Demeny (1983) model life tables. Table 11-1 shows the implied information for the !Kung, indicating that around 23 percent of the female population would have been postreproductive in a stationary population. Table 11-1 also presents data for the forest dwelling Aché (Hill and Hurtado, 1996), indicating that in a stationary female population, 28 percent would be postreproductive.[2]

Further evidence is summarized by Wilmoth (1995), who surveys a large number of estimated life tables for high-mortality populations and for each tabulates estimated life expectancy at birth and at age 50 (these are the only data he provides). Life expectancy at 50 is 2.5 to 3 years less than at age 45 in high-mortality populations (see Coale and Demeny, 1983), so we can adjust accordingly. Wilmoth reports values for 56 different life tables of which 26 have life expectancy at birth of less than 30 years. It is striking that of these 56, in only four tables was life expectancy at 50 at or below 10 years (plus one life table that gives a range of 9.5 to 12.5 years). The four exceptions are all for immigrants from the United States to Liberia. If the first year of experience in Liberia is included, life expectancies at birth were only 1.7 and 2.2 years (for males and females, respectively), but even in this case, life expectancy at age 50 was 7.9 and 6.6 years. These data for the first year of exposure to the West African disease environment can be dismissed as irrelevant in the present context. For those who survived the first year in Liberia, the corresponding figures are life expectancies at birth of 25.8 and 23.9 years, and at 50 of 9.6 and 8.3 years. Included in Wilmoth's table is a summary estimate for Stone Age populations, taken from Acsadi and Nemeskeri's (1970) history of the human life span; they estimate life expectancy at birth to be 21 years and at 50 to be 12 years.

Because women are still vigorous at age 45 and for many years after, it is also useful to consider the size of the elderly population, taking 65 as a convenient benchmark. Table 11-1 shows that although life expectancy for those reaching age 65 was probably 7-10 years, the population share of the elderly was probably in the range of only 1-8 percent.

In my view this evidence is quite persuasive: 15-45 percent of females in preagricultural societies would have survived to age 45, at which point their remaining life expectancy would have been more than 10 years and probably in the range of 12-25 years. Something like 10-30 percent of the stationary female population would have been postreproductive. If this view is right, then the prevalence of postreproductive human females in preagricultural populations would be similar to, or greater than, that for pilot whales.

---

[2]The life table gives values for l_x and for e_x. The product $l_x e_x$ gives T_x, the person years lived above age x in the stationary population; dividing this by e_0 gives the share of this age segment in the total population. Here, $0.463*22.1/37.1 = 0.276$ (see Hill and Hurtado, 1996:196-198). The proportion in a rapidly growing stable population such as that of the actual Aché would be much lower, but that is not the relevant number for the evolutionary long run in which populations have been close to stationarity on average.

It is also interesting to consider comparable figures for modern low-mortality populations, for which a female life expectancy at birth of 80 is not unusual. For the United States, we see in Table 11-1 that life expectancy at 45 is 36 years, and at 65 it is still 19 years. Forty-four percent of the female stationary population is postreproductive, and 20 percent is at or over age 65. Looking to the future, Table 11-1 also shows data projected to the year 2065, at which point the life expectancy at birth is 90 years, 50 percent of the stationary female population would be postreproductive, and 28 percent would be at or above age 65.

We can conclude that in our preagricultural past, postreproductive females probably made up a substantial proportion of the population. This leads us naturally to the question: what did these abundant older members of the population do? Were they a benefit or a burden for the younger members of the population? We turn now to consider a subset of the issues raised by this question.

THE ELDERLY AS REPOSITORIES OF KNOWLEDGE

"Knowledge, wisdom, and experience are social assets which normally accumulate with age and outlast physical stamina.... Those endowed with the art of writing and surrounded by printed documents can scarcely appreciate the inestimable value of an aged person possessing more knowledge than any other source within reach" (Simmons, 1945:131). Statements of this sort are frequently encountered and are certainly plausible. However, quantitative evidence is rarely available to support them. Fairbanks and McGuire (1986) have reported a striking inverse association of the mortality rates for young captive female vervets (small gray African monkey) with the presence of a grandmother.

It would be a simple matter to search for such associations in many preindustrial human populations using widely available survey data, but I am unaware of any such studies. However, an interesting study reported in Rosenzweig (1994) provides quantitative evidence on a related point. He notes that in India families farm the same plot of land for generations and there are important variations in the microclimatic and microagronomic conditions from plot to plot. Under these conditions, farmers accumulate much valuable information about their specific plots of land through experience over their lives, and the elderly have the most experience, sometimes of infrequent events such as serious droughts. Rosenzweig considers the extent to which farm profits decline under locally adverse weather conditions in two large samples of Indian farms for which longitudinal data are available. The findings are shown in Figure 11-1. Farm profits fell most when the eldest person present in the family was less than 40 years old; they fell less when the oldest was less than 60; and they fell only about half this much when the eldest was 60 or over. Having an eldest over age 60 appeared to reduce the losses to about half the level attainable through the presence of a local agricultural extension station or of electricity. A related

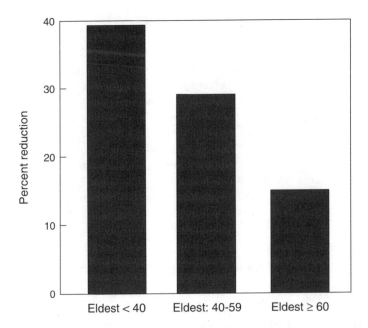

FIGURE 11-1 Percentage fall in profits due to bad weather, by age of eldest member. NOTES: These are households in which there is no extension aid. SOURCE: Based on Rosenzweig (1994).

analysis with a different data set for Indian farms showed similarly important effects of the years of experience of the most experienced worker on the farm, which appeared to raise average productivity and reduce the influence of adverse conditions on output (Rosenzweig, 1994:78).

It is important to realize that there are serious dangers in inferring causality from associations of this sort, whether for humans or for animals. If there were a genetic component to survival, then that component alone could account for a positive association of the survival of infants and grandparents, even if grandmothers had no effect on survival of their grandchildren. The same is true for any other source of variation in mortality that is specific to a particular family. For example, variations across families in the healthiness of the site they occupy could induce such a positive association. A spurious association might arise in other ways, as well. Causality might run from prosperity to coresidence of the grandparents, rather than the reverse, at least in human populations. Grandparents with a number of adult children might choose the most prosperous to live with, and grandparents might be sent away when food is inadequate to support them. Caution is necessary in interpreting data of this sort, intriguing as such data may be.

TRANSFER FLOWS TO AND FROM THE ELDERLY

"In summary, then, individuals everywhere seem to have become progressively dependent upon others for their food with the onset of old age" (Simmons, 1945:34-35).

An evolutionary perspective suggests that postreproductive and elderly humans would increase the reproduction or survival of their own children, as Kaplan (1994) argues. For toothed whales, discussed by Carey and Gruenfelder (in this volume) and Austad (in this volume), postreproductive females continue to lactate and thus transfer food to their young descendants. This view contrasts starkly with one of the best-known theories of fertility for traditional human societies (Caldwell, 1976). Caldwell's theory is based on the premise that in traditional societies, children transfer resources to their parents and are in other ways instrumentally useful to them:

> The key issue here, and, I will argue, the fundamental issue in demographic transition, is the *direction and magnitude of intergenerational wealth flows* or the net balance of the two flows—one from parents to children and the other from children to parents—over the period from when people become parents until they die.... In all primitive societies and nearly all traditional societies the net flow is from child to parent (1976:140).

Caldwell argues that a net upward transfer of resources provides the motivation for the high fertility typically observed in traditional societies until recently. Cross-cultural survey evidence confirms that in agricultural societies, parents do value children for their instrumental contributions—help around the house, in the fields, and support in old age. If Caldwell's argument is correct, then the behavior of elderly humans in preindustrial societies would present a strong contrast to the behavior of postreproductive elderly animals in nature, who typically transfer resources downward to their own adult offspring and to their grandchildren (as described by Carey and Gruenfelder, and by Austad, in this volume). If elderly humans in traditional societies are a drain on the resources of their adult children, receiving resources that might otherwise have been used for reproduction and child rearing, then it is hard to see how such behavior maximizes fitness, unless the elderly make sufficiently great contributions as stores of knowledge to warrant such support.

To shed light on these issues, I will review evidence on intergenerational transfers in human populations. There are two questions to address. (1) Is the general direction of transfers (intergenerational wealth flows, in Caldwell's terminology) upward from younger to older members of the population (as Caldwell asserts) or downward from older to younger members of the population? (2) Is there a stage in the life cycle when transfers flow upward from younger to older members of the population, particularly to elderly people, even if the net flow is downward over the whole life cycle? We will not be looking for individual cases of one kind of flow or another, because surely at one time or another, for one or another pair of individuals, one could find any kind and direction of flow. What does interest us is the broad pattern of flows, on average, in a population. The section concludes by discussing how selection could lead to upward transfers from children to parents while the parents are still in their reproductive phase.

While it would be instructive to have microlevel data showing who gave what to whom when, such comprehensive data are seldom, if ever, available, and partial data are of little use. The data more often available are aggregate average-age profiles of consumption and production by age. When capital markets and storable commodities are rare, mistrusted, or nonexistent, then differences between consumption and production are made up by transfers.

Formal modeling and analysis of populations in which there are interage transfer flows suggest some simple but useful measures (Willis, 1988; Lee, 1994a). (1) Simple inspection of the aggregate age profiles of consumption and production can be useful. (2) The population-weighted average ages of consumption, A_c, and production, A_y, are very informative. If $A_c > A_y$, then, on average, consumption in the population occurs later than production, and resources, on average, flow upward from younger to older. A simple arrow diagram, with a head at the average age of consumption and tail at the average age of production, is an effective way to display this information. The arrow then points in the direction of the transfers, and the arrow length indicates the degree to which these transfers flow either upward or downward. The position of the arrow shows the average ages. (3) In a stationary population, the product of the difference in average ages, $A_c - A_y$, and the average amount of consumption or production per capita in the population as a whole gives the total amount, W, that the average member of the population can expect to receive in net transfers, over the remainder of life.

If W is positive, the average person is expecting to receive more in future transfers than this person will give in transfers; transfers are upward from younger to older on net. If W is negative, transfers are downward. The diagram can be modified to incorporate the measure of W by thickening the arrow in proportion to per capita consumption. The arrow area then indicates the net future transfer to be received, W. (For a formal development of these ideas, see Lee, 1994a.) The thick arrows are most useful for comparing different kinds of transfer flows within the same population, such as child support, bequests, or a public sector pension system.

This diagrammatic approach provides a way to assess the overall direction of inter-age transfer flows in a population, thereby answering the first question about net direction of transfer flows in a population. For the second question—whether there is some life cycle stage when transfers flow upward from younger to older—either we can simply inspect the aggregate age profiles of consumption and production or we can explicitly evaluate flows between adult parents and their children, and between the elderly and their adult children, in a strictly intergenerational manner.

We can now look at some estimates of the overall direction of transfer flows for preindustrial societies. I have examined data on the following populations:

• Kaplan (1994) presents consumption and production data for three different groups of Amazon Basin hunter-gatherer-horticulturalists, including the Aché, and generously made these available to me for further analysis. The age profiles themselves show that people continue to be net producers throughout their adult lives, including in old age. The elderly clearly continue to transfer food to their children and grandchildren. The Aché practice gerontocide, particularly of females, once the elderly are no longer able to produce.

• Dodds et al. (1996) provide estimates for five other Amazon Basin hunter-gatherer-horticulturalist societies, based on time-use data combined with assumed age profiles of consumption and hourly productivity. In these data, the net direction of transfers is still clearly downward, but there is apparently a stage in which the elderly produce less than they consume. For Figure 11-2, I have pooled these data for all five societies.

• Stecklov (1995) presents data for rural Cote D'Ivoire and analyzes them using the framework outlined above. Here also the net direction of transfers is strongly downward from older to younger, but at the same time the elderly consume more than they produce, by virtue of transfers from younger members of the population.

• Mueller (1976) develops age profiles of consumption and production from a variety of broad-based estimates representative of Third World agricultural populations. These data clearly indicate a net downward flow of transfers in the population, but again the elders receive transfers that enable them to consume more than they produce.

Figure 11-2 presents arrows for these societies. They all point distinctly downward, indicating that the direction of transfer flows is, on net, from older to younger. This contradicts the statement from Caldwell quoted above, if his statement is taken to refer strictly to transfers of foods and other easily measured physical items. The horizontal position and length of these arrows reflect the average ages of making and receiving transfers, and the figures indicate the difference in these average ages.

The answer to the second question, more specifically about the elderly, is that in some societies average transfers are always downward, even in old age (Kaplan, 1994), whereas in other societies, perhaps the majority, the older population consumes more than it produces. In this connection, however, note that the elderly provide many useful functions besides directly producing food. As Rosenzweig's (1994) study indicated, and as suggested by the quote from Simmons (1945), the knowledge and experience of the elderly can contribute substantially to food production, even when their physical contribution is limited. Furthermore, they may contribute in other intangible ways through leadership, maintaining order, etc. Finally, they may contribute childrearing services that

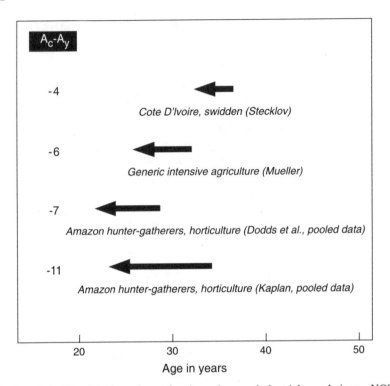

FIGURE 11-2 The direction of transfers in various preindustrial populations. NOTE: The tail of each arrow is located at the average age of producing in the population, and the head is located at the average age of consuming in the population. The length of the arrow is the number of years of age traversed by the average transfer. The thickness and vertical position of each arrow have no significance. A_c-A_y: difference between two average ages. SOURCE: Based on Lee (in press), Stecklov (1995), Mueller (1976), Dodds et al. (1996), and Kaplan (1994).

permit younger members of the population to be more productive, or they make tools for younger hunters (Hill and Hurtado, 1996:235-236).

For these reasons, some degree of upward-flowing physical transfers from adult children to elderly parents could be consistent with the demands of reproductive fitness. The same might also be true for other animals. If postreproductive female toothed whales provide fitness-enhancing childrearing services, including feeding and baby-sitting, then why should not their reproductive-age children or grandchildren render them some assistance through transfers of food, for example by sharing a kill? One could ask the same question about elephants, for whom elderly matriarchs appear to provide valuable services. Have such questions been addressed in field work?

Upward transfers of resources certainly do sometimes occur in nature, as in social insects, notably ants and bees. The queen, who is by far the oldest member of the population, produces no food and is herself fed and tended by younger members who are sterile. Following the analytic framework outlined above, there would doubtless be a strong downward transfer from worker bees to off-spring and another upward transfer to the queen. The net direction of flows is not apparent a priori. In any event, in these cases there is no puzzle about the relation of the upward transfers to reproductive fitness.

Upward transfer flows might also occur when generations share a domicile that includes a store of food, as happens when bannertail kangaroo rats permit one of their children to remain in the mound (as described by Austad, in this volume). Whether there is, in fact, any transfer, either upward or downward, through access to a common store of food, is not clear. A quote from Simmons (1945) is relevant: "... the aged among primitive peoples had greater opportunity for securing provisions from a common store in societies where group sharing of food was an established practice irrespective of age considerations than in societies where this was not the case."

As noted, the elderly may perform many services that enhance the reproductive fitness of their children and therefore of themselves but which escape an accounting of visible physical transfers. But it is also true, at least for humans, that the children may perform many valuable services for their parents that escape the measure of transfers. These services may involve low cost to the children, yet the services may be of high value to the older parents. Services of this kind include physical security for the household and its property arising from numbers of household members, care during occasional bouts of sickness or disability (risk spreading), political power in the community arising from kin networks, and so on. Some of these services may also be rendered to parents by children in nature. Such services make it very difficult to assess a broader version of Caldwell's theory, and clearly at times it is this broader version that Caldwell has in mind.[3]

So far I have discussed only preindustrial transfer flows. In the preindustrial societies for which I have presented data, the public sector was small, and its tax and transfer role was minimal. Financial institutions such as savings banks or stock markets were also of little relevance for the average person in the rural areas. Interage transfers took place almost entirely through the family, mainly in the form of childrearing or, in agricultural societies, through support for coresident elders. In the modern industrial state the situation is very different. Financial institutions are widespread, widely trusted, and widely used. I will not discuss their role here, however. Instead I will focus on three subjects: overall direction

---

[3]Children could also be viewed as providing a kind of insurance against the unlikely needs of survival to an incapacitated old age. Because of the rareness of the contingency, the average size of such upward flows in the population might be quite small, yet their insurance value to parents contemplating childbearing might be large. Such possibilities make it very difficult to test Caldwell's theory of fertility motivation in any definitive way.

of the transfer flow, transfers within the family, and transfers through the public sector.

Figure 11-3 shows arrow diagrams for transfers within the family in the United States, grouped into four kinds: (1) bequests to children at death of the parent; (2) interhousehold transfer flows between no-longer coresident parents and children; (3) parental costs of higher education; and (4) parental costs of child rearing, net of children's earnings as teenagers.

For each kind, the arrow is positioned as described earlier, and the thickness of the arrow represents the average size of the flow per person in the population (for details of estimation, see Lee, 1994b). All four kinds of familial transfers are downward. The area of each arrow indicates the expected value of net future receipts of transfers over the life cycle of the individual or the household. The average household expects a receipt of –$44,000 in bequests (data not shown); that is, the average household has received $44,000 in bequests already and anticipates leaving a similar amount to its heirs in the future. Bequests flow downward across age. Other interhousehold gifts and transfers are poorly measured in the data used for these calculations, but better data confirm the net direction of such flows. The average child receives about $81,000 in child-rearing expenditures (not counting parental time costs) and can expect to allocate a corresponding amount to each of its own children in the future, with the help of a spouse. There was an additional expenditure of about $6,000 per child for costs of higher education, which the child can also be expected to "repay" in the future. The figure shows massive downward transfer flows from parents to children within the family.

This pattern of downward familial transfers at all ages is consistent with Kaplan's (1994) measurements for the Aché and with the facts concerning post-reproductive toothed whales reported in Carey and Gruenfelder and in Austad (in this volume). However, the pattern is not consistent with the other agricultural and preagricultural societies for which data were earlier described; these commonly showed that the elderly received transfers from younger members of the population, enabling them to consume more than they produced. However, the net flows up to surviving elders are overwhelmed in value by the value of net flows downward from parents to children earlier in the life cycle, so the net direction of transfers flows overall is definitely downward, as shown earlier in Figure 11-2.

There is an obvious reason why the elderly in the United States continue to make net transfers to their adult children, in contrast to most preindustrial societies so far examined (except for those studied by Kaplan, 1994). The United States, like other industrial nations, has a well-developed system of transfers to the elderly through the public sector. These public transfers substitute for transfers to the elderly from their own children. Indeed, many elderly apparently believe that these public sector transfers go too far and offset the flows by private transfers in the opposite direction. Figure 11-4 shows arrows for public sector net

A. Interhousehold transfers

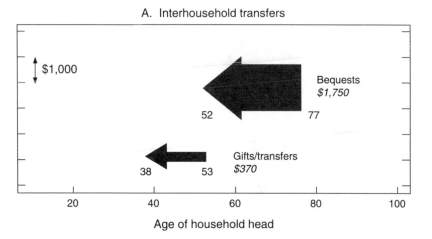

B. Within-household transfers (per child)

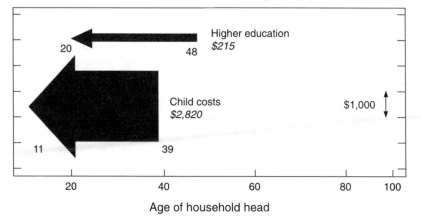

FIGURE 11-3 Familial transfers in the United States (data for the 1980s). NOTES: The four arrows represent bequests to children at death of parent; interhousehold transfer flows between no-longer coresident parents and children; parental costs of higher education; and parental costs of child rearing, net of children's earnings as teenagers. The top panel shows flows of transfers between households; the bottom panel shows flows of transfers within households. The tail of each arrow is located at the average age of making each kind of transfer in the population, and the head of the arrow is located at the average age of receiving each kind of transfer in the population. The thickness of each arrow represents the per capita (or per household) flow of each kind of transfer, indicated by the number below each label. The area of each arrow equals the average net transfer of each kind expected to be received by the average person or household over the remaining lifetime and is negative if the arrow points to the left. SOURCE: Based on Lee (1994b).

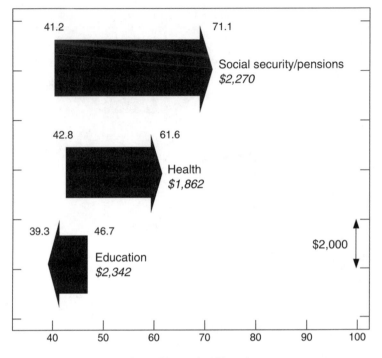

Age of household head

FIGURE 11-4 Public sector transfers to and from households in the United States (data for the 1980s). NOTE: See the note to Figure 11-3. The tail of the transfer is located at the average age of paying taxes in support of each kind of transfer, and the head at the average age of receiving each kind of transfer—in each case based on the age of the household reference person. Data combine federal, state, and local transfers. SOURCE: Based on Lee (1994b).

transfers for education, pensions, and medical care for the local, state, and federal levels combined. The areas of these arrows tell us the value of the expected net future transfer received per household, which is $69,000 for Social Security pensions; $35,000 for health care; –$17,000 for education (this negative sign means that the average household will pay more taxes in the future for education than it will receive in educational services, because educational services are received early in the life cycle of the average household and paid for through taxes later—the opposite to pensions and Medicare, for example). Clearly, on net, there are massive upward transfers through the public sector, even though educational transfers are, of course, downward. Indeed, when the upward transfers through the public sector are combined with the downward transfers through the family shown in Figure 11-3, the net direction of transfer flows is still upward, from younger to older. I think that this pattern would hold for other industrial countries as well. Data on interhousehold transfers support this speculation (see Lee, in press), although detailed analysis at the individual level has not yet been done except for the United States.

Caldwell (1976) argued that fertility is low in industrial societies because wealth flows have been reversed in these societies, with children now imposing substantial net costs on their parents rather than being the source of upward transfer flows. In fact, we have just seen that in the United States, net transfer flows are upward, not downward. However, we have also seen that it is the public sector transfers that are responsible for the upward direction, and the taxes in support of these transfers must be paid regardless of the number of children one has. For this reason, the net upward flows in the United States do not contradict Caldwell's ideas, and the downward flows we estimate within the family are consistent with his ideas.

The net upward direction of transfers in the United States and perhaps in other industrial societies is partly due to the changed demography (see Table 11-1). The proportion of elderly people in industrial societies is much higher than in traditional societies, due to lower mortality and lower fertility; moreover, their share in the population is destined to rise substantially in the coming decades. This transfer is also due to the relatively high consumption level (including health care) that the public sector transfers such as Social Security, Medicare, and Medicaid allow, together with home ownership, private savings, and private pensions.

I conclude this section by suggesting how evolution might lead in some cases to upward transfer flows from children to parents at some stage of the life cycle. Godfray (1995) reviews evolutionary theories of offspring-parent conflict, arising because the optimal parental investment in a child may be larger from the point of view of the child than the parent, so that generational interests diverge. A superficially related issue arises in analyses for humans of optimal parental investment in children's education, but with a more harmonious outcome than in the theories described by Godfray.

For humans, familial intergenerational transfers can be used to achieve the optimal investment in education from the child's perspective, even if this investment exceeds the optimal parental transfer to the child (Becker, 1988; Willis, 1994). The optimal investment in a child's education is such as to equate the rate of return from an incremental investment to the market rate of interest.[4] The child is unable to finance the education him/herself through credit markets, but

---

[4]I have simplified here. If the child has to pay for its education at the margin, then it will choose the amount described. If the education is received free from the parent, the child would like as much as possible. But given a total parental transfer in excess of the optimal educational amount (which equates the rate of return to the interest rate), the child would optimally take the amount in excess as a straight wealth transfer rather than an investment in education.

the optimal investment can nonetheless be achieved if the parents loan the child the incremental amount for education, in excess of the parental outright transfer. The child repays the parents later, in the form of old age support or perhaps assistance with the educational costs of younger siblings.

More generally, the parental investment t which maximizes the reproductive fitness of a given child is larger than the parental investment T which maximizes the reproductive fitness of the parent. In this circumstance, the reproductive fitness of both parent and child might be increased if the parent transferred outright the amount T to the child and then additionally "loaned" an amount of food or care to the child in excess of T, say $L = T - t$, with this amount L to be repaid by the child to the parent at a later life-cycle stage. The later repayment could take the form of assistance with a younger generation of the parent's children, as when adolescents help care for infants during a life-cycle stage in which they can generate a surplus to be transferred but are not yet capable of their own reproductive effort. Alternatively, the children could give food to their parent to replenish depleted reserves. Either way, parents could achieve more surviving offspring and greater reproductive fitness.

If a mutation should yield a gene that affected behavior so that children partially repaid parental investments in this way, the parents could then produce more surviving offspring by investing more in each or by having a greater number. Thus this gene would raise the reproductive fitness of those who had it, because it would be transmitted to their own children, who would behave similarly toward them. Furthermore, a gene for reneging would convey lower reproductive fitness in this example, because it also would be transmitted to offspring, and reproductive fitness would return to the original baseline level, which is by hypothesis lower than that with the repayment gene.

In this way, evolution could lead to life-cycle patterns of intergenerational transfers in which some parental investment in children is subsequently "repaid" by the child at a later life-cycle stage—that is, patterns in which transfers in both directions occur between parents and children, at different ages.

This theory has somewhat different implications than the inclusive fitness theory, according to which animals act to increase the reproductive fitness of those who share their genes. The repayment theory could explain such behavior independent of shared genes—for example, the behavior might be predicted to be as strong in relation to half siblings as to full siblings (if the exchange occurs with only one of the parents, rather than with both). At the same time, under the repayment theory and in contrast to the inclusive fitness theory, one would not expect any helpful behavior toward more distant relatives with whom a parent is not shared.

THE TRANSFER OF ASSETS: BEQUESTS

Austad (in this volume) discusses the transfer of assets from parents to their children. This transfer of a stock is usefully distinguished from transfer flows, such as routine feeding of children by their parents. The notions of assets and property rights for animals, and their transmissibility to offspring, at first seem odd and implausible to a social scientist. However, concrete examples make clear that these notions are indeed appropriate. Property rights do not seem to follow from a legal code or public sanctions, but rather from some aspect of the motivation of contestants, such that the defender of territory seldom loses a confrontation. Assets include territories, stores of food (seeds), and homes of various kinds such as burrows and mounds. Sharing the asset with a child during the parent's lifetime means that the child will inherit it on the death of the parent. Inter vivos bequeathal also occurs when the parent simply relinquishes the asset. Approximate ultimogeneture appears to be common, because parents are more likely to share their asset with a child when they are old and their life expectancy is short. According to Austad (in this volume), systematic study of the transfer of assets in relation to the aging of the parents is rare, and not much is yet known.

Transmission of assets among humans, and particularly bequest behavior, has been the subject of a great deal of study and literary effort. In parts of Europe, children could not marry until they inherited the family farm, creating a link between marriage, fertility, and mortality. Sometimes only one of the children was permitted to marry and reproduce, while the others might remain on the farm as unmarried servants or leave to become soldiers, emigrants, clerics, or servants elsewhere. In other parts of Europe, older parents might transfer ownership of the farm to a child, while continuing to live on the farm in an outbuilding; the child would then be obligated to feed and care for the parents until their death. Many other arrangements were also possible, including transmission of the rights to use land without outright ownership. The transmission of assets from parents to children was surrounded by elaborate strategic behavior on the part of both children and parents. Indeed, the ownership of property is one of the major ways in which elderly parents have induced their children to transfer flows of resources upward to them, as in the example given above in which inter vivos transfer of the farm to a child carried a contractual obligation on the part of the child to provide food for the elderly parents.

Because it appears from Austad (in this volume) that children who receive transfers of assets are at a real advantage in terms of reproductive fitness, it would be interesting to investigate whether the transmission of assets is also subject to strategic behavior on the part of either parents or, perhaps more likely, siblings. If it matters a lot who inherits the family mound, then there should be observable competition for the right to do so.

Austad (in this volume) suggests that "As a gross generality, males are more likely to be bequeathed valuable resources such as nests, dens, or territories in birds, whereas females are more likely to inherit such resources in mammals ...." It is interesting that Simmons (1945:49) also suggests a generalization, based on a statistical analysis of the practices of different societies: "... aged women, in contrast with men, have tended to acquire property rights more readily in simple societies characterized by collection, hunting and fishing, and also within the matrilineal type of family organization; while aged men have gained their greatest advantage in the control of property among farmers, and especially herders, as well as within the patriarchal system of family organization and amid social traits characteristic of more advanced cultures."

CONCLUSION

I will briefly summarize the main points that have emerged in the preceding discussion, including questions that might be addressed through animal studies:

- It is very likely that even in Stone Age populations, the life expectancy of females at age 45 was more than 10 years, and probably in the range of 12-25 years and that a substantial proportion of the female population, perhaps 10-30 percent, was postreproductive. The proportion of elderly at or above age 65 may have been very low, however.
- The average flow of net transfers within the family appears to be downward in all human societies so far examined, subject to the caveat that many studies measure mainly flows of food.
- There is often an upward net flow within the family from adult children to elderly parents, although this is always swamped by the magnitude of transfers downward through child rearing.
- There are many ways in which both human and animal elders can raise the reproductive fitness of their children, and therefore of themselves, beside the transfer of physical resources such as food. Such ways include leadership, storing knowledge, maintaining order, and so on.
- Widely available data would support the analysis of the effect on infant and child mortality of the presence of a grandparent in human agricultural households, if direction of causality can be established.
- Although upward transfer flows may be altruistic in humans, it is also possible that because the elderly can increase the reproductive fitness of their adult children, their children could enhance their own reproductive fitness by transferring resources to their parents. By a similar argument, one might expect sometimes to observe such transfers taking place, not only among humans but also among animals.
- It may be that upward transfers do occur sometimes in nature, and the possibility may be worth attention. Possible cases that come to mind include social insects (which are a very special case); stored food in shared dwellings, to which the elderly have access; kills which the elderly are permitted to eat; and general food sharing.
- Both humans and animals in nature sometimes bequeath valuable assets to their children. Among humans, control of these assets by the elderly, combined with declared plans to transfer the asset to a child at death, is often used to manipulate the favored child into supporting the elder through upward transfers.

Does such strategic use of valuable assets ever occur among animals? For example, do elders share in the stores accumulated by the coresident-favored offspring among bannertail kangaroo rats? And do animal children compete in some way for the right to inherit?

I have argued that postreproductive females and older males were quite prevalent in preagricultural human populations and that they probably raised the reproductive fitness of their children through leadership, knowledge, and food transfers. It is unknown, however, whether the longevity of humans can, in fact, be explained by the usefulness of older humans. The contribution of postreproductive humans to the reproductive fitness of their descendants is a necessary, but not sufficient, condition for the viability of an evolutionary explanation.

Austad (in this volume) concludes with the suggestion that if there is more field work linking transmission of assets to senescence in animals, then "a generalized theory of the ecology of resource transfer across generations may emerge." The study of the evolution of longevity together with a general study of intergenerational transfers does, indeed, appear to be a promising and fascinating area for further work.

ACKNOWLEDGMENT

I am grateful to Timothy Miller, Shripad Tuljapurkar, Kenneth Wachter, and two anonymous referees for comments during preparation of this chapter. Research for this paper was funded by a grant from National Institute on Aging (AG11761).

REFERENCES

Acsadi, G., and J. Nemeskeri
  1970   *History of Human Life Span and Mortality*. Budapest: Akademiai Kiado.
Becker, G.S.
  1988   Family economics and macro behavior. *American Economic Review* 78(1 March):1-13.
Bhat, M.P.
  1987   Mortality in India: Levels, Trends, and Patterns, Ph.D. dissertation, University of Pennsylvania.
Bongaarts, J.
  1983   The proximate determinants of natural marital fertility. Pp. 61-102 in R. Bulatao and R. Lee, eds., *Determinants of Fertility in Developing Countries Supply and Demand for Children*, Vol. 1. New York: Academic Press.
Caldwell, J.C.
  1976   Toward a Restatement of Demographic Transition Theory, *Population and Development Review*. Pp. 113-180 reprinted in (1982) J. Caldwell *Theory of Fertility Decline*. New York: Academic Press.
Carter, L., and R. Lee
  1992   Modeling and forecasting U.S. mortality: Differentials in life expectancy by sex. In D. Ahlburg and K. Land, eds., *Population Forecasting*, a special issue of *International Journal of Forecasting* 14(3):393-412.

Coale, A., and P. Demeny
    1983   *Regional Model Life Tables and Stable Populations.* New York: Academic Press.
Dodds, D., D. Friou, and C. Mason
    1996   Does wealth flow upward in lowland tropical America? A test of Caldwell's hypothesis.
            A paper presented at the 1996 annual meeting of the Population Association of America,
            New Orleans.
Ermisch, J.
    1989   Intergenerational transfers in industrialized countries: Effects of age distribution and
            economic institutions. *Journal of Population Economics* 1:269-284.
Fairbanks, L.A., and M.T. McGuire
    1986   Age, reproductive value, and dominance-related behaviour in vervet monkey females:
            Cross-generational influences on social relationships and reproduction. *Animal Behavior*
            34:1710-1721.
Godfray, H.C.J.
    1995   Evolutionary theory of parent-offspring conflict. *Nature* 376(July 13):133-138.
Hassan, F.A.
    1981   *Demographic Archeology.* New York: Academic Press.
Hill, K., and A.M. Hurtado
    1996   *Aché Life History.* New York: Aldine de Gruyter.
Howell, N.
    1979   *Demography of the Dobe !Kung.* New York: Academic Press.
Johnson, A.
    1975   Time Allocation in a Machiguenga Community. *Ethnology* 14:301-310.
Kaplan, H.
    1994   Evolutionary and wealth flows theories of fertility: Empirical tests and new models.
            Population and Development Review 20(4):753-791.
Lee, R.D.
    1994a   The Formal Demography of Population Aging, Transfers, and the Economic Life Cycle,
            Pp. 8-49 in L. Martin and S. Preston, eds., *The Demography of Aging.* Committee on
            Population, National Research Council. Washington, DC: National Academy Press.
    1994b   Population age structure, intergenerational transfers, and wealth: A new approach, with
            Applications to the U.S. In P. Gertler, ed., on *The Family and Intergenerational Rela-
            tions,* a special issue of *Journal of Human Resources* 29(4):1027-1063.
    In press A Cross-Cultural Perspective on Intergenerational Transfers and the Economic Life Cycle.
            Presented at IUSSP seminar, East West Center Population Program, Honolulu, September
            12-14, 1995. Forthcoming conference volume A. Mason, ed.
Lovejoy, C.O., R.S. Meindl, T.R. Pryzbeck, T.S. Barton, K.G. Heiple, and D. Kotting
    1977   Paleodemography of the Libben site, Ottawa County, Ohio. *Science* 198:291-293.
Mueller, E.
    1976   The economic value of children in peasant agriculture. Pp. 98-153 in R. Ridker, ed.,
            Population and Development: The Search for Interventions. Baltimore, MD: Johns
            Hopkins Press.
Preston, S.H., A. McDaniel, and C. Grushka
    1993   New model life tables for high-mortality populations. *Historical Methods* 26(4):149-159.
Rosenzweig, M.
    1994   Human capital development, the family, and economic development. Pp. 63-90 in S.
            Asefa and W.C. Huang, eds., *Human Capital and Economic Development.* Kalamazoo,
            MI: Upjohn Institute.
Simmons, L.
    1945   *The Role of the Aged in Primitive Society.* New Haven, CT: Yale University Press.

Stecklov, G.
1995   Intergenerational Resource Flows in Cote d'Ivoire: An Empirical Analysis, Presented at the annual meeting of the Population Association of America, San Francisco, May 1995.

U.S. Social Security Administration
1992   *Life Tables for the United States Social Security Area, 1990-2080.* Washington, DC: U.S. Department of Health and Human Services.

Weiss, K.M.
1973   Demographic models for anthropology. *Society for American Archaeology Memoirs* 27:1-186.

Willis, R.
1988   Life cycles, institutions and population growth: A theory of the equilibrium interest rate in an overlapping-generations model. Pp. 106-138 in R. Lee, W. B. Arthur and G. Rodgers eds., *Economics of Changing Age Distributions in Developed Countries.* New York: Oxford University Press.

1994   Economic analysis of fertility: Micro-foundations and aggregate implications. Pp. 139-172 in K.L. Kiessling and H. Landberg, eds., *Population and Economic Development and the Environment.* New York: Oxford University Press.

Wilmoth, J.R.
1995   The earliest centenarians: A statistical analysis. in Bernard Jeune and J.W. Vaupel, eds., *Exceptional Longevity.* Odense, Denmark: Odense University Press.

12

The Potential of Population Surveys for Genetic Studies

Robert B. Wallace

INTRODUCTION

Knowledge of the genetic causes of health conditions and age-related physiologic changes is growing rapidly. Much of the lore of genetics and health, in addition to basic genetic science and molecular biology, comes from the study of informative families and patient groups and, to some extent, from specifically designed population studies. Many populations have been surveyed in recent years to address general health issues, and many more are being surveyed for other important reasons, such as for testing social, economic, or political hypotheses. Among the sponsors of extensive population studies of many types, emphasizing older persons and their health and social needs, is the U.S. National Institute on Aging (NIA), part of the National Institutes of Health. With the emerging technology for conducting genetic studies, it is time to ask whether ways can be found to exploit these major population surveys to better understand the genetics of conditions important to public health. The methodologic challenges for marrying large population surveys to genetic hypotheses are complex and not easily solved, in part because each survey was thoroughly rationalized, scrutinized, and funded to address a set of important nongenetic scientific questions relating to general health, social behavior, and economics. However, given the substantial costs of these population surveys and the restricted availability of research funds, it is essential to at least explore possible intersections of genetic inquiry with existing and planned field studies. The purpose of this paper is to (1) catalog many of the important geographic surveys being supported and/or archived by

NIA, (2) describe selected, potential applications of these surveys for genetic study, (3) address the various modes of specimen collection applicable in population surveys, and (4) suggest a research agenda to realize these potential methodologic enhancements.

SUMMARY OF RECENT NIA POPULATION-BASED SURVEYS

Many population surveys are conducted in the United States and elsewhere; there is no clear way to identify all of them. Many of the NIA-sponsored surveys are extensive in scope and themes, and several are conducted outside of the United States. Information on a selection of these surveys, the basic characteristics of which are described in Table 12-1, was taken from the NIA document "Databases on Aging," a summary of surveys relevant to the demography, economics, and epidemiology of aging, published in February, 1996.[1] The surveys noted in Table 12-1 are not an exhaustive list of those available, nor does the table cite many of the survey data sets available in archive form for analysis. In some instances, the tabular information is simplified because of the complex, multiple sampling frames and the varied target populations and different survey intervals. On occasion, survey design and operational information were incomplete.

In summary, the survey study designs reveal the following: (1) the surveys vary dramatically in health-related content; many were intended largely to study behavioral, social, and economic issues; (2) most of the surveys are recent but inactive, and it is unclear whether participants could be located or recontacted to obtain additional information; (3) many of the surveys contain information on at least some family members, but sometimes this is limited to spouse pairs and the extent of documenting either nuclear or extended pedigrees is often limited or uncertain; (4) collection of bodily specimens—either blood or other tissues or fluids—is rare. In the few instances where specimens were collected, this was limited mostly to U.S. national samples and subsamples conducted by the U.S. National Center for Health Statistics; (5) follow-up rates for the longitudinal panels were generally quite good, including mortality follow-up when part of the protocol; and (6) the original investigators would almost always need to be contacted to explore further participant contact and any possibility of specimen collection, including the determination of ethical and administrative procedures. In general, this suggests that retrospective use of these surveys, particularly the inactive ones, would require additional resources and energy to suit them for genetic study, but nonetheless, a reasonable potential remains for exploitation of, at least, ongoing or planned surveys.

---

[1]Copies of this document may be obtained from Richard Suzman, Ph.D., National Institute on Aging, Gateway Building, National Institutes of Health, Bethesda, MD 20892, USA.

TABLE 12-1 Summary of Selected NIA-sponsored Population Surveys

Survey	Currently Active[a]	Country	Age Range	Family Data	Specimen Collection
Asset and Health Dynamics (N = 8,000)	Yes	USA	70+	Yes	No
Australian Longitudinal Study of Ageing (N = 2,087)	Yes	Australia	70+	Yes	No
Cross-sectional and Longitudinal Aging Study (N = 2,891)	Yes	Israel	75+	Yes	?
Established Populations for Epidemiological Study of the Elderly (N ≈ 14,000; four populations)	Yes	U.S.A.	65+	Yes	Yes
German Socio-Economic Panel (N ≈ 8,100 households)	Yes	Germany	All	Yes	No
Health and Retirement Survey (N = 12,600)	Yes	U.S.A.	51-61	Yes	No
Longitudinal Study on Aging (N ≈ 5,000)	No	U.S.A.	70+	No	No
Supplement on Aging II (Planning phase)	Yes	U.S.A.	70+	No	No
Luxembourg Income Study (Multiple databases)	Yes	Multiple	All	Yes	No
Second Malaysian Family Life Survey (N ≈ 6,000)	No	Malaysia	All	Yes	No
National Long-Term Care Survey (N = 6,393)	Yes	U.S.A.	65+	Yes	No
National Longitudinal Survey: Re-Survey of Older Males (N = 2,092)	No	U.S.A.	69-84	Yes	No
National Nursing Home Survey Follow-up (N ≈ 11,000)	No	U.S.A.	Older adults	No	No
National Survey of Families and Households Reinterview (N = 13,017)	No	U.S.A.	19+	Yes	No
New Beneficiary Survey and New Beneficiary Follow-up (N ≈ 16,000)	No	U.S.A.	60+	Yes	No
Panel Study of Income Dynamics (N ≈ 28,000)	Yes	U.S.A	All	Yes	No
Wisconsin Longitudinal Survey (N = 10,317)	Yes	U.S.A.	18-60	Yes	No

[a]Active as of December, 1995.

POTENTIAL APPLICATIONS OF POPULATION
SURVEYS FOR GENETIC STUDY

It is beyond the scope of this report to review advances in basic and clinical genetics and the relation of genetic structure and function to disease occurrence and outcome. For those involved in social surveys who are not schooled in genetics, a very brief discussion emphasizing the complexity of the situation may be of value. On 23 matched (except for the one pair of sex chromosomes) pairs of chromosomes in the nuclei of each human cell, the human genome contains about 100,000 genes, discrete functional and structural sites that interact with the internal cellular and external environment to direct basic cell growth, activity, and death and to transfer this information to the next generation. Each matched gene may vary somewhat from its mate and from the respective genes at the same site in other individuals. These structural variants, called alleles, may function somewhat differently from each other. The specific genetic makeup of an individual is called the genotype. The process of change in the structure of a gene, often accompanied by changes in function, is called mutation; mutation may occur spontaneously or be accelerated by external environmental forces. Mutations may be harmful or helpful to an organism or be biologically neutral. Not all human genes have yet been identified as to structure and function, but work is progressing rapidly. Determination of the structure and function of genes and the relation of altered gene structure to disease occurrence is made more complex by several recent observations: (1) some genes are not necessarily in one physical location on a chromosome; (2) to the extent that important chronic illnesses are gene-related, there are probably multiple genes involved; (3) the mechanisms of genetic regulation and how environmental factors alter that function are incompletely understood; and, (4) some genetic material (DNA) is located outside the nuclear chromosomes in the cytoplasm of the cell and is probably of maternal origin only. Thus, the search for gene-disease associations is clearly complex and difficult, although extremely important. However, as noted below, there are other potential genetically related applications of population studies.

To find potential applications of existing population studies for addressing genetic hypotheses, it is instructive to indicate some general categories of applications, temporarily leaving aside study methods and logistical issues. These categories are possible through the rapidly expanding ability to identify and characterize many genes within individuals and large population samples. However, as in all other fields of measurement, quality control in the laboratory determination of various alleles is essential, as substantial error can occur in laboratory procedures.

Given the emerging capacity to detemine alleles in population samples, the following is a selected list of general genetic research applications in population surveys, recognizing that specific studies have many scientific and methodologic contingencies:

Determination of Genotype Frequencies in Well-Defined Populations

A general survey application is to determine the distribution of various genes and alleles in defined populations. While it is an empirical question whether well-constructed and executed population samples will reveal estimates of genotype (allele) frequencies markedly different from more customary sources, such as volunteer populations, clinical populations, blood donors, and newborn screening samples, this use is probably one of the best applications for preexisting and planned general population samples. In addition to their specific sample representativeness, the NIA populations may be attractive because of their broad national coverage, multinational representation, and in some instances access to special populations such as the institutionalized elderly or the oldest old. This access would be particularly valuable as genes are discovered that are associated with late-onset diseases, given the age distribution of many NIA-sponsored survey participants. Several potential specific applications are presented, with examples from the recent scientific literature:

1. Identification of the age-specific prevalence rates for various alleles to explore hypotheses that these alleles are associated with longevity, at least in cross-sectional designs.

2. More precise estimation of rare gene/allele population prevalence, because many populations have thousands of participants. This would generally increase the ability to study the biologic behavior of putative, but rarely occurring, gene-disease associations. For an example in population genetic modeling, see Joyce and Tavare (1995). Another example is the population prevalence of the genetic variants of phenylketonuria, a condition that has a frequency of about 1:10,000 (Eisensmith and Woo, 1994).

3. Determination of allele frequency in multiple ethnic and national groups; this allows assessment of the genetic relatedness of such groups, as well as a comparison of gene frequencies with disease-occurrence rates (Gill and Evett, 1995).

4. Calculation of population inbreeding coefficients in selected populations to explore the emergence of recessive traits. If genetic determinations are done on available families ascertained from population surveys, it is possible to quantify the degree of population inbreeding, which positively correlates with the emergence rate of hidden (recessive) genetic conditions in that population. This value is sometimes a very important datum in understanding population disease rates (Gill and Evett, 1995).

5. Assessment of genetic relatedness of migrant and native ethnic, tribal, or national populations. Genetic tools may be useful for tracking the origins of population migration in prehistoric and early historic times (Kalnin et al., 1995).

6. Provision of high-quality population-referent genetic-marker data for forensic applications. The use of geographically defined populations may offer

greater precision in estimating genetic-marker prevalence, which has many medico-legal uses (van Oorschot et al., 1994).

7. Geographic searches for original or "founding" populations for various genetic diseases. Sometimes it is useful in understanding the population distribution of important genetic diseases to determine the historical source of the original mutations. This can often be difficult, but variation in allele frequencies among different ethnic groups in a population can offer useful clues, as in familial hypercholesterolemia, which is caused by a major gene (Rubinsztein et al., 1994).

8. Exploration for certain genes or alleles that may explain geographic differences in individual response to certain medications. For example, a particular allele that alters metabolism of a common class of antihypertensive drugs may be much more common in Chinese than in Caucasian populations (Lee, 1994). In an analogous manner, gene-directed alterations in the metabolism of toxic environmental chemicals may be used to explain population differences in disease risk associated with those exposures. Another example is the possibility of determining population differences in the risk of adverse reactions to blood transfusion based on the genetic characteristics of donor and recipient populations (Shivdasani and Anderson, 1994).

9. Determination of the risk of specific diseases in individuals. A major hope has been to use population studies to explore the role of various genetic determinations in disease risk for individuals. Earlier attempts at using measurable phenotypes (physical manifestations of gene function such as blood type or eye color) as risk factors for disease occurrence were only modestly successful. Even now, with a host of gene-measurement techniques, determining gene-disease associations in prospective population studies is probably inefficient, although perhaps useful for selected investigations. Most gene-disease associations are sought by other means, such as twin studies, segregation analysis of pedigrees, and case-control studies. Defined populations could also be used to verify gene-disease associations, discovered elsewhere, in a population context and to determine the sensitivity and specificity of particular alleles for predicting disease occurrence. One example is the recent association of the apolipoprotein E alleles with variation in the risk of dementia or cognitive change, which was seen in a cohort study (Hyman et al., in press). Other examples of genetic applications for determining disease risk in populations are the suggestion that there may be genes determining susceptibility to tuberculosis infection (Skamene, 1994) and the emerging demonstration of genetic forces in cardiovascular-disease risk factors, such as obesity and hypertension (Schork et al., 1994). Knowledge of population gene frequency for known disease-causing alleles is also quite useful for planning and executing population-based genetic screening programs, which are becoming more common as disease genes are discovered (Shickle and Harvey, 1993). However, regardless of whether genetic markers predict disease onset, they have other emerging uses, such as predicting the natural history and outcome

of diseases. For example, certain alleles predict whether young diabetic patients will acquire a certain severe form of retinal disease (Cruickshanks et al., 1992).

Many other applications exist, based on the population determination of genetic markers, but exploiting these opportunities requires dialogue and inter-disciplinary cooperation to identify and answer important scientific questions.

Unbiased Sampling of Families or Pedigrees to Ascertain Gene-Disease Associations

Currently, most gene-disease associations are explored in families. The basic logic is to ascertain whether certain genes (alleles) occur in the same members of genetically related families as does a medical condition of interest, called segregation analysis. Other general methods for studying gene-disease associations involve selected parts of family units such as siblings and cousins, or identical and fraternal twins. However, selecting these families (pedigrees) for study from clinical or volunteer populations may obscure some potential associations because of chance clustering of nongenetically related common diseases in these families, possibly leading to spurious negative findings. Sampling families from existing, defined general population surveys, particularly those with information on health and disease history, might be an effective way of unbiased pedigree sampling. The main obstacle may be that occurrence rates for most medical conditions are relatively low, even for population samples numbering in the thousands, and thus not all survey samples may be fully useful for identifying representative families with the multiple occurrence of various conditions. Panel (cohort) studies, as opposed to prevalence (cross-sectional) studies may be somewhat more valuable in this regard because over time additional cases of the study disease will occur and be monitored.

It is also possible, although somewhat inefficient, to ascertain certain family stuctures, such as twins, multiple siblings, or multiple cousins, from population surveys for further study.

Using Population Surveys for Estimates of Phenotypic Expression

Health-related population surveys have been determining disease and risk-factor occurrence in populations for many years. This fact is restated to emphasize that accurate data on the occurrence of nonfatal diseases and physiologic measures are surprisingly difficult to acquire in many national and regional populations, particularly when inferences from mortality statistics are unavailable. Potentially, social and economic surveys can collect basic health data in certain situations and these data will often contribute to knowledge on population health, as well as help assess the promise of that population for genetic study.

COLLECTING GENETIC INFORMATION
IN POPULATION SURVEYS

Genetic data can be divided roughly into two categories. The first category is the historical information obtained at interview, including family pedigrees with their biologic relationships, and the disease experience of those families both within and across generations. Standardized techniques exist for ascertaining and recording pedigree information (Bennett et al., 1995). The second category is the bodily specimens on which the genetic studies can be run. There are several general ways to acquire such specimens:

Venopuncture. The most effective way is to obtain blood at the time of survey, if resources allow. This procedure requires specific training of interviewers and use of equipment to store and transmit blood specimens. An alternative approach is to have a smaller number of trained venopuncturists visit the survey respondents later. This protocol would be particularly helpful when a willing primary respondent can gather available family members. Another approach that has been successful is to supply the study participant with blood vials, a prepaid mailing container, and a voucher to pay a local physician or clinic to obtain, process, and transmit the specimen. A less efficient but ancillary approach is to obtain a blood specimen that was stored for some other reason.

Hair follicles. In this technique participants are asked to supply a hair specimen that includes the follicular roots. We have less experience in obtaining such samples in the survey setting, but it may be worth pursuing.

Cheek swabs. This technique is noninvasive and offers promise where venopuncture is impossible. Processing specimens is more cumbersome and expensive, and a problem exists with contamination of the specimen by oral bacteria, food particles, etc.

Surgical specimens. A common technique in molecular epidemiology, particularly in the study of cancer occurrence and prognosis, is to acquire stored tissue specimens obtained at surgery, on which many genetic markers can be determined. These specimens will, of course, vary in availability, depending in part on the time interval since the operation, but they still may be an important source of markers—one that can be accessed by mail if participant and pathologist consents are obtained. A corollary approach is to obtain stored blood or tissue specimens that were obtained at autopsy. Unfortunately, autopsy rates are low and decreasing; this option will often be unavailable.

ETHICAL CONSIDERATIONS IN THE ACQUISITION AND
STORAGE OF GENETIC SPECIMENS

Although it is beyond the scope of this report to comprehensively review the ethical considerations of obtaining genetic markers, there are growing concerns and evolving regulations about the acquisition and disposition of these markers.

It is necessary for each investigator to ensure that appropriate consent procedures are followed for specimen acquisition, banking, and future applications. Particularly sensitive issues include: (1) accessibility of personal genetic information by other parties, such as family members or insurance companies, (2) accessibility of the specimens to other scientific laboratories, (3) ownership of potential commercial uses of biologic findings from collected specimens, (4) application of specimens for scientific determinations unplanned at the time of collection, (5) fear of discovering previously unreported paternity; and (6) disclosure of high levels of disease risk discovered after the main study has ended, including investigator obligation to maintain contact with participants after completion of the study. These and related issues have been recently discussed in depth, although not always with full resolution (Clayton et al., 1995; Wagener, 1995).

POTENTIAL ENHANCEMENTS TO NIA-SPONSORED SURVEYS TO IMPROVE APPLICATIONS TO GENETIC STUDIES

Given the apparent potential for amalgamating population surveys with genetic study, several possible enhancements to these studies might lead to improved applicability. These suggestions are intended for further discussion and research planning:

1. *Increase the number of studies in which biologic specimens with genetic material are routinely obtained.* This is, of course, both a logistic and a resource challenge. Surveys done over the telephone or over large geographic areas present substantial logistical difficulties, such as interviewer training and personal protection (the U.S. Occupational Safety and Health Administration has strict rules for persons handling blood and other biologic materials), specimen collection, and shipping. In addition, the prospect and burden of specimen collection may potentially decrease participation rates, possibly subverting survey success. However, as discussed, several alternative approaches exist to acquire specimens. Clearly, it is most efficient to consider appending genetic protocols to population surveys when the survey is being planned.

2. *Obtain informed consent, where possible, for future genetic studies in the event that they are executed.* As noted above, the ethical issues surrounding genetic determinations are complex and evolving. In recognition of investigator, institutional, and participant constraints, permission for future genetic determinations could be obtained as scientific issues emerge, perhaps offering with the consent procedures a set of guidelines about the type and disposition of studies possible in the future. Although this is being done presently, there are still numerous pitfalls, such as the action after identifiying a genotype associated with high risk of severe but preventable disease. An additional important element of informed consent is to document in advance who is to be contacted when a personally important genetic finding is discovered.

3. *Assemble an expert panel to develop a recommended, standard format for collecting pedigree information from participants in general health and social surveys, irrespective of any immediate need for the information.* This procedure would allow later reference to the pedigrees, both for sampling among them and for specific ascertainment if segregation analyses within a pedigree are being considered. Family structure and household rosters are sometimes collected as part of current social, economic, and demographic surveys, but a standardized format, easily displayed and in computerized form, would be very helpful. At a minimum, it would be essential to identify all first-degree relatives, their vital status, and location at the time of survey.

4. *Create a set of standard survey items that ascertain major conditions within families as part of routine survey procedures.* This would allow a standardized, general approach to cross-national and cross-cultural studies, where uniformity of morbidity and family data is a problem. There could also be sets of items that emphasize known or potential genetic and congenital diseases, allowing later restudy of the families or populations as candidate genetic markers emerge.

CONCLUSION

Both from substantive, methodologic, and ethical perspectives, study of the genetic causes of disease and dysfunction is advancing rapidly. Clearly, large-scale population surveys can be extremely informative on genetic issues if appropriate forethought accompanies the inception of these surveys. There is a need for multidisciplinary approaches, at the very least among social scientists, geneticists, epidemiologists, and survey researchers, to fully use the population-survey opportunity.

REFERENCES

Bennett, R.L., K.A. Steinhaus, S.B. Uhrich, C.K. O'Sullivan, R.G. Resta, D. Lochner-Doyle, D.S. Markel, V. Vincent, and J. Hamanishi
   1995   Recommendations for standardized human pedigree research. *American Journal of Human Genetics* 56:745-752.
Clayton, E.W., K.K. Steinberg, M.J. Khoury, E. Thompson, L. Andrews, M.J. Ellis Kahn, L.M. Kopelman, and J.O.Weiss
   1995   Informed consent for genetic research on stored tissue samples. *Journal of the American Medical Association* 274:1786-1792.
Cruickshanks, K.J., C.M.Vadheim, S.E. Moss, M.P. Roth, W.J. Riley, N.K. Macleran, D. Langfield, R.S. Sparkes, R. Klein, and J.I. Rotter.
   1992   Genetic markers associated with proliferative retinopathy in persons diagnosed with diabetes before 30 yr of age. *Diabetes* 41:879-885.
Eisensmith, R.C., and S.L. Woo
   1994   Population genetics of phenylketonuria. *Acta Paediatrica. Supplement* 407:19-26.

Hyman, B.T., T. Gomez-Isla, M. Briggs, H. Chung, S. Nichols, F. Kohout, and R. Wallace
In press   A population-based longitudinal study of the influence of apolipoprotein E genotype on the risk of cognitive impairment in the elderly. *Annals of Neurology*.

Gill, P., and I. Evett
1995   Population genetics of short tandem repeat (STR) loci. *Genetica* 96:69-87.

Joyce, P., and S. Tavare
1995   The distribution of rare alleles. *Journal of Mathematical Biology* 33:602-618.

Kalnin, V.V., O.V. Kalnina, M.I. Prosniak, I.M. Khidiatova, E.K. Khusnutdinova, K.S. Raphicov, and S.A. Limborska
1995   Use of DNA fingerprinting for human population genetic studies. *Molecular and General Genetics* 247:488-493.

Lee, E.J.
1994   Population genetics of the angiotensin-converting enzyme in Chinese. *British Journal of Clinical Pharmacology* 37:212-214.

Rubinsztein, D.C., D.R. van der Westhuyzen, and G.A. Coetzee
1994   Monogenic primary hypercholesterolemia in South Africa. *South African Medical Journal* 84:339-344.

Schork, N.J., A.B. Weder, M. Trevisan, and M. Laurenzi
1994   The contribution of pleiotropy to blood pressure and body-mass index variation: The Gubbio Study. *American Journal of Human Genetics* 54:361-373.

Shivdasani, R.A., and K.C. Anderson
1994   HLA homozygosity and shared HLA haplotypes in the development of transfusion-associated graft-versus-host disease. *Leukemia and Lymphoma* 15:227-234.

Shickle, D., and I. Harvey
1993   "Inside out," back-to-front: A model for clinical genetic population screening. *Journal of Medical Genetics* 30:580-582.

Skamene, E.
1994   The Bcg gene story. *Immunobiology* 191:451-460.

van Oorschot, R.A., S.J. Gutowski, and S.L. Robinson
1994   HUMTH01: amplification, species specificity, population genetics and forensic applications. *International Journal of Legal Medicine* 107:121-126.

Wagener, D.K.
1995   Ethical considerations in the design and execution of the National and Hispanic Health and Nutrition Examination Survey (HANES). *Environmental Health Perspectives* 103 (Supplement 3):75-80.

13

Comparative Perspectives on Plasticity in Human Aging and Life Spans

Caleb E. Finch

INTRODUCTION

Throughout the world, human life expectancy is increasing. Unprecedented numbers are reaching ages beyond the 10th decade and the maximum human life span is creeping up to break new records each year (Vaupel, Wilmoth, in this volume). I will discuss how these demographic shifts represent the plasticity found throughout the evolution of life histories. Similarly wide variations in life expectancy and maximum life spans are observed in animals and plants, within populations as well as between closely related species. The preceding chapters review the details of these increases and some of the mechanisms that may be involved. However, major unknowns remain about the nature of the aging process in humans and other organisms. The general information that is available from all sources gives a very limited basis for predicting further changes in human aging schedules and ultimate life spans.

The life history of multicellular organisms is built on the scheduling of functions during the life span. In sexually reproducing organisms, life history may be considered to begin with the gametes produced in the prior parental generation, which may exist for many decades before fertilization. Thus, the ova from which we arose were formed in our mothers' ovaries while she was a fetus in our maternal grandmothers' uterus, which allows environmental effects that span at least three generations in mammals (Finch, 1996; Finch and Loehlin, in press). Similarly, social insect queens store sperm acquired during their nuptial flights that remains viable for at least 7 years (Hölldobler and Wilson, 1990:146, 154). The prezygotic environment is a major unexplored domain of life history that could have profound influences on characteristics of one or more ensuing generations.

More conventionally, the analysis of life history emphasizes the zygote and subsequent developmental stages through maturation and later postmaturational stages. At later postmaturational ages, mammals typically show declining reproduction and slowly manifest increasing physiological and functional losses that, in association with increasing mortality risk, define the phase of senescence.

One measure of the rate of senescence is the rate of increase of age-specific mortality, $m(t)$. In many populations, $m(t)$ increases exponentially after maturity according to the Gompertz formula: $m(t) = \exp[\alpha(t)]$ (Finch and Pike, 1996; Finch et al., 1990; Mueller et al., 1995). A convenient basis for comparing mortality rate accelerations is the time required for mortality rates to double (MRDT = $\ln 2/\alpha$), which is about 8 years in humans and about 0.3 year in laboratory rodents (Finch et al., 1990).

A huge body of work demonstrates many ways in which the phenomena of senescence are highly plastic and subject to modifications through environmental parameters, for example diet, as discussed below. This plasticity challenges traditional beliefs that the life spans of higher organisms are rigidly preprogrammed by their genes. I use the plural, life spans, to emphasize that there may be many statistically distinct life-history trajectories within a given human population, which are subject to myriad gene-environment interactions, including lifestyle choices (Finch and Tanzi, 1997). The plasticity of life histories is generally consistent with an evolutionary basis for the numeric life span as a life-history trait. The vast range of schedules shown by multicellular organisms, as described next, implies that the plasticity in life-history schedules and phenotypes is itself a general outcome of evolution by allowing multiple alternative adaptive schedules.

THE MILLION-FOLD RANGE OF LIFE SPANS

The life expectancy of an individual in a population is not constrained by any known intrinsic feature of aging at the molecular or cellular level that is not open to evolution. As discussed by Tuljapurkar and by Rose (in this volume), for a species to survive, at least one of its populations must, on the average, maintain non-negative growth. This statistical outcome is achieved by balancing cumulative survival across adult ages by cumulative fecundity. The Euler-Lotka "equation of state" for population dynamics does not lead to any predictions about the duration of the developmental stages that precede reproduction. Although time is a necessary dimension in the parameters that are used to describe population growth, evolutionary biologists generally conclude that the magnitude of duration for any life-history stage is free to increase without constraint and that there is no biological limit to the maximum life span.

Nonetheless, phenomena of senescence leading to characteristic life spans in a population are expected to be the norm. Rose, Partridge, and Tuljapurkar (in this volume) summarize arguments from evolutionary theory that the force of natural selection diminishes at later ages, which therefore permits populations to accumulate germ-line mutations with delayed adverse consequences. This concept was developed in detail for sexually reproducing organisms (Haldane, 1941; Medawar, 1952; Hamilton, 1966; Williams, 1957; Charlesworth, 1994).

The plasticity of the life span was shown by artificial selection experiments in fruit flies. Life spans of outbred flies were lengthened during selection for individuals that could reproduce at later ages (see Rose, in this volume). Moreover, the increased life span could then be experimentally returned to starting values by selection for reproduction at younger ages. The rate of mortality acceleration (Gompertz coefficient α; see above) shows parallel changes to the maximum and median life spans in these genetic manipulations of the life span (Nusbaum et al., 1996). Because these bidirectional changes in life span and in reproductive history could be accomplished within 30 generations, it is likely that their genetic basis is shifts in genetic variations that pre-existed in the starting outbred population, rather than point mutations or chromosomal translocations. Natural populations of many organisms have genetic variations in neural and endocrine functions that regulate such quantitative life-history traits as the age at maturation and the frequency of reproduction (Finch and Rose, 1995). Indirectly, these parameters of the reproductive schedule are statistical determinants of the life span.

While the evolution of senescence in nonsexually reproducing organisms has been given less attention, clonal reproduction is well documented to coexist with senescence of the individual organism—e.g., two species of annelid worms (Martínez and Levinton, 1992). Mathematical modeling suggests that the evolution of senescence in organisms with the capacity for both sexual and clonal reproduction may depend on the age structure of the population (Orive, 1995) and the rates of sexual reproduction (Gardner and Mangel, 1997).

Existing organisms show a huge range in the life spans and reproductive schedules that implies the absence of evolutionary limits in life-history schedules, including the statistical life span in a population. The observed life spans in eukaryotes span a 1 million-fold range, with a short extreme from the 2-day life span of yeast cells (*Saccharomyces*) up to the $>1.8 \times 10^6$-day (5,000 year) life span of bristlecone pines (*Pinus aristata*) (Figure 13-1). Plant clones appear to exceed these examples severalfold—e.g., the "King clone" of the creosote bush (*Larrea tridentata*), which is estimated to be >10,000 years old (Vasek, 1980).

These examples suggest that it is the physiological architecture of the species that determines the life span (Finch and Rose, 1995). Thus, the allocation of resources for regeneration and repair or for hormone-behavior changes during reproduction are fundamental determinants of mortality, either through risky behavior or pathophysiological side effects that can influence the rate of senescence. In contrast, certain other cellular characteristics show weak correlation

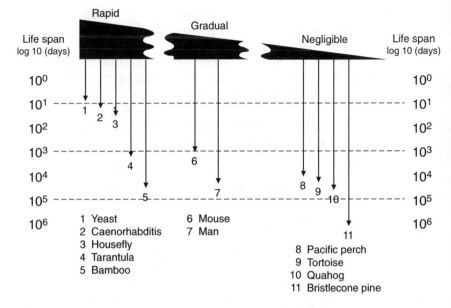

FIGURE 13-1   Life spans of sexually reproducing species rate of senescence in adult. Schema of the range of intensities of senescence on a spectrum from *rapid* to *gradual* to *negligible*, as indicated by thickness of the wedge. Durations of total life spans, embryo-to-adult life phase, are shown on the vertical scale as days in powers of 10. SOURCE: Life spans of individual organisms are taken from Finch (1990:chapters 2-4 and appendix I).

with life span—e.g., nuclear DNA content and neuron oxygen utilization differ by <10 percent in rodents and humans (Hoffman, 1983; Finch, 1990:260,283).

The bidirectional plasticity of life-history schedules that is shown experimentally for fruit flies is consistent with evolutionary changes that can, in part, be traced in the fossil record. A striking example is found in mayflies, which are famous for their adult phases lasting as little as a few hours to a few days, depending on the species. Their total life span, however, may extend for up to 5 years and commonly includes 10 or more instars. These ultrashort adult phases are a direct consequence of their physiological architecture, because mayflies from the 227-odd genera lack complete mouth parts as adults (Finch, 1990:49-50). Because mayflies cannot eat during the intense activities of reproduction that ensue upon eclosion, nutritional reserves accumulated before maturation are rapidly depleted. The trait of adult aphagy is almost certainly a derived trait—i.e., recently evolved—because fossils of mayflies from the Paleozoic Era, 300 million years ago, show mouth parts as adults that were well developed for chewing. Some ancient mayflies were giants relative to the present diminutive species. For example, *Bojophlebia* had an 18-inch wingspan and is thought to have been a fierce predator because of its well developed mandibles (Kukalova-Peck, 1985; Finch, 1990:583-584). Although it is not clear that the present mayflies have descended from gigantic ancestors, by the Eocene Epoch (57-36 million years ago) mayflies resembled those in modern families (Edmunds, 1972). The mayflies and many other examples are consistent with the idea that adult life spans, like adult body sizes, can become smaller as well as larger during evolution, depending on local ecological constraints.

Figure 13-1 also shows that nearly the same range of life spans is observed in sexual organisms that display very different rates of senescence and physiological characteristics. A scale of senescence is shown that approximates the rates of mortality acceleration in adults, ranging from rapid to gradual to negligible (Finch, 1990). *Rapid senescence* is observed in semelparous organisms that die within a year of maturation from causes that are typically relatively homogenous within the population. Typical mortality rate doubling times are less than 0.1 year. In these plants and animals, the very short adult phase is terminated by a rapid senescence after sexual reproduction that leads to death of the adult populations within one season. In general, such organisms display very similar pathophysiological changes that affect most members of the population, more-or-less concurrently (Finch, 1990:chapter 2; Finch, 1994). Rapid senescence is epitomized in the familiar example of spawning Pacific salmon, in which both genders rapidly develop symptoms like in Cushing disease that are caused by high blood cortisol levels. In marsupial mice (genus, *Antechinus* and *Phascogale*), males, but not females, show seasonal die-off soon after mating, also in association with elevated cortisol levels (Finch, 1990:95-97; Lee and Cockburn, 1985). The fruit fly *Drosophila* and the nematode *Caenorhabditis* are valuable laboratory invertebrate models for senescence, with life spans of up to several months that show extensive pathophysiological changes. Unlike the hyperadrenocorticism of Pacific salmon, however, no single pathophysiological trigger has been identified in the senescence of *Drosophila* or *Caenorhabditis*. Thus, the senescence of Pacific salmon may be atypical of the physiology of senescence in other animals.

Depending on the species, rapid senescence nonetheless can occur after very long total life spans, because of prolonged juvenile prereproductive phases before rapid senescence. Examples of this life-history type are shown by the thick-stemmed bamboo species in the genus *Phyllostachys* that, depending upon the species, grow vegetatively for several decades or for more than 100 years before flowering and dying in one season (Janzen, 1976; Finch, 1990:101). As another example with a different physiology, the male tarantula matures at about 10 years and dies a few months later with a shrinking abdomen that indicates cessation of feeding. In contrast, female tarantulas live at least 25 years (Baerg, 1920; Finch, 1990:67-68).

Gradual senescence represents the intermediate range in rates of senescence and probably represents the bulk of species among plants and animals with life spans of more than 1 year but that are more-or-less definite, depending on the population size and local conditions (Finch and Pike, 1996). Mortality rate doubling times range at least 100-fold, from about 0.3 year (mice, pond snail) to >27 years (river perch) (Finch, 1990:122-123). In general, gradual senescence is not associated with a homogeneous set of pathological changes throughout the population. Mammals have life spans ranging about 25-fold, from laboratory rodents with maximum life spans of about 5 years, to humans, presently at 122.4 years in the fleeting example of Jeanne Calment, who recently died. The increasing maximum life spans of humans from about 100 years in the best authenticated cases from the last century (Vaupel, in this volume) to the present >122 years may be considered as small relative to the full range of mammalian life spans.

In humans, midlife is marked by the increased incidence of numerous diseases (cancer, hypertension, vascular conditions, type II diabetes, etc.) that are major factors in the acceleration of mortality. Although the burden of various diseases may be associated with varying degrees of frailty and dependence, the presence of numerous sources of morbidity does not constitute a *senium*, or demarcated phase of morbidity during old age that precedes death, as once believed. For example in one population, >50 percent of those aged 65 of older were in apparent good health up to 1 year before their death (Brock et al., 1992). With the clear exception of the ovary (vom Saal et al., 1994), there is no general failure of cells throughout the body at a particular age. The dogma that mammals lose neurons throughout life during normal aging is being sharply challenged in studies of rodents and humans (Gallagher et al., 1996). Moreover, recent studies demonstrate that age-related dysfunctions in memory can occur without loss of neurons in the hippocampus (West, 1993; Rasmussen et al., 1996) and that impairments of hypothalamic control of gonadotrophins can occur without loss of gonadotropic-releasing-hormone neurons (Hoffman and Finch, 1986). The example of Madame Calment implies that the duration of functions of most organs do not have a predetermined upper age limit to functioning that would precipitate a general senile involution. At 122 years, she was, of course, postreproductive and recently became nearly blind and deaf. Yet, she was living independently until 10 years ago and showed no indications of dementia (informal accounts communicated to me by local observers).

Laboratory rodents have undergone increase in life spans during the past 50 years that parallel those of humans. Russell (1966) summarizes survival curves for highly inbred strains of mice—e.g., C57BL/6J strain—which was established in 1936 and has been since inbred for more than 100 generations. Several cohorts at the Jackson Laboratory showed progressive improvement in adult survival between 1948 and 1962, when the mean life span increased from about 560 days to 700 days, and maximum life spans increased from 800 to 900 days. Another cohort of this strain obtained from Jackson Laboratory by this author a few years later had markedly greater life spans, with a mean of 900 days and a maximum of 1460 days (Finch, 1971; Finch et al., 1969). The basis for this increased life span is almost certainly not genetic in view of the extensive inbreeding and includes such environmental factors as improved nutrition and husbandry, particularly the major decreases in the incidence of *Salmonella* and other infections.

Chronic moderate food restriction, 10-50 percent ad libitum, can increase rodent life spans even more. Food-restricted rats lived up to 45 months in 1943 (McCay et al., 1943), whereas present food-restricted rodents (note, not the same genotype) can live at least 8 months longer than they did 50 years ago. The present record maximum life spans are 1742 days in mice (Harrison and Archer, 1987) and about 1600 days in rats (Sprott and Austad, 1996). Ongoing studies of food-restricted rodents may lead to even greater life spans. It might be informative to analyze historical trends for mortality rates and life spans of laboratory rodents since the beginnings of modern small animal husbandry. A midcentury segment of this history was helpfully summarized by Russell (1966).

At the further extreme of senescence (Figure 13-1) are even slower aging patterns that I have provisionally called *negligible senescence*. In these species, there is no evidence of physiological dysfunctions at advanced ages, no acceleration of mortality during adult life, and no recognized characteristic limit to life span (Finch, 1990:chapter 4). Although the demographic analyses by Promislow and colleagues identified some mammalian species that did not show the expected increase of mortality with adult age (Gaillard et al., 1994), these cases need further study for physiological and pathological traits of aging before it can be concluded that these species or populations lack senescence. This category of life histories warrants caution and unremitting scrutiny, because few individual organisms of authenticated great ages have been rigorously examined.

A promising example of negligible senescence from the vertebrates is the rockfish genus *Sebastes,* a scorpaenid with several species that achieve ages greater than 100 years. The age is estimated from measurements of otolith rings in conjunction with natural radioisotopes (Finch, 1990:217; Chilton and Beamish, 1982; Mulligan and Leaman, 1992; Leaman, 1991). The age-specific fecundity increases progressively during continued body growth after maturation at about 20 years. In remarkable contrast to mammals (vom Saal et al., 1994), there is no evidence of reproductive decline in males or females by 55 years or more. At necropsy, a few older fish (*Sebastes aleutianus* aged 50-80 years) appeared healthy on gross examination; their ovaries contained the usual seasonal complement of mature eggs by histological studies (X. de Bruin, R. Gosden, C. Finch, and B. Leaman, unpublished work). In *Sebastes*, the oldest fish are generally not the largest in the population, implying size-selective mortality—e.g., from predation or interactions of growth rate and mortality. Although the numbers of fish aged over 50 years are few, the statistical procedure of Mueller et al. (1995) might be used to evaluate the stability of mortality rates at advanced ages.

In contrast to *Sebastes*, the much shorter-lived fish *Cynolebias*, shows considerable gross pathology during aging under laboratory conditions in association with accelerating mortality rates during its 2- to 3-year life span that approximate the schedule of senescence in laboratory rodents (Finch, 1990:137-138; Liu and Walford, 1969). *Cynolebias* is a cyprinodont from a different order than the scorpaeniform *Sebastes* (both belong to the same taxon of bony fishes, the superorder Acanthopterygii). Because *Cynolebias* shows age-related changes that are heterogeneous in the population with respect to the time of onset and the variations among individuals, we observe here a different phenomenon than the nearly synchronous senescence of spawning Pacific salmon. Although little is known about the age-related pathology of long-lived fish species, evidence like this does indicate a very wide range of phenomena.

Other examples of fish with very slow aging are the cod and sturgeon, which show increasing fecundity with age (Finch, 1990:chapter 4). Certain turtles also achieve life spans of at least 100 years. However, detailed microscopic or biochemical examination of tissues are lacking for any older specimens of very long-lived fish or other animals except for mammals. While these observations are consistent with very slow aging, much further work is needed to evaluate biochemical markers from mammals that are sensitive to slowly accumulated chemical changes in molecules with long life spans. Biochemical markers for future study could include the "I-spot" adducts formed on brain DNA nucleotides (Randerath et al., 1993) and the pentosidine glycooxidation products found on collagen from cartilage and skin (Miyata et al., 1996; Sell et al., 1996). Until we have data on such biochemical markers on aging and detailed histological studies, we should not assume that certain animals escape aging, even if senescence is not obvious. That is, age-related molecular damage could be slowly accumulated that might *not* be sufficient to cause age-related dysfunctions recognized as senescence. Whatever the future findings, some organisms clearly show even more gradual forms of senescence than observed in humans.

The putative category of negligible senescence merits a great deal more attention than given it so far because of its apparent challenge to the evolutionary theory that "senescence must always creep in" (Hamilton, 1966; Rose, in this volume). Important opportunities for study of life spans in natural populations are rapidly disappearing because of environmental disruptions from human population growth and, in the case of *Sebastes* and many other long-lived fish, because of commercial exploitation. The preservation of natural age-structured populations with multiple coexisting generations should be considered as a crucial aspect of the efforts to protect endangered species and biodiversity (Finch and Ricklefs, 1991). Investigators will encounter special statistical problems of sampling the few individuals of advanced ages to obtain estimates of the distribution of life spans and of age-related diseases. The size of later age groups will likely be small and could have different mortality characteristics from younger age classes, as observed for humans after 85 when mortality rates decline. For such subgroups, the population size will have a greater influence on estimates of apparent maximum life span than for the estimates of mean life span (Finch and Pike, 1996).

PLASTICITY IN SENESCENCE

Three Examples from Semelparous Animals

The rapid senescence of Pacific salmon can be prevented by blocking reproduction—e.g., by castrating juvenile kokanees, which then survive to 8 years, or about twice the usual life span associated with spawning (Robertson et al., 1961; Finch, 1990:90-92). A similar example is the extension of life in the normally semelparous male marsupial mice by castration before mating (Finch, 1990:97; Lee and Cockburn, 1985). Moreover, a segmented worm, the polychaete *Nereis,* was recently shown by experimental interventions to be capable of living twice its usual life span. When worms mature at 2 years of age, they stop feeding, lose the ability to regenerate ablated segments, and die soon after spawning (Golding and Yuwono, 1994). However, these changes can be postponed by transplanting cerebral ganglia from immature donors into adults; the worms then begin to feed and recover the ability to regenerate; the transplantation was repeated, thereby doubling the usual maximum life span. For other examples of life-span extension from postponed reproduction in animals and plants, see Finch (1990:chapters 2 and 10; Finch, 1994) and Golding and Yuwono (1994).

These striking experiments demonstrate that somatic cells have a great deal more potential for function than available in the usual life span. In fact, the evolutionary theory of senescence does not require that the leading causes of death during senescence be synchronized with other aging processes (Rose, 1991:167).

This view is consistent with the historical trends for lengthened life spans in humans but without the compression of morbidity at later ages predicted by Fries (1980). Moreover, each species must be considered in terms of the physiological architecture that reflects its unique evolutionary history. For example, in blood-cortisol elevations common in vertebrates during reproductive stress, there may be a wide quantitative range of cell responses to a given elevation of blood cortisol, which result in different degrees of cell damage and its reversibility (C.V. Mobbs and C.E. Finch, unpublished work). Endocrine manipulations give a valuable experimental approach to resolving gene-environment interactions that trigger senescence in some semelparous and iteroparous species.

Examples from Mammalian Life Histories

Mammalian life histories are also subject to alternative schedules in the timing and rate of events and age changes, particularly through nutritional influences on the reproductive schedule. In laboratory rodents, food restriction to 10-

50 percent of ad libitum intake slows many age-related changes (Weindruch, 1996; Weindruch and Walford, 1988; Finch, 1990:506-536; Hopkin, 1995; Roth et al., 1995)—e.g., the mortality-rate doubling time, mean life spans, and maximum life spans of rodents are extended by 30 percent or more. Genotype-specific tumors are delayed, e.g., in the p53 "knock-out" mouse strain, which has a very high incidence of malignancy (Hursting et al., 1994). At necropsy, some very old food-restricted rats (nonmutant strains) lacked any display of gross pathology that could be assigned as a cause of morbidity or mortality (Maeda et al., 1985; Weindruch and Walford, 1988; Finch, 1990:518-519). The causes of death in these rats could include transients in blood pressure, cardiac rhythms, and blood glucose, which might not lead rapidly to gross organ pathology.

Food restriction also delays puberty and slows the age-related loss of ovarian oocytes in laboratory mice (Nelson et al., 1985). When mice are fed ad libitum, fertility recovers and is maintained to later ages than in fed controls. The effects of food restriction extend to delaying age-related impairments in key neuroendocrine functions, such as the preovulatory surge of gonadotrophins (McShane and Wise, 1996) and the pulsatile release of growth hormone (Sonntag et al., 1995). The ad libitum food intake of laboratory rodents may be atypical, because food resources are subject to seasonal and other fluctuations in natural populations. This plasticity in the reproductive schedule is hypothesized to be adaptive, because it would coordinate reproduction with food availability (Holliday, 1989; Harrison and Archer, 1989; Graves, 1993). In particular, Graves (1993) argues that these responses to food restriction demonstrate tradeoffs between energy expended on survival versus reproduction.

The generalizability of these effects of food restriction to humans is not clear. In ongoing studies with rhesus monkeys, chronic food restriction had effects on metabolism that, in part, resembled those observed in rodents. Food restriction decreased both blood glucose and insulin, (integrated 24-hour levels) and increased insulin sensitivity (Roth et al., 1995). This change might be expected to oppose the age-related trend in humans for subtle, but persistent, decreases in insulin sensitivity during aging, in association with age-related trends for increased levels of fasting blood glucose (Rowe et al., 1983; Harris et al., 1987).

I suspect that gene-environment interactions will eventually be identified that lead to vulnerability of particular organ systems for degeneration during aging, but that a great deal of plasticity will be observed in the age when a particular degree of impairment is manifested. A potential example of this is the strong statistical association of higher education with a lower incidence of Alzheimer disease at later ages, which is observed in five human populations on three continents (Katzman, 1993). Education, of course, may be a proxy (surrogate) variable for other primary environmental factors. The existence of at least four genetic risk factors for Alzheimer disease gives a basis for evaluating how education and other environmental factors influence these risk factors at different ages.

CELL PROLIFERATION AND LIFE-HISTORY PLASTICITY

Against the above examples, we must also consider if there are changes at cellular and molecular levels that may not be readily reversible or open to intervention. The Hayflick phenomenon, or the limited proliferative life span of diploid human fibroblasts in serial culture, is often cited as an example of a built-in aging clock (Hayflick, 1977, 1994; Fries, 1980). In parallel with the loss of proliferative capacity, there is a loss of telomeric DNA at the ends, or telomeres, of chromosomes (Martin, 1994; Harley and Villaponteau, 1996). Telomere DNA loss during replicative senescence has been demonstrated so far only in human cells and in some ciliated protozoans. The enzyme telomerase that maintains telomere DNA is not found in most somatic cells but is expressed in malignant cells. These phenomena are manifested during aging in vivo—e.g., telomere loss is detected in cells cloned from blood vessels of older humans in which there has been local endothelial cell proliferation (Chang and Harley, 1995). A major question is the relationship between proliferative limits and telomere shortening. The impact of telomere shortening on the proliferative potential of bone marrow cells is unclear but may be pertinent to immunoproliferative responses and red blood cell production at later ages.

In contrast to these widely appreciated phenomena, a fundamental fact is less well known—that cell death does not ensue simply because fibroblasts have stopped dividing (Campisi, 1997). There is no general failure of biosynthesis of RNA and protein at the time when DNA synthesis ceases in fibroblasts, despite their unhealthy appearance with accumulations of lipids and pigments. In particular, postreplicative fibroblasts can still support full viral infections with undiminished yield of infective progeny (Tomkins et al., 1974; Holland et al., 1973). In view of the fact that neurons in our brains have been postreplicative for decades without detectible cell death (see above), it is not surprising that postreplicative fibroblasts can live for at least 3 years in culture if properly cared for (Smith and Pereira-Smith, 1996). The capacity for functional survival of postreplicative fibroblasts is well known to investigators of in vitro models for aging but is less known outside of this research community.

Another feature of cell proliferation in life histories is the unlimited somatic cell proliferation demonstrated by many species of animals and plants that can propagate by vegetative or asexual reproduction. Familiar examples are the vegetative propagation of plants by shoots and cuttings and the asexual propagation of flatworms by fission. This capacity, while widespread among plants, is scattered among the animals. Depending on the species, vegetative reproduction may be the primary mode, as well as an alternate life-history strategy. From its distri-

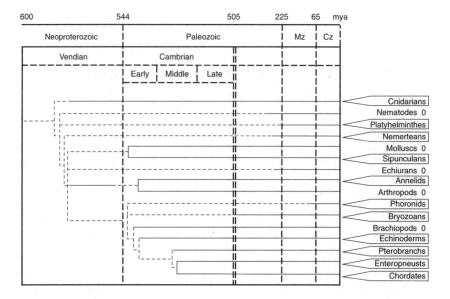

FIGURE 13-2 Schema showing distribution of phyla containing species that manifest vegetative reproduction in at least one species of a subphylum or order, as shown in boxes. Vegetative reproduction includes reproduction from somatic cells by budding or segmentation. In many examples, vegetative reproduction can prevail for many successive generations, without a required intermediate cycle of sexual reproduction. For examples, see Buss (1987) and Finch (1990:chapter 4). This capacity for extensive vegetative reproduction depends on an unlimited capacity for proliferation of somatic cells. Davidson et al. (1995) proposed that the evolution of animal development depended on an unlimited capacity for proliferation of embryonal cells. These phenomena markedly diverge from the finite proliferation of mammalian fibroblasts during serial culture, the "Hayflick limit." The phylogenetic tree shows the depth of the fossil record (solid lines) and the minimum age of divergence; Mz, Mesozoic; Cz, Cenozoic; mya, million years ago. In the early-to-middle Cambrian, when most extant phyla are represented in the fossil record, one can find lines of descent that lead to phyla that show both the presence and absence of vegetative reproduction, as denoted by the *boxes* (report of at least one species showing vegetative reproduction in adults) or by *O* (its apparent absence). For example, annelids (*box*) and arthropods (*O*) diverged by the early Cambrian Period. Among chordates, urochordates (tunicates) (*box*), e.g., *Botryllus* (Grosberg, 1982; Sabbadin, 1979) and vertebrates (*O*) may also have diverged by the early Cambrian Period. It is likely that vegetative reproduction is a primitive trait in the animal phyla and that its absence, in any phylum, is a derived trait. These perspectives imply that finite clonal proliferation of diploid mammalian fibroblasts is also a derived trait. SOURCE: The phylogenetic tree is adapted from Davidson et al. (1995).

bution across all grades of organization, vegetative reproduction would appear to have existed in the earliest multicellular organisms (Figure 13-2).

An important example is found in the tunicates (urochordates), which have two-chambered beating hearts, a notochord, and a complex neural network. This lineage separated from other chordates about 500 million years ago. *Botryllus*, in particular, develops from a tadpole-like free-swimming larva, which settles down to form a sessile colony that can reproduce sexually or asexually, depending on the local conditions (Buss, 1987; Grosberg, 1982, 1988; Finch, 1990:106-108). Asexual reproduction by budding from the body wall of adult animals (e.g., Chang and Lauzon, 1995) has been observed as the exclusive mode of propagation for hundreds of vegetative asexual generations in the laboratory (Sabbadin, 1979), with no signs of a proliferative limit analogous to the Hayflick phenomena. Neighboring colonies of *Botryllus* and other tunicates may display asexual reproduction concurrently with sexual semelparity and iteroparity. *Botryllus* is also being studied as a model for synchronized apoptosis (Chang and Lauzon, 1995).

In animal embryos, an unlimited capacity for proliferation of undifferentiated cells is thought to be the basis for the development of larger structures from small initial numbers of cells (Davidson et al., 1995). A well-studied case of this is the vast proliferative capacity of larval fruit fly cells: after serial transplantation of imaginal discs for hundreds of doublings, exposure to ecdysone induces morphologically normal differentiated adult organs (Hadorn, 1966, 1968). During development in mammals, there may be a marked reduction of proliferative capacity during early development, since mouse blastocyst cells can be serially cultured from >250 cumulative doublings, or about 10-fold more than obtained with mouse fibroblasts derived from later-stage embryos (Suda et al., 1987). "Progenitor" cells from adult rat brains can be grown in culture for >2 years and >33 passages, when fibroblast growth factor (FGF-2) is present (Gage et al., 1995; Suohonen et al., 1996). During serial culture, the homogenous-appearing cells had doubling times of 2 days and then differentiated into several types of neurons when transplanted into adult brains. While each of these studies could involve extensive selection of minor cell subpopulations with very high proliferative capacity, there was no indication of a culture crisis or proliferative limit.

Provisionally, the acquisition of finite proliferative capacity as epitomized by mammalian fibroblasts may be regarded as a specialized, or evolutionarily derived, feature of cell differentiation, rather than a fundamental limitation of animal cells to which germ cells are an exception. Ongoing work may demonstrate whether the immortality of germ-cell lineages is an exclusive property of these special cells. From a comparative perspective, the plasticity of the human life span should not depend as much on the proliferative capacity of somatic cells as on changes in hormones and growth factors that modify cell functions.

The huge proliferative capacity of mouse cells when obtained from blastocysts before the germ cells had differentiated (Suda et al., 1987) recalls Weissman's concept of "disposable soma" from the last century (Kirkwood and Cremer, 1982; Martínez and Levinton, 1992). According to the disposable soma concept, natural selection protects the immortality of the germ cells but does not protect against the evolution of somatic senescence. The capacity for indefinite somatic proliferation during asexual or vegetative reproduction weakens this dichotomy, because in these examples a subpopulation of somatic cells are equivalent to germ-line cells. However, the capacity for vegetative reproduction does not exclude somatic senescence, as observed in tunicates (see above), annelids, and flatworms (Martínez and Levinton, 1992).

If proliferative limits are considered as an aspect of organismic senescence, then it would be important to observe the timing during development of acquisition of finite cell proliferation in relation to germ-cell differentiation. However, cell differentiation does not confer inevitable proliferative senescence, as shown above by Hadorn's example of vast proliferation of imaginal discs in fruit flies: although these cells do not terminally differentiate until exposed to ecdysone, they were already differentiated by their capacity for hormonal responses.

There is no close link between the timing of germ-cell differentiation and the onset of somatic senescence. On one extreme are female mammals, in which germ-cell differentiation and proliferation are complete before birth (vom Saal et al., 1994). Ovarian senescence can be said to begin in utero, because the numbers of ovarian oocytes and primary follicles decrease exponentially after birth, so that more than half are lost by puberty. Eventually, the loss is complete at menopause, leading to decreases of estrogens that increase the risk of mortality from osteoporosis, vascular disease, and Alzheimer disease (e.g., Holinka, 1994; Schneider and Finch, 1997).

At the other extreme are flowering plants and some animals, in which germ-cell differentiation is delayed until just before reproduction, whether a species is semelparous or perennial (Finch, 1990:239-240). Bony fish give an important counter-example to mammals. Although their germ-cell differentiation begins early in development, as in mammals, unlike mammals, bony fish maintain de novo oogenesis as adults (vom Saal et al., 1994)—for example, the new seasonal stocks of oocytes found in chronologically old *Sebastes* that do not show indications of somatic or ovarian senescence, as described above.

MOLECULAR AGE CHANGES AND PLASTICITY

At a molecular level, long-lived proteins and DNA are subject to diverse changes that may ultimately limit the plasticity of the life span. Proteins such as collagen and elastin slowly accumulate oxidative damage from a variety of chemical processes, including the formation of oxidation productions from glucose. The advanced glycation end-products or glycooxidation products arise from spontaneous (nonenzymatic) additions of glucose and other reducing sugars to free amino groups, with the subsequent formation of pentosidine and other condensation products that can cross-link adjacent protein molecules (Cerami, 1996; Baynes, 1991; Sell and Monnier, 1995). Several different types of advanced glycation end-products have been shown to accumulate progressively, with a nearly linear time course from birth onward. In the skin, for example, pentosidine accumulates in skin collagen, at rates that are in proportion to the life spans of humans and other mammals of short- and intermediate life spans (Sell et al., 1996). In the human eye, a different oxidation product, LM-1, a blue fluorophore covalently associated with lens crystallins, accumulates linearly with age; in this case, the reducing sugar may be ascorbic acid rather than glucose (Nagaraj and Monnier, 1992). These examples suggest the complexity of the biochemistry of aging, where there are important variations between tissues and multiple substrates from intermediary metabolism.

Certain targets in tissues of glycoxidation by glucose and other reducing sugars can be modified through diet and drugs. For example, glycooxidation is accelerated by chronic elevations of blood glucose, as in diabetes (Schnider and Kohn, 1980). Correspondingly, food restriction, which lowers blood glucose, has been shown to decrease oxidative damage to proteins in rats (Reiser, 1994; Youngman et al., 1992). This finding points to the potential impact of nutrition across the life span on amount of damage that may accumulate in slowly replaced molecules. The nontoxic antioxidant aminoguanidine appears to block glycooxidation in animal studies and is in clinical trial (Cerami, 1996). Because minimum levels of blood glucose and other reducing sugars found both extra- and intracellularly are essential to physiological function, it would appear that glycooxidative damage to long-lived proteins may set some ultimate limit on plasticity of human life histories. The high blood sugar of birds (5- to 10-fold that of mammals) would predict intense glycooxidative damage to proteins (Monnier et al.,1990; Finch, 1990:405; Holmes and Austad, 1995). In view of their long life spans, special antioxidant mechanisms must have been evolved during the evolution of birds.

DNA damage from oxidation and a variety of other mechanisms is also observed in chromosomal and mitochondrial DNA of tissues with little cell replication like brain and muscle (Linnane et al., 1989; Randerath et al., 1993; Fraga et al., 1990; Soong et al., 1992; Mecocci et al., 1993). The age-related accumulation of mutations during aging is of unquestionable importance to one or more steps in malignant transformation and may be important to other dysfunctions of nondividing as well (Finch and Goodman, 1997).

Recent findings from van Leewen's group indicate that some mutational processes are under physiological control. The Brattleboro rat carries a germ-line mutation causing a frame-shift in the vasopressin gene. Remarkably, about one hypothalamic neuron per day reverts to acquire the normal vasopressin peptide; the reverted neurons accumulate in an age-related schedule from birth onward—

at least beyond middle age (Finch and Goodman, 1997; Evans et al., 1995). The molecular analysis so far shows that the reversions result from clustered replacements of amino acids. Moreover, if the mutant rats are given vasopressin hormone replacements, then the rate of reversion is slowed. Ongoing studies are evaluating whether other genes show these processes. The present findings point to an utterly different form of plasticity in molecular aging processes, which suggest that physiological manipulations could be used to intervene and reduce mutational changes in DNA.

PROSPECTS FOR A GENETICS OF LONGEVITY

Many laboratories are actively pursuing genes that influence life spans in short-lived animal models of aging, particularly nematodes (Johnson and Shook, in this volume), fruit flies (Rose, in this volume) (reviewed in Finch and Tanzi, 1997). Efforts to breed long-lived mice by selecting for reproduction at later ages are showing some success (Ngai et al, 1995) in parallel with similar studies on fruit flies (Rose, in this volume). In humans, genes that cause specific age-related diseases that shorten the life span are continuing to be identified, as in familial breast cancer, vascular disease, and Alzheimer disease. One of the progerias, Werner syndrome, which is characterized by intensified atherosclerosis and malignancy (both proliferative disorders), has been mapped to a gene predicted to encode a helicase, an enzyme that, by modifying DNA structure, may alter telomere replication (Yu et al., 1996).

The genetics of centenarians promises to reveal alleles that may favor extreme longevity, including the apoE2 allele (Schächter et al., 1994) and certain HLA haplotypes (Schächter, in press). There may be other general classes of genes that promote longevity through similar physiological mechanisms in widely different organisms, so-called "longevity assurance genes" or "gerogenes" (Jazwinski, 1996; Johnson and Shook, in this volume). One class of such genes may prove to reduce the effects of oxidative damage, a challenge to all organisms that exist in an oxidizing atmosphere and must cope with the myriad by-products of oxidative metabolism, including the continuing production of free radicals through oxidative phosphorylation. Atmospheric oxygen concentration increased steadily, if not monotonically, during the great radiations of the extant animal phyla more than 550 million years ago (Figure 13-2) and progressed to a maximum of 35 percent during the late Paleozoic Era (Graham et al., 1995). The machinery for combating oxidative stress was presumably subject to strong evolutionary pressures long before ancestors of the present long-lived birds and mammals had evolved in the Mesozoic Era. There is every reason to expect a continuing parade of genes controlling such protective mechanisms from diverse organisms that can shorten or lengthen life span.

At present, we do not understand the basis for the striking recent historical trends in increased life expectancy at the oldest ages in humans. It is unlikely that this can be attributed to a genetic change in chromosomal genes because of its broad occurrence throughout the world. Nonetheless, the role of outbreeding through migration and the impact of social changes on the degree of consanguineous marriage has not been systematically evaluated. Outbreeding could contribute to increased adult life spans through hybrid vigor, as observed, for example, in the offspring of laboratory inbred rats and mice (Storer, 1978; Finch, 1990:321-324). Moreover, the evidence for the roles of older individuals in socially organized long-lived mammals (Carey and Gruenfelder, in this volume), as well as humans (Kaplan, in this volume) give a basis for discussing whether genes that are permissive of long life spans in some environments might be subject to kin selection mechanisms. Nonetheless, the most obvious alternative causes of increased longevity are improvements in public health, including nutrition, reduction of infectious disease, and other aspects of medical technology. Intriguing questions remain open about whether these environmental advances can account for the increased numbers of centenarians in rural China (Yi, in press) as satisfactorily as they appear to account for increases of centenarians in North America. Increased population size is certainly another factor. Although population size does not have a major effect on maximum life span during the Gompertz acceleration of mortality, when mortality accelerations slow at very advanced ages, population size will be a greater determinant of maximum life span (Finch and Pike, 1996).

In conclusion, the biology of human aging allows few predictions about the ultimate limits to life spans in different environments. The available evidence from different species shows that organisms of whatever body construction have the potential for widely varying patterns of senescence, with respect to the intensity of any particular pathophysiological age change and its time course of occurrence. This enormous plasticity is completely consistent with the recent increases of human life spans.

ACKNOWLEDGMENT

This research was supported by a grant to C.E.F. from the National Institute on Aging (K07-AG-00729).

REFERENCES

Baerg, W.J.
    1920   The life cycle and mating habits of the male tarantula. *Quarterly Review of Biology* 3:109-116.
Baynes, J.W.
    1991   Role of oxidative stress in development of complications in diabetes. *Diabetes* 40:405-412.

Brock, D.B., M.B. Holmes, D.J. Foley, and D. Holmes
1992   Methodological issues in the last days of life. Pp. 315-332 in *The Epidemiologic Study of Aging*. New York: Oxford University Press.
Buss, L.W.
1987   *The Evolution of Individuality*. New York: Princeton University Press.
Campisi, J.
1997   The biology of replicative senescence. *European Journal of Cancer* 35:703-709.
Cerami, A.
1996   Hypothesis. Glucose as a mediator of aging. *Journal of the American Geriatrics Society* 33:626-634.
Chang, E., and C.B. Harley
1995   Telomere length and replicative aging in human vascular tissues. *Proceedings of the National Academy of Sciences U.S.A.* 92:11190-11194.
Chang, W-T., and R.J. Lauzon
1995   Isolation of biologically functional RNA during programmed death of a colonial ascidian. *Biological Bulletin* 188:23-31.
Charlesworth, B.
1994   *Evolution in Age-Structured Populations*. Cambridge: Cambridge University Press.
Chilton, D.E., and R.J. Beamish
1982   Age determination methods for fishes studied by the groundfish program at the Pacific biological station. *Canadian Special Publication of Fisheries and Aquatic Sciences* 60.
Davidson, E.H., K.J. Peterson, and R.A. Cameron
1995   Origin of bilaterian body plans: Evolution of developmental regulatory mechanisms. *Science* 270:1319-1325.
Edmunds, G.F.
1972   Biogeography and evolution of Ephemeroptera. *Annual Review of Entomology* 17:21-42.
Evans, D.A.P., J.P.H. Burbach, and F.W. van Leeuwen
1995   Somatic mutations in the brain: relationship to aging? *Mutation Research* 338:173-182.
Finch, C.E.
1971   Comparative biology of senescence: Evolutionary and developmental considerations. Pp. 47-67 in *Animal Models for Biomedical Research IV*. Washington, DC: National Academy of Sciences.
1990   *Longevity, Senescence, and the Genome*. Chicago: University of Chicago Press.
1994   Commentary: Latent capacities for gametogenic cycling in the semelparous invertebrate *Nereis*. *Proceedings of the National Academy of Sciences U.S.A.* 91:11769-11770.
1996   Biological bases for plasticity during aging of individual life histories. Pp. 488-512 in D. Magnusson, ed., *The Lifespan Development of Individuals: Biological and Psychosocial Perspectives, a Synthesis*. Cambridge: Cambridge University Press.
Finch, C.E., J.R. Foster, and A.E. Mirsky
1969   Aging and the regulation of cell activities during exposure to cold. *Journal of General Physiology* 54:690-712.
Finch, C.E., and Goodman, M.F.
In press   Relevance of adaptive mutations arising in non-dividing cells in microorganisms to neurobiological systems. *Trends in Neuroscience*.
Fince, C.E., and J. Loehlin
Iin press   Environmental influences that may precede fertilization: A first examination of the prezygotic hypothesis from maternal age influences on twins. *Behavior Genetics*.
Finch, C.E., and M.C. Pike
1996   Maximum lifespan predictions from the Gompertz mortality model. *Journal of Gerontology* B183-B194.

Finch, C.E., M.C. Pike, and M. Witten
   1990   Slow mortality rate accelerations during aging in animals approximate that of humans. *Science* 249:902-905.
Finch, C.E., and R.E. Ricklefs
   1991   Age structure of populations (letter). *Science* 254:799.
Finch, C.E., and M.R. Rose
   1995   Hormones and the physiological architecture of life history evolution. *Quarterly Review of Biology* 70:1-52.
Finch, C.E., and Tanzi, R.E.
   1997.   Genetics of aging. *Science.*
Fraga, C.G., M.K. Shinegaga, J.W. Park, P. Degan, and B.N. Ames
   1990   Oxidants, antioxidants, and the degenerative diseases of aging. *Proceedings of the National Academy of Sciences U.S.A.* 87:4533-4537.
Fries, J.F.
   1980   Aging, natural death, and the compression of morbidity. *New England Journal of Medicine* 303:130-135.
Gage, F.H., P.W. Coates, T.D. Palmer, H.G. Kuhn, L.J. Fisher, J.O. Suhonen, D.A. Peterson, S.T. Suhr, and J. Ray
   1995   Survival differentiation of adult neuronal progenitor cells transplanted to the adult brain. *Proceedings of the National Academy of Sciences U.S.A.* 92:11879-11883.
Gaillard, J., D. Allaine, D. Pontier, N.G. Yoccoz, and D.E.L. Promislow
   1994   Evolutionary patterns among measures of aging. *Evolution* 48:509-516.
Gallagher, M., P.W. Landfield, B.S. McEwen, M.J. Meaney, P.R. Rapp, R.M. Sapolsky, and M.J. West
   1996   Hippocampal neurodegeneration in aging. *Science* 274: 484-485.
Gardner, S.N., and M. Mangel.
   1997   When can a clonal organism escape senescence. *American Naturalist.*
Golding, D.W., and E. Yuwono
   1994   Latent capacities for gametogenic cycling in the semelparous invertebrate. *Proceedings of the National Academy of Sciences U.S.A.* 91:11777-11781.
Graham, J.B., R. Dudley, N.M. Aguilar, and C. Gans
   1995   Implications of the late paleozoic oxygen pulse for physiology and evolution. *Nature* 375:117-120.
Graves, J.L.
   1993   The costs of reproduction and dietary restriction: Parallels between insects and mammals. *Growth, Development and Aging* 57:233-249.
Grosberg, R.K.
   1982   Ecological, Genetical, and Developmental Factors Regulating Life History Variation Within a Population of the Colonial Ascidian *Botryllus schlosseri* (Pallas) Savigny. Unpublished Ph.D. dissertation, Yale University.
   1988   Life history variation within a population of the colonial ascidian *Botryllus schlosseri* I: The genetic and environmental control of seasonal variation. *Evolution* 42:900-920.
Hadorn, E.
   1966   Konstanz, Wechsel, und Typus der Determination in Zellen aus mannlichen Genitalanlagen von *Drosophila melanogaster* durch Dauerkulter in vivo. *Developmental Biology* 13:424-509.
   1968   Transdetermination in cells. *Scientific American* 219:110-114.
Haldane, J.B.S
   1941   *New Paths in Genetics.* London: Allen and Unwin.
Hamilton, W.D.
   1966   The moulding of senescence by natural selection. *Journal of Theoretical Biology* 12:12-45.

Harley, C.B., and B. Villeponteau
1996   Telomeres and telomerase in aging and cancer. *Current Biology* 5:249-255.
Harris, M.I., W.C. Hadden, W.C. Knowler, and R.L. Bennett
1987   Prevalence of diabetes and impaired glucose tolerance and plasma glucose levels in U.S. population aged 20-74 yr. *Diabetes* 36:523-534.
Harrison, D.E., and J.R. Archer
1987   Genetic differences in effects of food restriction on aging in mice. *Journal of Nutrition* 117:376-382.
1989   Natural selection for extended longevity from food restriction. *Growth Development and Aging* 53:3-6.
Hayflick, L.
1977   The cellular basis for biological aging. Pp. 159-188 in C.E. Finch and L. Hayflick, eds., *Handbook of the Biology of Aging*, 1st ed. New York: Van Nostrand.
1994   *How and Why We Age*. New York: Ballantine Books.
Hoffman, M.A.
1983   Energy metabolism, brain size, and longevity in mammals. *Quarterly Review of Biology* 58:495-512.
Hoffman, G.E., and C.E. Finch
1986   LHRH neurons in the female C57BL/6J mouse brain during reproductive aging: No loss up to middle-age. *Neurobiology of Aging* 7:45-48.
Holinka, C.F.
1994   Aspects of hormone replacement therapy. *Annals of the New York Academy of Sciences* 734:271-284.
Holland, J.J., D. Kohne, and M.V. Doyle
1973   Analysis of virus replication in aging human fibroblasts. *Nature* 245:316-318.
Hölldolber, B., and E.O. Wilson
1990   *The Ants*. Cambridge, MA: The Belknap Press of Harvard University Press.
Holliday, R.
1989   Food, reproduction, and longevity: Is the extended lifespan of calorie-restricted animals an evolutionary adaptation? *Bioessays* 10:125-127.
Holmes, D.J., and S.N. Austad
1995   Birds as animal models for the comparative biology of aging: A prospectus. *Journal of Gerontology and Biological Science* 50A:B59-B66.
Hopkin, K.
1995   Aging in focus: Caloric restriction may put the brakes on aging. *Journal of NIH Research* 7:47-50.
Hursting, S.D., F.N. Perkins, and J.M. Phang
1994   Calorie restriction delays spontaneous tumorigenesis in p53 knock-out transgenic mice. *Proceedings of the National Academy of Sciences U.S.A.* 91:7036-7040.
Janzen, D.H.
1976   Why bamboos wait so long to flower. *Annual Review of Ecological Systems* 7:347-391.
Jazwinski, M.
1996   Longevity-assurance genes and mitochondrial DNA alterations: Yeast and filamentous fungi. Pp. 39-54 in E.L. Schneider and J.W. Rowe, eds., *Handbook of the Biology of Aging*, 4th ed. San Diego: Academic Press.
Katzman, R.
1993   Education and the prevalence of dementia and Alzheimer's disease. *Neurology* 43:13-20.
Kirkwood, T.B.L., and T. Cremer
1982   Cytogerontology since 1881: A reappraisal of August Weismann and a review of modern progress. *Human Genetics* 60:101-112.

Kukalová-Peck, J.
1985 Ephemeroid wing veination based on new gigantic Carboniferous mayflies and basic morphology, phylogeny, and metamorphosis of pterygote insects (Insecta, Ephemerida). *Canadian Journal of Zoology* 63:933-955.

Leaman, B.M.
1991 Reproductive styles and life history variables relative to exploitation and management of *Sebastes* stocks. *Environmental Biology of Fishes* 30:253-271.

Lee, A.K., and A. Cockburn
1985 *Evolutionary Ecology of Marsupials.* New York: Cambridge University Press.

Linnane, A.W., S. Marzuki, T. Ozawa, and M. Tanaka
1989 Mitochondrial DNA mutations as an important contributor to ageing and degenerative diseases. *Lancet* 1:642-645.

Liu, R.K., and R.L. Walford
1969 Laboratory studies on life span, growth, aging, and pathology of the annual fish, *Cynolebiasbellottii* Steindachner. *Zoologica* 54:1-16.

Maeda, H., C.A. Gleiser, E.J. Masoro, I. Murata, C.A. McMahan, and B.P. Yu
1985 Nutritional influences on aging Fischer 344 rats. 2. Pathology. *Journal of Gerontology* 40: 671-688.

Martin, G.M.
1994 Genetic modulation of telomeric terminal restriction-fragment length: relevance for clonal aging and late-life disease. *American Journal of Human Genetics* 55:866-869.

Martínez, D.E., and J.S. Levinton
1992 Asexual metazoans undergo senescence. *Proceedings of the National Academy of Sciences U.S.A.* 89:9920-9923.

McCay, C.M., G. Sperling, and L.L. Barnes
1943 Growth, ageing, chronic diseases, and life span in rats. *Archives of Biochemistry* 2:469-479.

McShane, T.M., and P.M. Wise
1996 Life-long moderate caloric restriction prolongs reproductive lifespan without interrupting maintenance of regular estrous cyclicity in rats: Evidence for central mechanisms. *Biology of Reproduction* 54:70-75.

Mecocci, P., U. MacGarvey, A.E. Kaufman, D. Koontz, J.M. Shoffner, D.C. Wallace, and M. Flint Beal
1993 Oxidative damage to mitochondrial DNA shows marked age-dependent increases in human brain. *Annals of Neurology* 34:609-616.

Medawar, P.B.
1952 *An Unsolved Problem of Biology.* London: H. K. Lewis

Miyata, T., S. Taneda, R. Kawai, Y. Ueda, S. Horiuchi, M. Hara, K. Maeda, and V.M. Monnier
1996 Identification of pentosidine as a native structure for advanced glycation and products in beta2-microglobulin-containing amyloid fibrils in patients with dialysis-related amyloidosis. *Proceedings of the National Academy of Sciences U.S.A.* 93:2353-2358.

Monnier, V.M., D. R. Sell, S. Miyata, and R.H. Nagara
1990 The Maillard reaction as a basis for a theory of aging. Pp. 393-414 in P.A. Finot, ed., *Advanced Life Sciences, Proceedings of the Fourth International Symposium on the Maillard Reaction.* Basel: Birkhausert-Verlag.

Mueller, L.D., T.J. Nusbaum, and M.R. Rose
1995 The Gompertz equation as a predictive tool in demography. *Experimental Gerontology* 30:553-569.

Mulligan, T.J., and B.M. Leaman
1992 Length-at-age analysis: Can you get what you see? *Canadian Journal of Fisheries and Aquatic Science* 49:632-643.

Nagaraj, R.H., and Monnier, V.M.
1992   Isolation and characterization of a blue fluorophore from human eye lens crystallins: In vitro formation from Maillard reaction with ascorbate and ribose. *Biochimica Biophysica Acta* 1116:34-42.

Nelson, J.F., R.G. Gosden, and L.S. Felicio
1985   Effect of dietary restriction on estrous cyclicity and follicular reserves in aging C57BL/6J mice. *Biology of Reproduction* 32:515-522.

Ngai, J., C.Y. Lin, and M.P. Sabour
1995   Lines of mice selected for reproductive longevity. *Growth, Development and Aging* 59:79-81.

Nusbaum, T.J., L.D. Mueller, and M.R. Rose
1996   Evolutionary patterns among measures of aging. *Experimental Gerontology* 31:507-516.

Orive, M.E.
1995   Senescence in organisms with clonal reproduction and complex life histories. *American Naturalist* 145:90-108.

Randerath, K., K.L. Putnam, H.H. Osterburg, S.A. Johnson, D.G. Morgan, and C.E. Finch.
1993   Age-dependent increases of DNA adducts (I-compounds) in human and rat brain DNA. *Mutation Research* 295:11-18.

Rasmussen, T., T. Schliemann, C. Sorensen, J. Zimmer, and M. J. West
1996   Memory impaired aged rats: No loss of principal hippocampal and subicular neurons. *Neurobiology of Aging* 17:143-147.

Reiser, K.M.
1994   Influence of age and long-term dietery restriction on enzymatically mediated crosslinks and nonenzymatic glycation of collagen in mice. *Journal of Gerontology* 49:B71-B79.

Robertson, O.H., B.C. Wexler, and B.F. Miller
1961   Degenerative changes in the cardiovascular system of the spawning Pacific salmon (*Oncorhynchus tshawytscha*). *Circulation Research* 9:826-834.

Rose, M.R.
1991   *The Evolutionary Biology of Aging.* New York: Oxford University Press.

Roth, G.S., D.K. Ingram, and M.A. Lane
1995   Slowing ageing by caloric restriction. *Nature Medicine* 1:414-415.

Rowe, J.W., K.L. Minaker, J.A. Pallotta, and J.S. Flier
1983   Characterization of the insulin resistance of aging. *Journal of Clinical Investigation* 71:1581-1587.

Russell, E.S.
1966   Lifespan and aging patterns. Pp. 511-519 in E.L. Green, ed., *Biology of the Laboratory Mouse,* 2nd ed. New York: McGraw-Hill.

Sabbadin, A.
1979   Colonial structure and genetic patterns in ascidians. Pp. 433-444 in G. Larwood and B.R. Rosen, eds., *Biology and Systematics of Colonial Organisms.* New York: Academic Press.

Schächter, F.
In press Chronos Project in *Longevity: To the Limits and Beyond.* Foundation IPSEN: Paris, France.

Schächter, F., L. Faure-Delanef, F. Guénot, H. Rouger, P. Froguel, L. Lesueur-Ginot, and D. Cohen
1994   Genetic associations with human longevity at the ApoE and ACE loci. *Nature Genetics* 6:29.

Schneider, L.S., and C.E. Finch
1997   Can estrogen prevent neurodegeneration? *Drugs and Aging* 11:87-95.

Schnider, S.L., and R.R. Kohn
1980   Glucosylation of human collagen in aging and diabetes mellitus. *Journal of Clinical Investigation* 66:1179-1181.

Sell, D.R., M.A. Lane, W.A. Johnson, E.J. Masoro, O.B. Mock, K. Reiser, J.F. Fogarty, R.G. Cutler, D.K. Ingram, G.S. Roth, and V.M. Monnier
    1996   Longevity and the genetic determination of collagen glycoxidation kinetics in mammalian senescence. *Proceedings of the National Academy of Sciences U.S.A.* 93:485-490.

Sell, D.R., and V.M. Monnier
    1995   Aging of long-lived proteins: Extra-cellular matrix (collagens, elastins, proteoglycans) and lens crystallins. Pp. 235-305 in E.J. Masoro, ed., *Handbook of Physiology Section 11, Aging.* New York: Oxford University Press.

Smith, J.R., and O.M. Pereira-Smith
    1996   Replicative senescence: Implications for in vivo aging and tumor suppression. *Science* 273:63-67.

Sonntag, W.E., X. Ziaowei, R.L. Ingram, and A. D'Costa
    1995   Moderate caloric restriction alters the subcellular distribution of somatostatin mRNA and increases growth hormone pulse amplitude in aged animals. *Neuroendocrinology* 61:601-608.

Soong, N.W., D.R. Hinton, G. Cortopassi, and N. Arnheim
    1992   Mosaicism for a specific somatic mitochondrial DNA mutation in adult human brain. *Nature Genetics* 2:318-323.

Sprott, R.L., and S.N. Austad
    1996   Animal models for aging research. Pp. 3-23 in E.L. Schneider and J.W. Rowe, eds., *Handbook of the Biology of Aging,* 4th ed. San Diego: Academic Press.

Storer, J.B.
    1978   Effect of aging and radiation in mice of different genotypes. Pp. 55-71 in D. E. Harrison and D. Bergsma, eds., *Genetic Effects on Aging.* New York: Liss.

Suda, Y., M. Suzuki, Y. Ikawa, and S. Aizawa
    1987   Mouse embryonic stem cells exhibit indefinite proliferative potential. *Journal of Cell Physiology* 133:197-201.

Suohonen, J.O., D.A. Peterson, J. Ray, and F.H. Gage
    1996   Differentiation of adult hippocampus progenitors into olfactory neurons *in vivo. Nature* 383:624-626.

Tomkins, G.A., E.J. Stanbridge, and L. Hayflick
    1974   Viral probes of ageing in the human diploid strain, WI-38. *Proceedings of the Society of Experimental Biology and Medicine* 146:385-390.

Vasek, F.C.
    1980   Creosote bush: Long-lived clones in the Mojave Desert. *American Journal of Botany* 67:246-255.

vom Saal, F.S., C.E. Finch, and J.F. Nelson
    1994   The natural history of reproductive aging in humans, laboratory rodents, and selected other vertebrates. Pp. 1213-1314 in E. Knobil, ed., *Physiology of Reproduction,* 2nd ed., Vol. 2. New York: Raven Press.

Weindruch, R.
    1996   Caloric restriction and aging. *Scientific American,* 274(1):46-52.

Weindruch, R.H., and R.L. Walford
    1988   *The Retardation of Aging and Disease by Dietary Restriction.* Springfield, IL: C.C. Thomas.

West, M.J.
    1993   Regionally specific loss of neurons in the aging human hippocampus. *Neurobiology of Aging* 14:287-293.

Williams, G.C.
    1957   Pleiotropy, natural selection, and the evolution of senescence. *Evolution* 11:398-411.

Yi, Z.
In press　Han Chinese mortality at older ages and Chinese centenarians. In *Longevity: To the Limits and Beyond*. Paris, France: Foundation IPSEN.
Youngman, L.D., J-Y.K. Park, and B.N. Ames
　1992　Protein oxidation associated with aging is reduced by dietary restriction of protein or calories. *Proceedings of the National Academy of Sciences U.S.A.* 89:9112-9116.
Yu, C-E., J. Oshima, Y-H. Fu, E.M. Wijsman, F. Hisama, R. Alisch, S. Matthews, J. Nakura, T. Miki, S. Ouais, G.M. Martin, J. Mulligan, and G.D. Schellenberg
　1996　Positional cloning of the Werner's syndrome gene. *Science* 272:258-262.

Glossary

Aché. Hunting and gathering group of subtropical Paraguay

Adaptation. The condition of showing fitness for a particular environment, as applied to characteristics of a structure, function, or entire organism; also the process by which such fitness is acquired

Allele. One of two or more alternate forms of a gene found at the same location (locus) in homologous chromosomes

Altruism. Self-destructive behavior performed for the benefit of others; any form of nonselfish behavior

Antagonistic pleiotropy. Multiple gene effects, such that alleles that improve fitness in early life have detrimental effects later in life

Apoptosis. Programmed death of cells during embryogenesis and metamorphosis or during cell turnover in adult tissues

Chromosome. A DNA-containing body in the nucleus of the cell observed during the mitotic phase of cell replication; the carrier of the (nuclear) genes

Cloning. Growing a colony of identical cells or organisms in vivo; a recombinant DNA technique used to produce millions of copies of a DNA fragment. The fragment is spliced into a cloning vehicle (such as a virus, plasmid, or bacteriophage). The cloning vehicle penetrates a bacterial cell or yeast (the host), which is then grown in vitro or in an animal host

Complementation. The restoration of wild-type function by two different mutations brought together in the same cell

Congenic. Referring to members of the same genus

Conspecific. Referring to members of the same species

Cumulative density function. Probability that a variable takes on a value less than a given number; for example, the probability that an individual dies before passing age x

Dominance. Determination of the phenotype of a heterozygote by one allele. Dominant alleles suppress the effects of recessive alleles when the latter are also present in diploid organisms

DNA. Deoxyribonucleic acid; the molecular basis of heredity

Ecdysone. The hormone produced in insects that induces molting and metamorphosis

Electrophoresis. A technique used to separate mixtures of ionic solutes by differences in their rates of migration in an applied electric field

Ethological. Behavioral

Ethology. The scientific study of animal behavior, particularly under natural conditions

Eukaryote. Organism whose cells have a true nucleus (one bound by a nuclear membrane) within which are the chromosomes

Eusociality. Social system in which certain individuals enhance their fitness by aiding their collateral kin to rear their offspring. For example, sterile female worker bees may rear the offspring of their fertile sister queens

F_2. Second filial generation; all of the offspring produced by the mating of two individuals of the first filial generation

Fecundity. Ability to produce offspring rapidly and in large numbers. In demography of human populations, the physiological ability to reproduce, as opposed to fertility

Fertility. Reproductive potential. In demography, the number of births per year divided by the number of women of childbearing age, expressed as a rate

Fibroblast. Connective tissue cell that can differentiate into other blastic cells to form fibrous tissues; a fiber-producing cell widely distributed in tissues

Fitness. The ability of a genotype to reproduce its alleles in a particular environment or after some environmental change

Free radical. A highly reactive chemical moiety characterized by unpaired electrons, which can damage the cell fabric and other biological macromolecules.

Gamete. Egg or sperm cell; germ cell

Gene. A unit of inheritance coded by DNA, carried on a chromosome, transmitted from generation to generation by the gametes, and controlling the development and characteristics of an individual

Genetic drift. Genetic changes in populations caused by random phenomena rather than by selection

Genetic marker. A gene mutation that has phenotypic effects useful for tracing the chromosome on which it is located

Genotype. Genetic makeup of an organism or group of organisms, with respect to a single trait or a group of traits; sum total of genes transmitted from parents to offspring

Genome. The total set of genes carried by an individual or cell

Gerontogene. Gene affecting longevity, either reducing average lifespan of the organism (e.g., as a result of antagonistic pleiotropy) or increasing average lifespan. "Longevity assurance gene" is often used for genes that promote survival at older ages. See chapter 7 for discussion.

Germ cell. The egg or sperm cell

Gompertz model. Class of statistical models first proposed by the nineteenth-century British actuary Benjamin Gompertz, in which the hazard rate for death rises exponentially with increasing age of the organism (at least after an initial period of high risk of mortality in infancy and much lower risk in late childhood and adolescence)

Grandmother hypothesis. By ceasing to reproduce, old people (and by extension, old members of other species) can use their time and resources to invest in the survival and reproduction of kin

Hayflick limit. An experimental limit to the number of times a diplosomatic cell is capable of dividing during serial cell culture

Hazard function. Probability that an individual surviving to age x will die at that age. Ratio of the probability density and survival functions; also called "the force of mortality"

Hiwi. Hunting and gathering group of the Venezuelan savanna

Homeostasis. Self-regulation that tends to restore the conditions existing before a disturbance or shift

Homologous. Corresponding in structure and position; allelic chromosomes are homologous. Also, referring to structures or processes that have the same evolutionary origin though their functions may vary widely (as opposed to analogous, referring to structures having a different evolutionary origin but performing the same function)

Inbreeding. Crossing with genetically similar individuals, particularly with close relatives

Iteroparity. The state in an individual organism of reproducing repeatedly or more than once in a lifetime

!Kung San. Hunter and gathering group of the Kalahari in Africa who now practice a mixed economy of hunting, gathering, farming, and wage labor

Knock-out mutation. Deletion of a gene or a portion of a gene from the genome

Life expectancy. Mean life span remaining for individuals of a given age

Life history. Combination of age-specific survival probabilities and fertilities characteristic of a type of organism; the time table of development and aging for each species (for example, puberty, menopause, and longevity in humans)

Life span. Age of death (for individual); maximum potential length of life for most robust member(s) of the species (for species)

Limit-distribution hypothesis. There exists a limiting distribution that mortality curves may approach but not surpass

Limited-life-span hypothesis. There exists some age beyond which there can be no survivors

Linkage. Occurrence of genes on the same chromosome. The closer the genes are, the more tightly they are linked—that is, the less likely that crossing over will separate them

Locus, pl. loci. The set of homologous parts of a pair of chromosomes that may be occupied by allelic genes; the locus thus consists of a pair of locations (except in the X chromosome of males)

Longevity genes. Genes that promote survival; most fixed genes are presumed to be of this type

Lotka equation. An identity from mathematical demography developed by Alfred J. Lotka that defines the built-in long-term or "intrinsic" rate of natural increase of a population when age-specific fertility and survivorship rates are held constant

Meiosis. Two consecutive special cell divisions in the developing germ cells characterized by the pairing and segregation of homologous chromosomes; the resulting gametes will have reduced, or haploid, chromosome sets

Mortality trajectory. Plot of death rate against age group over time

Niche. The set of environmental factors into which a species fits; its specific way of using its environment and pattern for association with other species

Oocyte. The developing female gamete before completion and release

Out-crossing. Breeding with genetically different, not closely related individuals, particularly with members of different populations

Phenotype. Physical manifestation of gene function

Pleiotropy. Multiple effects of one gene; the capacity of a gene to affect several aspects of the phenotype

Polygenic. Relating to a normal characterisitic or hereditary disease controlled by the added effects of genes at multiple loci

Polymorphism. Simultaneous occurrence of several discontinuous phenotypes or genes in a population, with the frequency even of the rarest type higher than can be maintained by recurrent mutation, typically > 1%

Positional cloning. A genetic technique for determining the location of a mutation in a small area of the genome

Preadaptation. Presence of previously existing structure, physiological process, or behavior pattern already functional in another context and available as an aid to attainment of a new adaptation

Progeria. A syndrome in which certain characteristics of senescence are compressed. In Werner syndrome, the defect is in gene repair

Quantitative trait. A trait for which phenotypic variation is continuous (rather than discrete)

Quantitative trait locus. One of a group of genes specifying any particular quantitative trait

Recessive gene. Gene that fails to express itself in the phenotype of the heterozygote; that is, its effect is masked in the presence of its dominant allele

Recombinant. Having altered DNA resulting from insertion into the chain by chemical, enzymatic, or biologic means of a sequence not originally present in the chain; an offspring that has received chromosomal parts from different parental strains

Recombination. Reshuffling of parental genes during meiosis due to crossing over, or induced in a test tube by enzymes

Semelparity. A life-history pattern that is characterized by only one burst of reproductive activity and rapid aging

Senescence. Deterioration in performance seen later in the adult life span, associated with increasing mortality rates

Senility. A general term for a variety of mental disorders occurring in old age, consisting of two broad categories, organic and psychological disorders

Somatic. Relating to the body; of cells that are not germ cells

Somatic cell. Any body cell except a germ cell

Speciation. The splitting of a phyletic line; the process of the multiplication of species; the origin of discontinuities between populations caused by the development of reproductive isolating mechanisms

Stochastic. Involving a random variable; involving chance or probability

Survival function. Probability that an individual is still alive at age x

Telomere. Specialized gene sequences found at the ends of chromosomes, which tend to shorten in diploid cells

Territoriality. Occupation of an area that usually contains a scarce resource either by overt defense or advertisement

Wild type. The allele that is most frequent in natural populations, often indicated by the symbol +; this term cannot be applied for a locus that has undergone mutation

Zygote. The cell resulting from the union of a male and female gamete until it divides; the fertilized ovum

Index